LIVESTOCK SERIES

HORSE DISEASES

FULLY REVISED EDITION

H. G. BELSCHNER, ED, DVSc, HDA, FACVSc
Formerly Assistant Director of Veterinary Services, First Cavalry Division, Australian Military Forces —Eastern Command; Chief, Division of Animal Industry, Department of Agriculture, New South Wales and Senior Lecturer in Animal Management, University of Sydney.

REUBEN J. ROSE, BVSc, Dip VetAn, PhD, MACVSc, MRCVS
Senior Lecturer in Veterinary Clinical Studies (Surgery), University of Sydney.

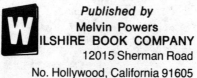

Published by
Melvin Powers
WILSHIRE BOOK COMPANY
12015 Sherman Road
No. Hollywood, California 91605
Telephone: (213) 875-1711 / 983-1105

ANGUS & ROBERTSON PUBLISHERS
London • Sydney • Melbourne • Singapore • Manila

First published by Angus & Robertson Publishers, Australia, 1969
Revised edition 1974
Reprinted 1976
This revised edition 1982

National Library of Australia
Cataloguing-in-publication data.

Belschner, H.G. (Herman Godfrey), 1895–1976
Horse diseases.

Rev. ed.
Bibliography.
Includes index.

1. Horses – Diseases. I. Rose, R.J. II. Title.
636.1'089'6

Typeset in 10 pt Plantin

Printed in the United States of America
ISBN 0-87980-302-9

Contents

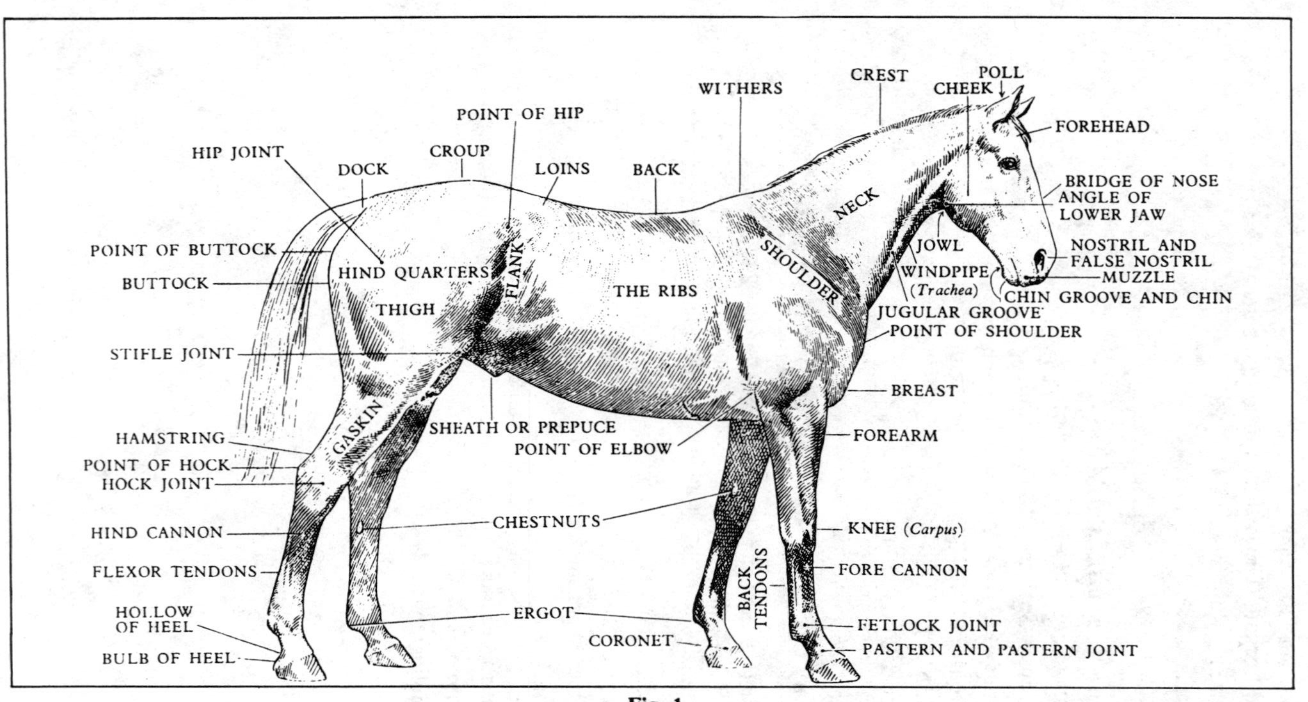

Fig. 1
The points of the horse.
(after Miller and Robertson)

Preface

Since the first edition of *Horse Diseases* in 1969 there has been a remarkable increase in knowledge concerning the causes and treatment of horse diseases. Increased research into this area has been prompted by a greater interest in use of the horse for sport, pleasure and work. This revised edition of Dr Belschner's book has been considerably expanded, with emphasis on those aspects of horse diseases of particular concern to horse owners. In addition, it is hoped that this new book will provide the type of material necessary to satisfy special needs of the new horse diploma courses at various advanced colleges of education.

Most horse owners today have the services of a veterinary surgeon readily available, even in more remote areas. The focus of this book then is to assist owners in understanding the types of disorders in their horses and to enable veterinary attention to be sought where appropriate.

I would like to thank Mr J. Kohnke for providing some of the illustrations.

R.J. ROSE
Department of Veterinary Clinical Studies,
The University of Sydney,
New South Wales.

ABORTION

Normal pregnancy in the mare lasts between 325 and 355 days. If the foetus is expelled prior to these times this is termed abortion. Most twins are aborted before full term and abortion can occur at any time between the first and tenth months of pregnancy. Foals born before 325 days of gestation rarely survive and those born before 300 never survive.

Causes There are many causes of abortion in mares, many of which are not completely understood. The most common cause of abortion in mares relates to infection of the uterus (womb). Bacteria, fungi and viruses may all cause infection and abortion; however, in more recent times virus abortion has been the most common type encountered. A virus known as equine herpes type 1 or *equine viral rhinopneumonitis* is the virus which has been isolated in many cases of abortion within the last few years. This virus causes an initial respiratory tract infection in mares and this infection may be very mild. Later the virus infects the uterus and causes abortion of the foetus. The abortion of the foetus frequently takes place several months after the initial respiratory tract infection and commonly results in the foetus being expelled alive. Another virus infection which is not yet present in Australia, called *equine viral arteritis,* has been responsible for severe outbreaks of infective abortion in mares in the United States of America.

Abortions with no apparent cause do occur as well and may be a consequence of hormonal imbalance, poor nutrition and other as yet undefined factors.

Symptoms Abortions are frequently associated with metritis (inflammation of the uterus) and in this respect the symptoms are similar to brucellosis in cattle. A sticky rust-coloured discharge may be noticed a few days before the act of abortion and this continues after the abortion has occurred. Early abortions may take place without any warning symptoms, and may not be seen. In such cases, the first indication that this event has taken place is that the mare comes in season again. With early abortions, the membranes are usually discharged with the foetus. When they occur in the later months of pregnancy, the placenta or portion thereof may be retained, to be followed by a severe metritis with persistent discharge from the vulva. Other than by microscopical examination of smears from discharges, or by blood or other tests, it is not possible to say whether the abortion has been due to a specific infection. If abortions have occurred in a number of mares, suspicion would be aroused.

Treatment Mares showing indications of having aborted or of impending abortion should be immediately isolated. The foetus, its membranes and any discharges should be collected so that post-mortem examination can be made and diagnostic tests performed by a veterinarian. A veterinarian should also examine the mare to determine if any metritis is present, so that treatment can be instituted. The affected mare or mares will require good nursing, and the strictest sanitary measures should be practised. The mare should not be served again until it has been established by taking bacteriological swabs that no infection persists.

ABSCESS

An abscess is a localised collection of pus which may occur anywhere on the body and is sometimes deep seated. Internal abscesses also occur. An acute abscess is a hot painful swelling which develops rapidly with formation of pus. The swelling gradually increases in size, comes to a head and bursts. A chronic abscess is one which takes a long time to develop, is frequently deep seated and seldom bursts unless near the surface. Examples of chronic abscesses are those seen in poll evil and fistulous withers.

Cause Generalised infection, which occurs in certain specific diseases such as strangles in the horse, or infection of a wound (for example, nail prick in the foot) by various types of bacteria are the main causes of abscesses. More recently abscesses have been seen at the site of injections, which have been improperly administered by laymen using dirty syringes and needles.

Symptoms The first symptom is a hot, painful swelling which rapidly increases in size over 1 to 2 days. If the abscess is localised it will eventually burst and discharge pus to the exterior. Where internal abscesses occur, for example in the chest or abdomen, the only symptoms may be poor appetite, failure to thrive and a consistently high temperature. Abscesses of the roots of the molar (cheek) teeth may occur and result in discharging pus over the lower or upper jaw, depending on which teeth are involved.

Treatment The treatment for an acute external abscess is to hasten its ripening by warm fomentation. Once localised, the abscess becomes soft and should be surgically opened to allow drainage. After allowing the pus to drain, the cavity of the abscess should be syringed out with some weak antiseptic solution. This should be repeated twice daily until no more discharge appears from the drainage site. It is important to keep the

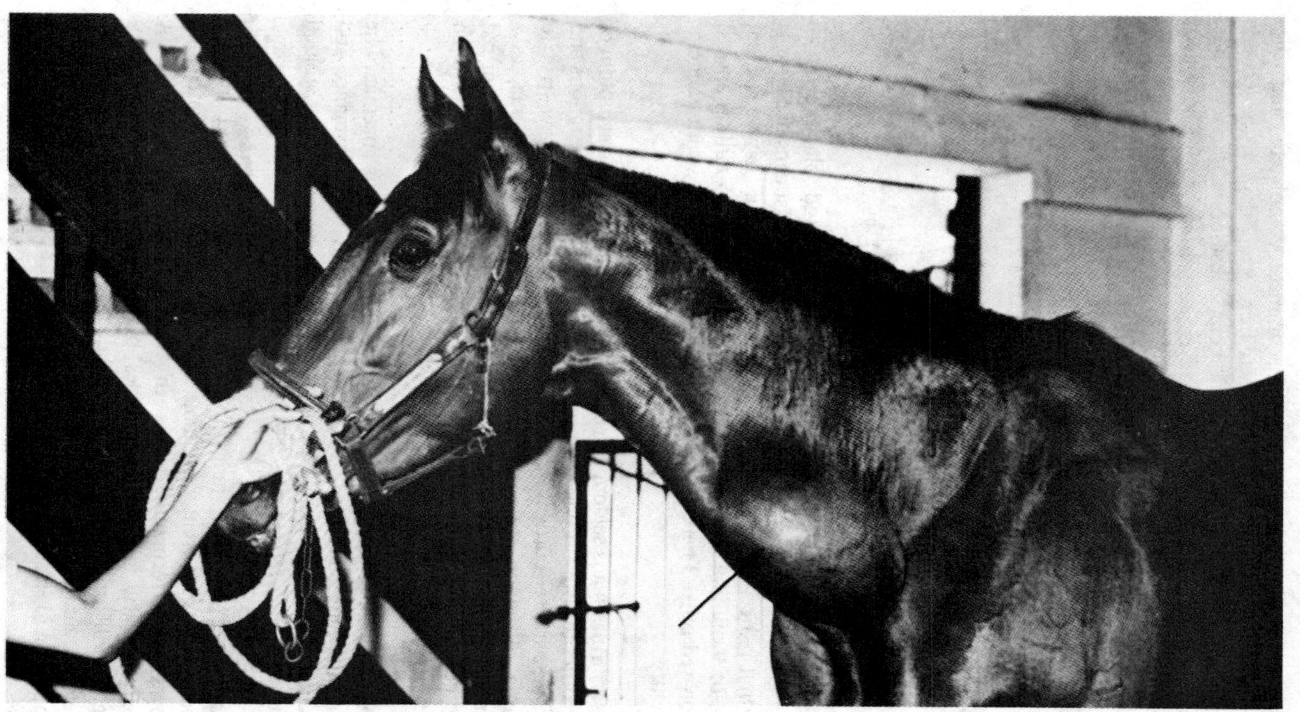

Fig. 2
Abscess (arrow) in the neck of a horse resulting from injection of material with an unsterile needle.

wound open until the cavity has drained completely and the infection is under control. This may take from 3 to 7 days. If the wound is allowed to close early the abscess will recur. Most local abscesses do not require the use of antibiotics. However, in chronic or deep-seated abscesses, particularly those which may involve the chest abdominal cavities, a veterinary surgeon will be required to examine the horse and then select the appropriate antibiotic therapy.

AGE BY THE TEETH

See *Dentition and Ageing*

ANAEMIA

Anaemia is a term applied to a deficiency of red blood cells or haemoglobin in the blood. In defining anaemia we must consider what is a normal red cell count. Whereas an average horse may have a red cell count of 9 million, the normal range will lie between 6 million and 12 million red cells. Therefore, it can be seen that there is a wide range of normality.

Cause Anaemia is seldom a primary disease, but usually a symptom of some other disorder. Long-term infections, severe worm infestations and external parasite burdens are all conditions which may give rise to anaemia. Although there are many possible causes of anaemia, as a general rule all causes result in either an inadequate production of red blood cells by the bone marrow or an increased loss of red cells through either haemorrhage or red cell destruction.

Symptoms Frequently it is difficult to tell if a horse is anaemic. The main symptoms commonly relate to a reduction in performance and stamina. A definitive diagnosis can only be made by performing a blood count.

Treatment A wide range of injectable vitamin and mineral preparations are currently available and are widely used by owners and trainers of performance horses in the mistaken belief that these preparations will improve their horses' blood count. Most horses in this category will have blood counts that fall within the normal range and, therefore, cannot be said to be anaemic. If a horse is truly anaemic then it is important to establish the cause of the anaemia and to treat this primary cause.

ANTHRAX

Anthrax is an acute infectious disease of a septicaemic nature which may affect any animal. The disease is of world-wide distribution and is more commonly seen in herbivorous animals including the horse. Man is also susceptible and may contract the disease at a post-mortem examination.

Cause The disease is caused by a specific organism, *Bacillus anthracis,* gaining entrance to the body.

Symptoms The initial symptoms are high fever, general depression, and frequently, especially in the horse, severe pains resembling those of colic or acute enteritis. Later, swellings may occur on different parts of the body including the neck, throat, chest, along the abdomen and on the legs. There may be a blood-stained discharge from the nose and anus, but usually this is not shown until after death. Horses commonly exhibit a longer course of the disease than other animals, but death usually occurs in 1 or 2 days.

Treatment There is no treatment. If the disease is suspected it should be reported immediately to the nearest veterinary inspector or other authority.

The disease is confirmed by microscopic examination of a blood smear from the affected animal. The sick horse should be placed in isolation and fowls and dogs kept away. If the animal dies before the authorities arrive, no attempt should be made to carry out a post-mortem examination, as it is very dangerous to open the carcase. A tarpaulin or bags should be thrown over the carcase to cover it and all discharges completely. Subsequently the carcase should be burnt or deeply buried and covered with a thick layer of unslaked lime. The authorities will advise concerning any disinfection of premises which may be necessary.

ANTIBIOTICS

Since the first usage of penicillin in the horse after the second world war, a number of antibiotics have become available which allow the effective treatment of certain bacterial diseases in the horse. Antibiotics have no effect against diseases caused by viruses, for example, most respiratory tract infections. It is important for the correct selection and usage of antibiotics to be undertaken as their inappropriate usage has resulted in widespread resistance by bacteria to effects of the antibiotics. Some antibiotics also have severe side effects, such as diarrhoea, shock and even death, following inappropriate administration in some horses.

Therefore, it is important to obtain skilled veterinary advice before using antibiotics to treat any disease condition in horses.

APPETITE — "DEPRAVED"

Sometimes a horse will eat earth, cinders, stones, plastic, bark of trees, dung and other rubbish. This is referred to as "pica", which means a depraved appetite for unnatural food, and varies from licking to actual eating. However, foals will normally eat their mother's faeces.

Bark-eating is a fairly common habit amongst horses in certain districts, and is a cause of some concern to owners. The horses strip off the bark sometimes to the extent of ring-barking the tree. No ill effects may result if the bark is not eaten to excess, but it can cause serious digestive upsets and obstruction of the bowels, as can the ingestion of other foreign matter.

Cause It is not always easy to determine the many causes of depraved appetite, but there may be some type of mineral deficiency involved. Boredom may also result in this form of behaviour.

Prevention Quite often the habit of bark-eating in particular can be prevented by feeding liberal amounts of good quality lucerne chaff or lucerne, which is a fodder rich in both protein and calcium. Other than this, a change of environment sometimes helps.

ARTHRITIS

Arthritis is a wear and tear disease commonly involving the highly mobile joints such as the carpus (knee), fetlock and hock. As a result of the stresses involved the cartilage lining the ends of the bones becomes thinned.

Causes Conformational faults such as upright pasterns and calf knees can result in arthritis. It is a condition most commonly found in racehorses, where stresses on the limbs are greatest.

Symptoms The most common symptom involved in arthritis is lameness of the affected leg. Depending whether the injury and reaction involved is recent or long standing, there will be a variable amount of swelling around the affected joint. Horses will also show pain when the involved joint is flexed, so that pressure is put on the joint.

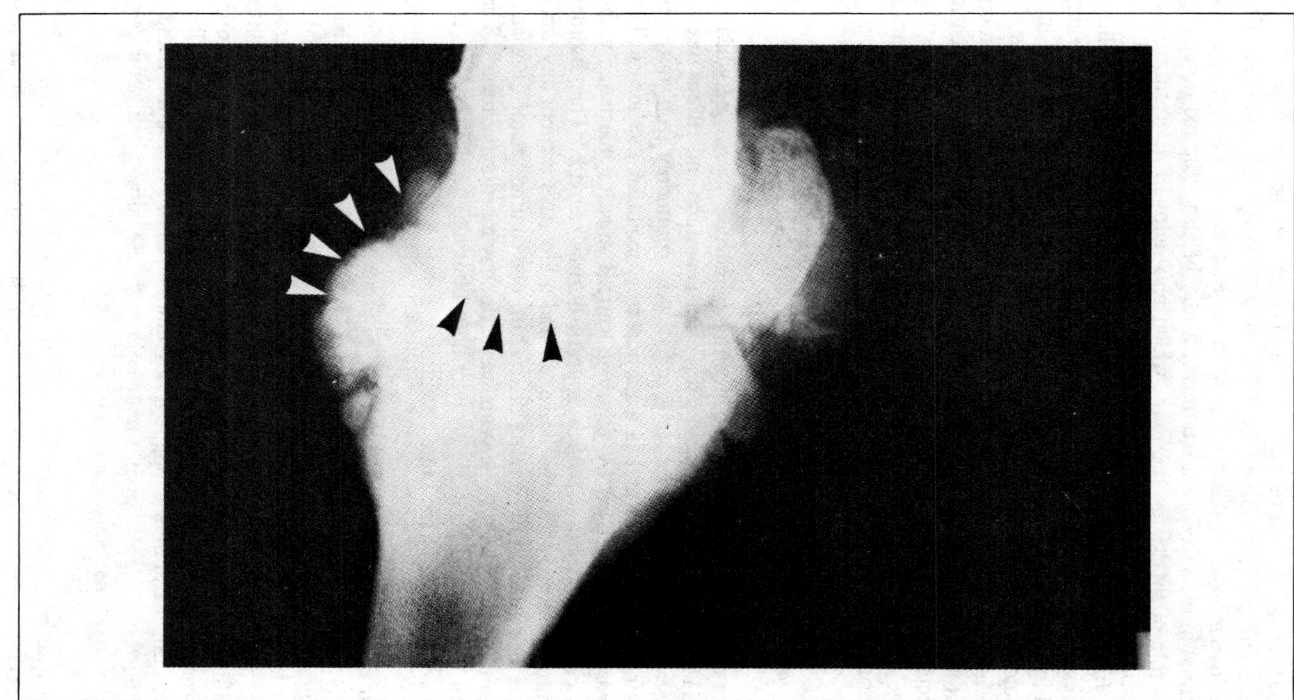

Fig. 3
X-rays showing severe arthritis of fetlock joint with collapse of joint space (black arrows) and new bone production (white arrows).

Treatment To correctly assess and diagnose the damage to the affected joint it is important for the horse to be x-rayed. This enables the veterinarian to assess the duration of the disease and its severity, which is essential in the subsequent treatment. It may be also indicated to remove a sample of fluid from the joint, which also helps in determining the duration and severity of the condition.

In early acute sprains involving a joint with much heat and swelling it is essential to use anti-inflammatory measures such as cold water hosing and ice packs to the affected area, followed by bandaging the joint. This should be done twice a day for 3 to 4 days. Anti-inflammatory drugs such as *phenylbutazone* and *corticosteroids* may be indicated and consultation with a veterinarian is essential before their use. A newer drug which is injected directly into the involved joint, called *Healon*, acts to restore some of the lubricating properties which are lost in joints affected with arthritis.

AZOTURIA AND "TYING UP SYNDROME"

This disease, the modern name of which is *rhabdomyolysis* and which is also referred to as *myoglobinuria*, was once a common and serious disease in working draught horses. It is not now so commonly seen, but does occur in light horses and is a particular problem in racehorses. The disease is characterised by injury to certain muscles, particularly the muscles in the rump, which appears during exercise. The disorder commonly occurs after the horse has had a few days without any work while being fed a full working diet. Thus, one common name associated with this disorder for some years was "Monday morning sickness". The term "tying up syndrome", or describing a horse as being "tied up", is a less severe form of the same condition.

Cause The exact cause of the disease is not known but the conditions under which it occurs are well defined, as referred to above. It has been suggested that when horses accustomed to regular work are allowed to rest for several days on full rations, some derangement in the process of conversion of carbohydrates in tissues occurs with the accumulation of lactic acid in the tissues and blood. This produces a myopathy or muscle disease. When the horse works after being spelled, the muscle fibres break down and muscle pigment is liberated, passes into the blood and is excreted by the kidneys. It is not a kidney disease, although in some cases the kidneys may subsequently be involved.

Symptoms The symptoms seen will vary with the severity of the muscle damage. In the severe condition the horse will be reluctant to move, show trembling and pain in the muscles, usually lameness in one or both hind limbs and profuse sweating, panting and crouching. A dark-coloured urine will usually be passed in these cases and the horse will eventually go down on the ground and be unable to rise. After the onset of this condition the muscles will become very hard and almost board-like over the rump region. In the less severe condition of tying up the horse may show some degree of hind leg lameness and stiffness following a work programme. This will usually become worse as the horse's work is continued. It may also be noticed that the horse has a painful area and swelling around the muscles of the rump and in some cases a darker-coloured urine may be passed. However, in most cases of tying up there is no change in colour of the urine.

Treatment In severe cases of *rhabdomyolysis* veterinary attention should be sought as soon as possible. Until the veterinarian arrives there should be no attempt made to keep the horse walking about but it should be kept warm and quiet. If the horse has to be moved then this should be done using a horse float. The horse should also be encouraged to drink as much water as possible.

The muscle pigment released into the blood can damage the kidneys and therefore the veterinarian will give intravenous fluid solutions to help prevent this complication. In the less severe form of the condition, that is tying up, treatment may not be required. Various drugs, including vitamin B1, sodium bicarbonate, vitamin E, and selenium have all been used to try to prevent the disorder from recurring. However, in many cases the condition will recur despite any form of treatment. A change in training programme may be necessary and a change in diet. This should consist of an elimination of any grain in the horse's diet and a programme of graded exercise starting with walking and trotting for the first 1 to 2 weeks, followed by a gradual increase in the amount of exercise over the next 2 to 3 weeks and a gradual introduction of grain back into the horse's diet.

It can be helpful to have blood samples taken by a veterinarian to determine the levels of muscle enzymes in the blood. These muscle enzymes will increase with muscle damage and as the condition improves the enzyme parameters will return to normal.

There is a sex difference in the occurrence of the disorder with mares and fillies being approximately 3 times as commonly affected as geldings and stallions.

BACK DISORDERS

Injuries to the back may be either congenital or acquired. Congenital

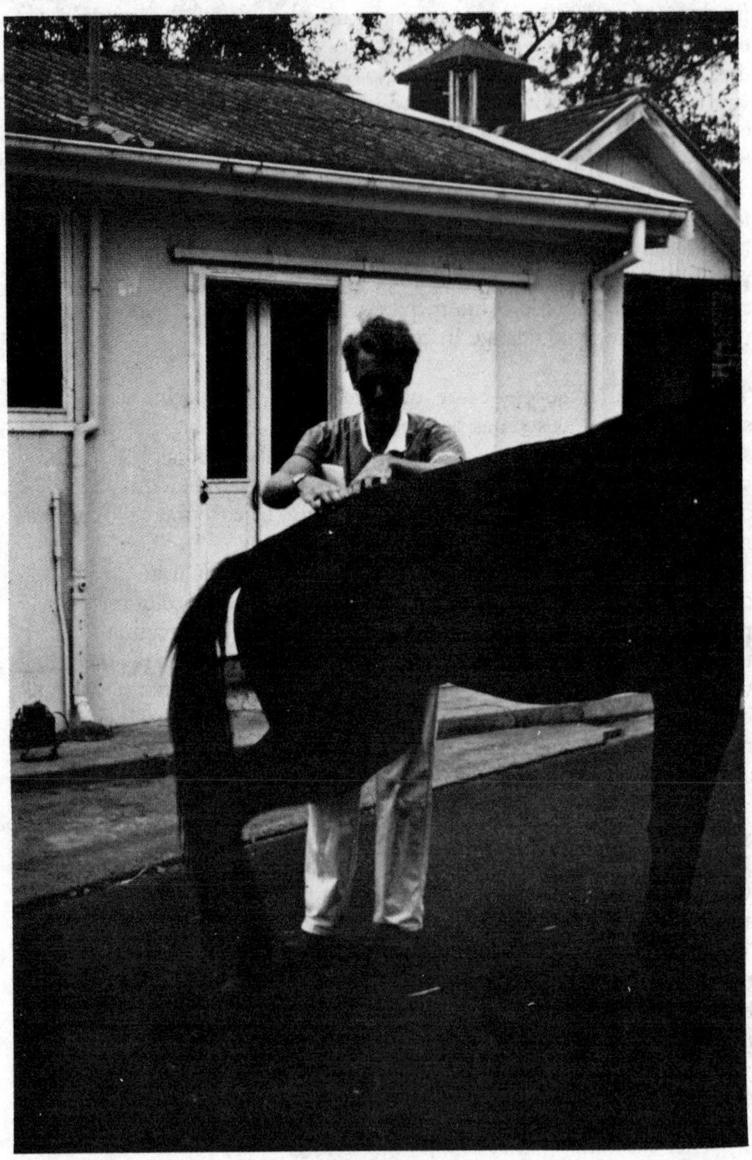

Fig. 4
Sacro-iliac back pain, with the horse showing extreme reaction on mild pressure over the sacral prominences.

disorders (those that the horse is born with) are usually associated with malalignment of the vertebrae. These conditions can result in obscure hind limb lameness problems as well as changes in temperament of the animal.

Causes There are a variety of causes of back problems in horses. Initial deformity of the vertebral column (spine) may result in pain and problems within the back. Slipping and falling in the horse may result in soft tissue damage to muscles and ligaments around the back or even in fractures and other bony damage. In trotters and pacers sacroiliac pain is a very common condition and this seems to be the result of the natural gait of these horses leading to stresses in the upper part of the back.

Symptoms The symptoms of back disorders vary depending on the location and damage involved, and in many cases it is difficult to determine exactly where the problem lies. The most common symptoms relate to a change in temperament of the horse, in particular when the rider gets on the back. Many horses will resent the presence of a rider and will tend to crouch away when the rider becomes seated in the saddle. Other horses will shake their head, buck, kick and show general signs of irritability. In other cases the only change seen may be an alteration in performance with horses showing poor performance on the flat or over jumps. Painful areas may be found along the back and in some cases there may be lumps and bumps present along the vertebral column.

Treatment The most important consideration in treatment of horses with back disorders is the establishment of a correct diagnosis. This is possible by having a veterinarian examine the horse, where he may take blood samples to aid in diagnosis. More recently, powerful x-ray machines have allowed x-rays to be taken of the back and visualisation of bony damage is possible. Many horses may show an improvement on anti-inflammatory drugs such as *phenylbutazone;* however, in most cases a long spell of up to 12 months is required to help resolve back disorders.

BARK-EATING

See *Appetite — "Depraved"*

BIG HEAD (Osteomalacia)

Osteomalacia is a general term used to describe softening of the bones and is sometimes referred to as "*adult rickets*". In cattle more particularly, the bones of affected animals become swollen, soft and spongy and are easily broken. In horses the bones of the skull are often involved and the head shows a grossly swollen appearance, hence the common name "big head". It occurs chiefly in mature animals.

Cause The cause of the disease is not fully understood, but it appears to be associated with either a deficient intake or absorption of calcium or phosphorus, or to increased excretion of either of these elements, or to a calcium-phosphorus imbalance. A deficiency of vitamin D or trace elements may contribute to the condition.

Symptoms Swelling of bones of the face, generally midway between eyes and nose and under the surface of the jaw. There is usually no pain, but the teeth may be loosened.

Treatment Unless the specific dietary deficiencies can be determined it is impossible to treat the animal intelligently. Change of feed and locality sometimes arrests the condition. Lucerne hay or lucerne chaff should be added to the ration, or 40 g of finely-ground limestone supplied daily in the feed.

BIRDSVILLE DISEASE

See *Kimberley or Walkabout Disease*

BLADDER — INFLAMMATION OF (Cystitis)

Inflammation of the bladder is mostly caused by bacterial infection. The presence of large or irregular shaped calculi ("stones") in the bladder sometimes causes inflammation of the wall of the bladder. It is uncommon to find cystitis in the horse, but if seen it requires prompt veterinary attention.

Symptoms The symptoms are repeated efforts to urinate and slight or severe colicky pains. The urine, which is passed in small quantities, may be clear or red or more commonly flocculent. The urine comes in spurts and is accompanied by signs of pain, which persists after the discharge, as shown by continued straining, groaning, and sometimes by movement of the feet and tail. The animal may kick at the abdomen, look around at the flank and lie down and rise frequently. When the condition is due to bacterial infection there is commonly a rise in temperature and accelerated pulse and respiration. The presence of calculi may be differentiated from cystitis due to infection by having a veterinarian palpate the bladder via the rectum where the calculus may be felt.

Treatment If cystitis is suspected then it is important to obtain a sterile specimen of urine from the horse to allow the veterinary surgeon to test the specimen for the presence of bacteria. Once bacteria are isolated, then a rational selection of antibiotic may be made. If a calculus is present then this will require surgery to allow its removal.

BLEEDING FROM NOSE (Epistaxis)

Nose bleeding is a symptom of a number of diseases in horses. It may arise from damaged blood vessels in the back of the nose or rupture of blood vessels within the lungs.

Symptoms In racehorses nose bleeding is usually seen after stressful exercise (swimming or galloping) and the amount of blood may vary from a teaspoonful to a bucketful. Most of these cases are due to haemorrhage from the lungs. Recent research has shown some mild haemorrhage to be present in the windpipe of as many as 60 per cent of normal horses following racing. Other causes of nose bleed include tumours and infections at the back of the nose. These cases can usually be differentiated from lung haemorrhage as bleeding can occur at rest. Incorrect passage of a stomach tube can result in nose bleed by damaging the thin bones within the nose.

Treatment The treatment for simple bleeding from the nose consists of keeping the horse quiet and under observation for 1 to 2 hours. Treatment is seldom needed as bleeding usually stops spontaneously within 15 to 30 minutes.

In racehorse bleeders treatment is seldom successful and all that can be done is to rest the horse for between 6 and 9 months. It is important to differentiate this condition from other causes of bleeding. This can be done by a veterinary surgeon carrying out certain diagnostic tests, which include blood counts and biochemical profiles as well as the use of a special instrument called a rhinolaryngoscope, which allows the veterinarian to examine the back of the nose and throat.

BLEEDING FROM VEINS

Bleeding or venesection was at one time employed in the treatment of a great many diseases of horses, and was also adopted in human medicine. It is now seldom carried out, although there are occasions, such as in the case of infertility, *polycythaemia* (increased red cell count) or acute laminitis (founder), when it is occasionally used. The blood letting is usually from the jugular vein, by distending the vein with pressure from the fingers or the use of a cord around the neck, and withdrawing the blood with a bleeding needle. It is essential for bleeding to be undertaken by a veterinary surgeon as close monitoring of the horse's cardinal signs is important. Usually 4 to 6 litres can be safely removed from an average-sized horse.

Accidental bleeding from veins as a result of injury is usually not serious. Pressure within the veins is quite low and the blood flow generally stops spontaneously. Arteries, on the other hand, have a much higher pressure as they take blood away from the heart and if cut can result in more severe blood loss. It is usually possible to differentiate arterial blood which is bright red and tends to spurt out, from venous blood which is darker in colour and generally has a lower flow. The best means of stopping bleeding is by pressure, which may be carried out by tight bandaging over a pad of clean cotton wool or a folded clean cloth. Bleeding stops because blood clots in the damaged vessels due to the pressure of the bandage.
See also *Wounds*

BLISTERING

Blisters are applied directly to the skin for counter-irritation exernally and vary from mild applications of liniments containing ammonia and oil of turpentine, to the more severe blistering ointments which contain cantharides, red iodide of mercury (red precipitate ointment), and other materials. The object of counter-irritation is to set up a new inflammatory process in an area, which stimulates it to continue the work of healing and repair. Although this is the aim, it is doubtful whether blisters are really effective. Most blisters simply result in irritation to skin over the damaged area and there are now more effective treatments for most conditions where a blister was formerly used.

BLOOD COUNTS

Blood counts are nowadays widely used as a diagnostic aid in a number of disease conditions. In addition it is common for racehorses in training to have blood counts taken at regular intervals to help in the assessment of fitness. It is important when taking a blood sample from the jugular vein that the horse be completely quiet, otherwise a false result may be obtained. There are a wide range of tests to which the blood sample may be subjected following its removal. These include tests for muscle function, kidney, liver and heart function, as well as examinations of various salts and electrolytes, which are an important part of normal body processes. Blood counts can also detect the presence of infection and may be used to monitor the progress of a particular disease. There is wide variation in normal blood counts from horses of varying breeds and uses. It must also be remembered that within a breed there will be a range of normality. These factors should be remembered when assessing an individual horse's blood count, and it should also be known that the measurement techniques for performing blood counts have up to a 6 to 10 per cent error involved.

Typical blood counts from a fit racehorse, endurance horse and trotter are given below. These should be used only as a guide to normality and the veterinary surgeon is trained to interpret results of the blood count, given the animal's age, training and possible disease process.

		Thoroughbred Racehorse	Standardbred Racehorse	Endurance Horse
Packed cell volume	(1/1)*	0.44	0.38	0.34
Haemoglobin	(g/1)	159.00	135.00	120.00
Red blood cells	(x10^{12}/1)	10.00	8.80	7.40
Mean corpuscular volume	(fl)	43.00	42.00	46.00
White blood cells	(x10^{9}/1)	8.80	8.50	9.60
Total plasma protein	(g/1)	68.00	64.00	65.00

*l = litre

These blood counts taken from fit horses of each type show that thoroughbreds usually have higher red blood cell counts, haemoglobin and packed cell volume than standardbreds, which, in turn, have higher blood counts than endurance horses. The figures provided here give only a guide and more complete analysis, including the types of white cells, provides the veterinarian with additional information.

BLOOD POISONING (Septicaemia)

The popular term "blood poisoning" means a general infection of the bloodstream by various types of bacteria. This may be of a specific nature such as in the case of anthrax, or may be the result of infection of wounds by bacteria of the "gas gangrene group", which thrive in the absence of air, or other organisms which need air for best growth. Pyogenic (pus-forming) bacteria circulating in the blood usually cause abscess formation in various parts of the body.

Causes When not due to a specific infectious disease, septicaemia usually results from wound infection, especially puncture wounds in the feet of horses and elsewhere on the body; extensive wounds or inflamed areas; bone and joint injuries; difficult parturition, or following operations such as castration, extraction of teeth and bleeding.

Symptoms All forms of septicaemia are serious. It is not uncommon for a horse to die suddenly, the only signs observed being a very high temperature and loss of appetite. In other cases there is shivering, fever, laboured respiration and increased heart rate.

Treatment Treatment of septicaemia involves identification of the specific bacteria involved and then selection of the correct antibiotic by a veterinarian. It is important that good general nursing care be applied and this involves keeping the horse warm and making sure that the horse does not become dehydrated.

BONE — INFECTION OF (Osteomyelitis)

Many bones in the lower limbs of horses are very superficial and therefore cuts and injuries may result in damage and subsequent local infection of bone.

Cause Cuts and injuries can result in introduction of bacteria and local infection of bone. In young horses infection can also result from spread by the bloodstream to rapidly growing areas of the bone, such as growth plates.

Symptoms The most common symptom is a chronic discharge of pus from the leg following a local wound. There may be no lameness involved, but there is usually some pain on palpation of the affected area.

Treatment Antibiotics seldom resolve *osteomyelitis* as infected areas of bone are usually deficient in blood supply. Surgery is usually required to remove infected and dead pieces of bone and to establish drainage to the area.

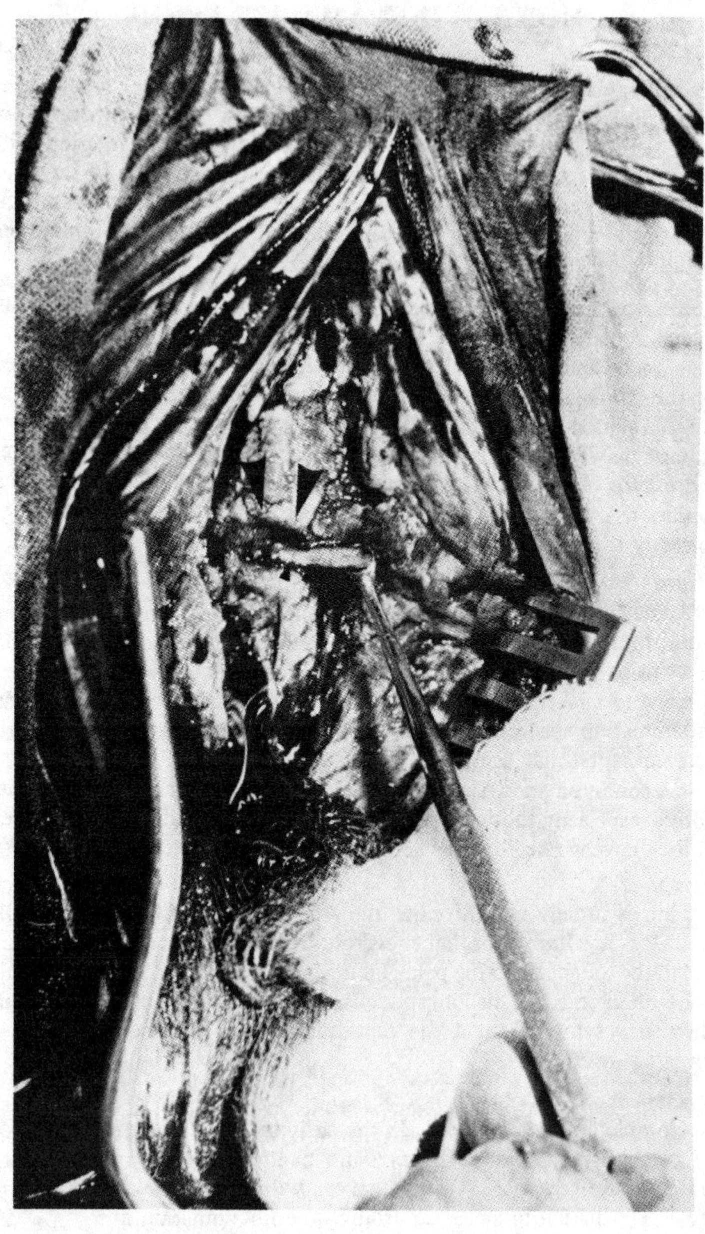

Fig. 5
Surgical treatment of *osteomyelitis*. Arrows point to infected area of bone.

BONE — INFLAMMATION OF

Probably bone diseases are responsible for more unfitness of horses than any other type of ailments. The usefulness of large numbers of racehorses, trotters and other light horses is often temporarily or permanently lost through some bone affection, which may interfere with the movement of a joint. In addition, acute inflammation of the bone which commonly results from some external violence, such as a kick, often results in at least temporary unfitness and may lead to complications including exostosis (extra deposit of bone.)

Acute inflammation Bones are covered with a fibrous membrane known as the periosteum, except at the points of tendinous and ligamentous attachment and on the articular surfaces where cartilage is substituted. On those bones which are not deeply seated, as in the legs, the periosteum is easily injured by a blow and the result is very painful. Acute inflammation of bone may be divided into *periostitis* (inflammation of the periosteum), and *osteitis* or *ostitis* (inflammation of the bone substance itself). These conditions may progress so that extensive new bone growth occurs, unless correctly treated early.

Cause

Acute inflammation usually arises from external injuries which result from stumbling, falling, being kicked, striking hurdles and so on. It may arise from constitutional disturbance. Injury frequently involves some damage to ligament or tendon sheaths at points along their course, with inflammation spreading to the periosteum in the near vicinity. Bacterial contamination may aggravate the condition.

A condition known as "sore shins" affects the cannon bones of young horses, especially thoroughbreds when their training has been too severe or they have worked on very hard ground. This is ascribed to a *periostitis*.

Symptoms

Pain is usually evident when the affected part is handled and, if the trouble is in a limb bone, lameness results. The area is at first swollen and hot to the touch. Later the pain and heat are less but the thickening on the bone often remains for long periods. Very mild cases of *periostitis* may show few symptoms and the condition is often overlooked until it is revealed by *exostosis*.

Treatment

Complete rest is essential. In the early stages, the use of an ice pack or cold hosing, followed by pressure bandage is essential to limit the inflammatory response. Drugs such as *phenylbutazone* may be prescribed by a veterinarian to aid in controlling the inflammation.

Exostosis An *exostosis* or outgrowth of bone tissue not uncommonly follows upon a *periostitis*. Long continued irritation to a part may cause bony growths, and concussion in some form or other is a common cause of *exostosis*. Among the more common forms of *exostoses* are splints, spavin, ringbone and some sidebones.

The treatment of these various conditions is dealt with under the respective headings.

BOTS

The "bot", as found in the stomach of the horse and commonly seen in the dung, is an intermediate stage in the life cycle of the horse bot fly (*Gastrophilus spp.*). There are several species of these flies and their larvae are the parasitic "bots" of horses which inhabit the stomach for a time.

Horse bot flies are yellowish to dark-coloured, hairy, bee-like flies which are not seen throughout the whole year, having a well defined seasonal occurrence which varies according to climatic conditions and according to the species. In Australia the common bot fly worries horses from January to April. It deposits its eggs on the long hairs of the forelegs just below the knee and elsewhere on the legs, on the mane, chest and shoulders. Other species of bot flies deposit their eggs on the hairs of the jaw, throat and chest, while others leave their eggs on the long hairs of the lips and sometimes on the nostrils. The female fly hovers near the horse, darts in rapidly and deposits an egg which is cemented to a hair. This process is repeated. The adult female does not feed and lives from a few days to a fortnight solely for the purpose of laying eggs.

Horses resent the presence of the flies and kick or run away. This has given rise to the idea that the flies bite or sting, which however, is not the case. The eggs of the common bot fly hatch in about 7 to 10 days and the emerging larvae cause some slight irritation which makes the horse lick or bite at the part and so the larvae reach the mouth. Here they make their way into the mucous membranes of the lips, tongue and cheek where they wander for several days. After leaving these tissues they may attach to the pharynx for a short time and eventually are swallowed and attach themselves to the stomach wall where they remain to maturity. The larvae of other species behave somewhat differently, but finally attach themselves to the stomach wall. Maturity of the larvae or bots is reached in 8 to 12 months, when they detach themselves from the stomach wall and are passed out with the dung, where they are commonly seen. Pupation occurs in the soil and the adult fly emerges in 3 to 10 weeks depending on temperature.

Ill Effects of Bots There is considerable controversy among horse owners as to the ill effects of the bots on horses. Actually their presence in

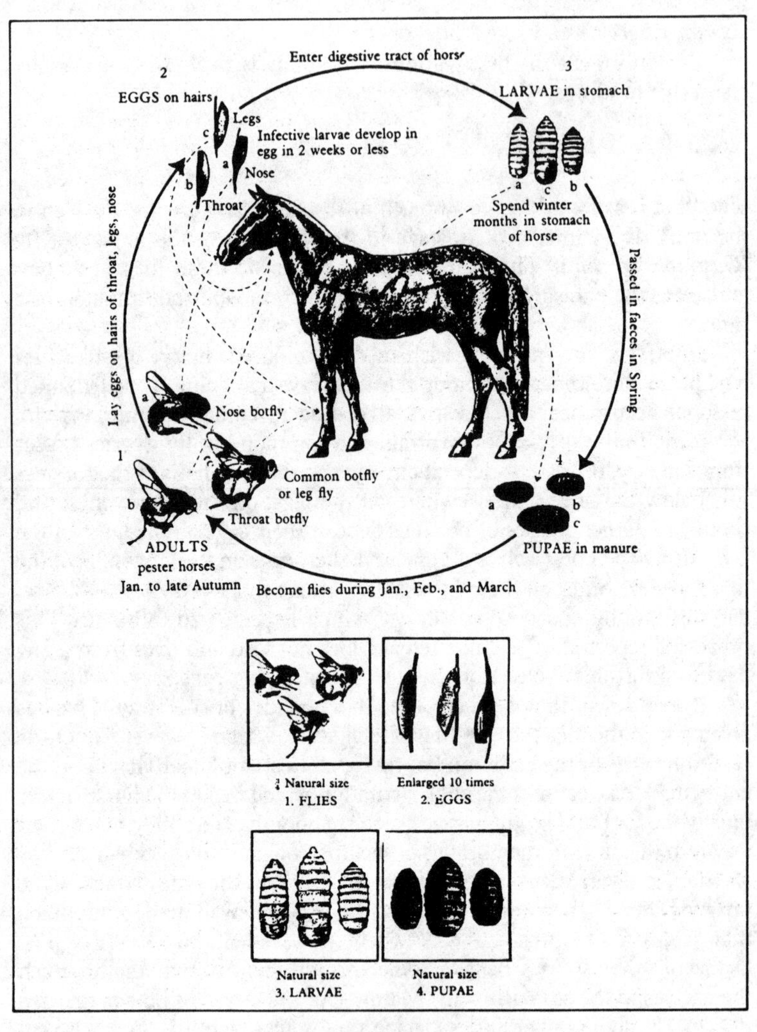

Fig. 6
Life history of bot flies.

(F. Thorpe and R. Graham, University of Illinois, College of Agriculture)

the horse's stomach does not cause as much trouble as is commonly attributed to them. It is probable that they are harmful to young horses when present in the stomach in large numbers. Further, in horses of any age, the accumulation of bots in the pyloric region of the stomach near the duodenum can cause mechanical obstruction or irritation leading to closure of the pylorus. Occasionally bots may weaken the wall of the stomach where they are attached, leading to ulceration, abscess formation and toxaemia and, on still rarer occasions, bots have been known to penetrate the stomach wall and deaths have occurred from peritonitis. Heavy infection with bots may cause digestive upsets and unthriftiness.

Bots do not eat away portions of the stomach wall, as is commonly thought by some horsemen who have conducted a post-mortem examination and examined the stomach. The left half of the stomach into which the gullet enters is lined with a white mucous membrane. Contrasting sharply with this—with no gradual transition—is the reddish-brown mucous membrane of the right half of the stomach. This contrast is so remarkable that a person without knowledge of the anatomy of the horse is naturally inclined to believe that one half of the mucous membrane is wanting as a result of some disease, or, when bots are found in the stomach, to assume that the membrane has been eaten away by the bots.

It is important to remember that unthriftiness in horses is more likely to be due to other much smaller internal parasites than bots, such as red worms, which cause a lot of trouble and are not seen in the droppings as are bots.

Treatment An old and effective treatment for bots in the stomach of the horse is the administration of a gelatine capsule of carbon bisulphide in the correct dose according to body weight. As carbon bisulphide is very irritant and unpleasant, it must be given in a capsule as a "ball" or by stomach tube. The dose rate on the basis of 5 ml per 50 kg body weight is — foals 10 ml, yearlings 10 to 15 ml, adults 20 ml. The maximum dose for a large draught horse should not exceed 30 ml. The horse should be starved for 18 hours before treatment and for 4 hours afterwards but may be given access to water. Subsequently a light diet should be given for several feeds. Under no circumstances should a purgative drench, such as oil, be given following the administration of carbon bisulphide as this is dangerous. Other methods of treatment under veterinary supervision include the use of *Neguvon*, which has been found to be safe and effective.

Prevention The protection of horses from the egg-laying activities of the female bot flies is difficult. The flies dislike shade and are not inclined to enter stables. With horses at grass, the provision of shelter trees or sheds into which horses may go during periods of fly activity is beneficial. It is not possible to protect the areas where the more common bot fly lays its eggs, but when the throat bot fly is prevalent, the under surface of the jaws and the jowl can be protected with sacking or cloth attached to a headstall. In this way the flies are prevented from laying eggs on these favourite sites and this may reduce the extent of bot infection. Washes of various insecticides are of little value in preventing the fly laying its eggs. Perhaps the soundest measure is thorough grooming through the dangerous summer and autumn months to remove all visible eggs. Singeing is also quite sound, if well carried out. Frequent vigorous scrubbing of the areas where the eggs are deposited with hot water (35 °C) is also effective. This stimulates mass hatching and rapid death of the young larvae. No satisfactory repellent is known which will keep the female fly away from the horse.

BOTULISM (Forage Poisoning)

Botulism is a type of food poisoning caused by the ingestion of a powerful toxin produced by an organism known as *Clostridium botulinum.* It differs from other bacterial diseases in that it is an intoxication and not an infection, and therefore is neither infectious nor contagious. For the disease to occur the toxin must be present in the feed before it is eaten. The botulism organism exists as a spore in the surface layers of the soil from which it gains access to hay, silage, dry tussocky grass, vegetables and stagnant shallow water containing decomposing organic matter. In such situations, and subject to certain suitable conditions, the organism multiplies and elaborates its toxin. The conditions necessary are moisture, warmth and the absence or restriction of air. Moisture and warmth also favour the development of mould and, whereas ordinarily *Cl. botulinum* can grow only in the absence of air, it can grow in fodder exposed to air if it has a mould growing over it. Thus mouldy fodders are liable to contain the botulism organism. In a hay stack or chaff silo the fouling caused by mice or mice carcases is not infrequently responsible for the toxin in only a portion of the stack or silo. Grain may be similarly contaminated. In the case of silage, botulism spores may be blown into the silo and remain dormant until conditions such as mould formation favour their development. This is one reason why mouldy fodder should not be fed to horses or other stock. The organism may grow in dry tussocky grass clumps and commonly develops in carrion, including rabbits, birds and rodents. If this occurs near or in shallow stagnant water, it may be "poisoned" by the toxin and if animals drink this water it may be responsible for the disease. Toxic fodders are usually palatable and will be eaten by animals to which they are offered. Likewise, stock may graze closely on new shoots of grass over dead tussocky clumps in which toxin has developed.

There are five principal types of *Cl. botulinum* known as types A, B, C, D and E, and, although the symptoms produced by all types are similar, the fact that differences exist in the toxin produced is important in relation to prophylactic vaccination. A vaccine prepared from one type will not protect against another type.

Briefly then the condition of botulism is produced by the presence in and the absorption from the intestines of a toxin produced by the organism *Cl. botulinum.*

Symptoms The symptoms of botulism in horses, as in other animals, are those associated with the action of the virulent toxin on the nervous system. At first there is lassitude, drooling of saliva, a peculiar slow and very persistent movement of the jaws, and unsteady gait. Inability to swallow food is soon manifest. Eating becomes progressively difficult and drinking is only carried out with great difficulty. Often partially chewed food will be dropped or becomes lodged at the base of the tongue. As the disease progresses, the tongue hangs from the mouth and there is a mucous discharge from the nostrils. The horse stands in one place and there is slight swaying of the body and sometimes twitching of the muscles. Abdominal type respiration occurs due to paralysis of the chest muscle. The animal loses co-ordination of the limbs and finally goes down. There are no manifestations of pain but the horse struggles ineffectually to regain its feet, these efforts utimately passing to a paddling action with both fore and hind limbs. The temperature is usually below normal except when the animal has become distressed from struggling, and is never high. Death usually occurs in from 1 to 4 days after the commencement of the illness. Some chronic cases last longer but very seldom does recovery occur. No characteristic changes are seen on post-mortem examination. The slight abnormalities which may be observed, such as congestion of the lungs and even congestion of the mucous membranes of the intestinal tract and abnormal conditions of the heart, are not due to the effect of the toxin. It is not uncommon to find food plugged at the base of the tongue.

Treatment Little can be done in the treatment of horses affected with botulism. Skilled veterinary attention in the early stages of cases which develop slowly may effect a cure. Quick acting purgatives are given in an attempt to remove the toxin from the alimentary tract, and central nervous stimulants are given. Stomach tube feeding and good nursing are also recommended in mild cases of the disease.

Prevention It is possible to immunise stock against the disease with a type-specific toxoid, which is a vaccine prepared from the particular type of organism present in the fodder. This is, of course, difficult to determine.

Mixed type immunising toxoids are available but are seldom used due to the infrequency of the disease. Generally, the main method of prevention of this disease is by careful feeding of horses and the discarding of all damaged or mouldy fodder, whether hay, chaff, grain or silage.

BOWELS — IMPACTION

See *Colic*

BOWELS — INFLAMMATION OF (Enteritis)

Inflammation of the intestines (enteritis) is a fairly common disease condition, and generally results in diarrhoea.

Causes In horses it is often associated with errors in diet leading to irritation of the mucous membranes of the bowels and infection with organisms which are common in the intestinal tract. Other causes include unrelieved impaction of the bowels or obstruction by calculi, eating of sand, indiscriminate dosage with irritant drugs and ingestion of irritant poisons. Foals are commonly affected, when the disease is mainly of dietary origin and frequently occurs during the mare's "foal heat". Enteritis is frequently accompanied by gastritis (inflammation of the stomach) and may occur secondarily to some infectious diseases. One of the more common bacteria causing diarrhoea is salmonella.

Symptoms The symptoms vary considerably, depending on the extent of the inflammation and also the age of the animal. Foals, for example, are very dull, disinclined to suck, exhibit a foetid diarrhoea which may contain mucous, have colicky pains and raised temperature and become dehydrated. Older horses may show similar signs to colic, that is paw the ground, look anxiously around, lie down and roll and when dehydrated will have an increased pulse and may be cold in the limbs and ears. When diarrhoea results, the massive loss of fluid involved can result in shock.

Treatment Enteritis is frequently fatal in the horse if professional attention is not obtained as quickly as possible. In the meantime the horse should be isolated from others and placed in a well ventilated stable or shed and kept warm. The horse should be starved pending the arrival of the veterinarian, but allowed access to water. Chlorodyne in 7 g doses in 600 ml of water may be given and repeated every 4 to 6 hours if necessary. In the case of young foals the most frequent cause is a change in the milk associated with the mare's "foal heat". This seldom requires any treatment and will usually resolve within 24 to 28 hours. If diarrhoea is still present after this time complete withholding of milk for 24 to 48 hours and substitution with boiled water containing 30 g of glucose per 600 ml of water every 4 hours is often sufficient to effect a cure. Dehydration and shock may happen very quickly in severe diarrhoea in foals and, therefore, veterinary attention should be sought to administer intravenous saline type solutions or plasma.

BRAIN — INFLAMMATION AND DISEASES OF

The brain may be affected by infectious diseases which directly attack and inflame the substance of the brain itself, or the covering membranes. This may be from bacterial or viral disease, but fortunately few of these horse diseases are likely to be experienced in Australia. Infectious diseases primarily affecting other parts of the body may spread to the brain and cause inflammation or abscesses. In some cases, toxins from infectious processes in other parts of the body may cause brain damage. Toxic materials found in some plants also have specific effects on the brain.

Depending on the area of the brain affected, and the extent of the damage, symptoms may vary from coma, drowsiness or paralysis, to loss of co-ordination, twitching or violent spasms and convulsions.

Other conditions may be caused by tumours, injuries, heat exhaustion or congenital abnormalities.

It will be appreciated that inflammation and diseases of the brain and central nervous system are exceedingly difficult conditions to diagnose and to treat and must be left to a veterinarian.

Certain of these diseases are discussed briefly in their appropriate alphabetical order.

BRAN MASH — PREPARATION OF

Because a properly prepared bran mash will be eaten readily by most sick horses and is therefore of importance in general nursing, details of preparation are now given.

Take a clean iron bucket and scald it; throw away the water. Then place 1.5 kg of bran and 30 g of salt in the bucket, add 1.5 litres of boiling water, stir well, cover with a folded bag and allow to stand for a quarter of an hour. Give when sufficiently cool.

BREEDING

See *Parturition, Pregnancy*

BROKEN-WIND

The term "broken-wind" is applied by horsemen to 2 quite different diseases. It is used to describe horses that make a respiratory noise ("roaring") during exercise. This condition is generally found in large horses, 16 or 17 hands high, and usually becomes noted between the ages of 3 and 5 years. The other condition for which the term broken-wind is used is when the horse has a chronic cough and difficulty in breathing. This is also termed the "heaves". These conditions are discussed separately under *Roaring* and *Heaves.*

BRUSHING

The terms "brushing" or "cutting" refer to an injury to or near the inside of the fetlock joint caused by the inside of the opposite foot striking these parts. The injury may be on the inside of the coronet.

Cause The trouble is seen mainly in young horses which tire easily, or in old and out-of-condition horses. Some cases result from bad shoeing, especially the fitting of too wide a heel on the inside, or it may be due to the conformation of the legs, particularly if the toes are turned outwards from the fetlocks. The fetlock of a horse which turns his toe out is bent inwards as well as backwards when the weight is passing over the leg, and is thus brought nearer to the other leg, the foot of which may strike it in passing. The liability is greatest when the horse is fatigued.

Horses may "brush" with both fore and hind legs, but the trouble is more serious in the fore limbs as the horse is apt to stumble and may fall. Regardless of whether the "brushing" is slight, perhaps only to the extent of rubbing off the hair, or whether it is sufficiently severe for skin to be cut by the edge of the shoe, the cause should be ascertained and an attempt made to prevent it.

Treatment and Prevention The wound itself usually requires but slight attention, provided the cause is removed and the place protected from further injury. If infection is controlled, such a wound only becomes serious when from constant repetition of the blow, the part thickens. If this happens on the inside of the fetlock, it may result in an enlarged joint.

Protective boots and pads may be purchased, or a pad may be made from a piece of folded rug or blanket tied or strapped around the leg above the fetlock, care being taken not to adjust it too tightly. When turned-out toes are responsible for the brushing, special shoes should be fitted, of which many types have been recommended, the pattern depending largely on the type of work the horse is required to perform.

Special care should be taken with young horses shod for the first time and they should not be required to do fast work or be over-extended until they have become accustomed to their shoes and have obtained hard condition. Over-exertion of horses at any time should be avoided, especially if they are in poor condition.

CALCULI

A calculus is a solid stone-like concretion composed usually of mineral substances and found in ducts, passages and hollow organs throughout the body.

Common calculi which occur in the horse are discussed under their appropriate headings.

See *Colic*—Obstruction Colic (intestinal), *Salivary Calculi* (cheek stone), *Urinary Calculi* (kidneys, ureters, bladder)

CANCER

Cancer is the term popularly used for any malignant tumour or neoplasm. It is characterised by a rapid growth of certain cell types, resulting in destruction of normal tissue at the site of the growth and spread to adjacent lymph glands and deeper structures. Malignant neoplasms spread to other parts of the body via the bloodstream or lymph vessels setting up secondary growths (metastases) in new organs or tissues, including vital organs such as lungs, liver, spleen and kidneys.

In horses cancer is uncommon and many tumours are slow growing and metastasise relatively late in their course.

The most common type of tumour in the horse is the *sarcoid.* It usually occurs following cuts to the legs or other areas of the body and results in proliferation of granulation tissue ("proud flesh"). Although *sarcoids* can grow quite large they do not spread to other areas of the body or metastasise to vital organs.

Another common neoplasm in the horse is the *squamous cell carcinoma.* This is a more malignant neoplasm than the sarcoid and usually involves areas such as the third eyelid or the penis and can result in spread to local lymph glands and other areas of the body. In grey horses *melanomas* are very common and are found around the anus and vulva, just under the tail. Unlike *melanomas* in man, *melanomas* in horses are usually slow spreading.

Cause It is not known what causes most forms of cancer, but *sarcoid* formation is thought to be the result of a particular virus.

Treatment Radiation therapy with radioactive cobalt or randon seeds is effective for treatment of *squamous cell carcinomas* if used early in their course. Recently, good results have been reported in the treatment of *sarcoids* by use of cryotherapy or freezing. If seen early in their development *melanomas* can be surgically removed.

CANKER

The term "canker" is applied to a chronic moist softening of the horn of the horse's foot, starting at the frog and slowly extending to the sole and wall of the foot. This condition results from an inflammatory change in the horn-forming tissue which causes secretion of a serous fluid instead of the normally produced cells.

Cause While the exact cause of canker is not understood, the predisposing causes which lead to the condition are generally known. Continued standing in dampness and filth, general neglect and injury to the foot, and faulty shoeing that removes frog pressure are some of the important predisposing causes of the disease.

Symptoms The symptoms of canker are frequently not observed until considerable damage has been done and the disease is far advanced. The main signs of the condition are the offensive odour from the foot, the liquid secretion from the cleft and sides of the frog and the rotting away of the horn of the frog and sole. Eventually the frog and even part of the sole may be separated from the underlying sensitive tissue. Instead of normal horn being produced, there is often a fungoid mass. Deep in the tissues there is frequently a foetid cheesy material. As a result of the fungoid growth, the horny sole and frog and sometimes the entire foot become deformed.

Treatment The cure of canker is no easy task, especially if the condition is well advanced. Surgery is indicated to remove the fungoid growths and decayed horn. A hot searing iron is sometimes used, but the knife is preferable. When the condition is extensive, this treatment should be carried out under a general anaesthetic by a veterinary surgeon.

Antiseptic dressings are useless without first removing the diseased tissues. The surgery involves cutting away or stripping all the diseased horn and some of the healthy horn. The foot must be dressed regularly for some considerable time until it is certain that the new growth of horn is healthy. After the foot operation, the walls of the foot should be shortened and a broad plain shoe nailed on, which can later be used to hold dressings in place. The foot should now be held in a foot bath of 60 g of bluestone dissolved in 4.5 litres of water for an hour. It should then be allowed to dry thoroughly, following which one of a number of astringent antiseptic dressings may be applied by dipping cotton wool or gauze into same and packing it over the affected area. A pad of oakum sufficiently thick to cause considerable pressure is placed over the dressing and held in place by pieces of tin fitted to slip under the edge of the shoe. The dressing should be changed daily, and the horse kept in a clean dry stall or yard and given light exercise daily on dry ground. The persistent application of simple remedies and great cleanliness are more important than any particular drug. Subsequently, care should be taken to see that the horse is properly shod to ensure ground pressure to the frog.

CAPPED ELBOW (Shoe Boil)

Capped elbow is an inflammatory swelling of the tissues between the skin and the bone at the point of the elbow.

Cause The injury is caused by a bruise at the point of the elbow usually by pressure when the horse is resting on hard ground, sharp stones, or in a stable where there is inadequate bedding. It may also be caused by the heel of the shoe.

Symptoms Inflammation of the skin and rapid swelling, usually with a quantity of fluid beneath, are the early symptoms observed. This does not as a rule cause lameness, but the swelling may extend so that it not only covers the point of the elbow but extends to the armpit when there may be difficulty in moving the leg. The swelling usually subsides or becomes more circumscribed after a few days and may even eventually disappear. On the other hand, especially if the condition has occurred several times, a firm fibrous capsule may form and a pendulous sac may remain. In severe cases there is abscess formation.

Treatment Early cases will respond to constant cold water applications, which may be given with a hose. These should be followed by the use of astringent lotions, mild absorbent liniments and gentle

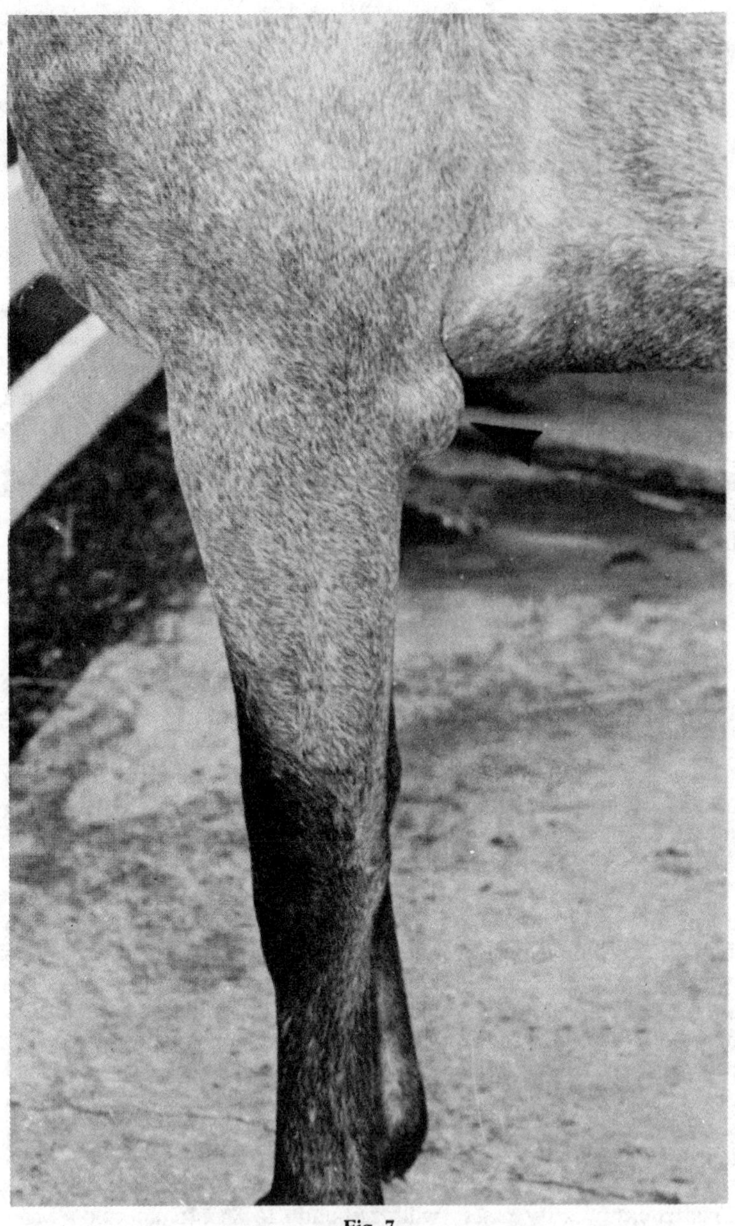

Fig. 7
Capped elbow ("shoe boil"). Swelling (arrow) over the point of the elbow due to trauma.

massage. If the swelling does not subside and continues to increase in size, aseptic aspiration of the fluid at the lowest point of the swelling is indicated. This should be left to a veterinarian who will also syringe out the cavity and may inject a corticosteroid preparation. In long standing cases surgical removal of the swelling may be the only feasible treatment.

In order to prevent recurrence of the condition, extra bedding should be provided in the stall. In the case of a horse kept in the open, a small sausage-shaped pillow about 10 cm in diameter may be attached around the pastern to prevent the elbow touching the ground when the horse is lying down.

Old chronic enlargements become very hard but although they are unsightly, do not necessarily interfere with the utility of the horse.

CAPPED HOCK

The condition of capped hock is similar to that of capped elbow. It consists of a swelling over the point of the hock. Two forms of capped hock are recognised, the common one being due to distension of a subcutaneous or false bursa covering the point of the bone. The second form is due to swelling of the tendon sheath and serous bursa, more deeply seated in the hock.

Causes As in the case of capped elbow, the injury is caused by a bruise at the point of the hock produced by blows, kicks or striking against hard objects. In stabled horses the damage is usually self-inflicted. Capped hocks are not common in unstabled horses.

Symptoms Swelling over the hock is readily recognised, especially if the hock is seen from the side. In the more common form, usually designated as "true capped hock", the swelling lies just under the skin, is soft and freely movable. When there is distension of the tendon sheath, the swelling is firm and less mobile. Lameness seldom occurs in the common form of capped hock and, in spite of quite a large swelling, which is unsightly, the usefulness of the horse is generally not affected. When there is inflammation of the tendon sheath or of its bursa, there may be difficulty in movement and lameness is evident.

Treatment This follows the same general lines as for capped elbow. Cold applications with a hose or ice packs, astringent lotions, absorbent liniments and gentle massage will reduce the swelling in many cases, but it is often impossible to effect complete reduction. If the swelling is fluid filled, aspiration should be performed by a veterinarian and a corticosteroid injected. If this is followed by a pressure bandage, resolution often occurs.

CATARACT

Cataract is an opacity or opaque condition of the crystalline lens of the eye or its capsule, which more or less obscures vision. Opacities of the lens are commonly observed in old horses and may gradually progress until the horse is blind. On the other hand, the cataract may only partly occlude the lens and have little effect on vision. White spots or opacities of various shapes occurring on the front of the eye, due to scars of wounds which have generally resulted from external violence, are commonly thought by horse owners to be cataract. This is incorrect as cataract is confined to the lens. Cataract is not a growth but a biochemical change in the lens, and there are many causes. Although cataract occurs more commonly in old horses, it may be congenital and therefore seen in newborn foals.

Cataract is a serious defect in horses and is regarded as an unsoundness, although small cataracts may cause very little interference with vision. A veterinary surgeon is able to diagnose and determine the extent of a cataract with the electric ophthalmoscope, and this is important.

Whereas in man and dog very effective surgery can be carried out in the treatment of cataract, this surgery is not usually effective in the adult horse. Congenital cataracts in foals can be removed with some success.

CATARRH (Rhinitis) ("Colds")

Catarrh is an old term once widely used to describe inflammation of mucous membranes, particularly those of the air passages of the nose and throat and associated with a copious secretion of mucus. Today, inflammation of the mucous membranes of the nose is more correctly referred to as rhinitis. Acute rhinitis or coryza occurs in the common "cold", and is frequently accompanied by pharyngitis and laryngitis.

Cause The cause in most cases is due to a virus infection. The disease is very contagious and, although horses of all ages are affected, it occurs more commonly in foals and yearlings. The disease is more prone to occur in the autumn and winter.

Symptoms The mucous membranes of the nose are at first dry and congested. This is followed by a watery discharge from the nostrils and

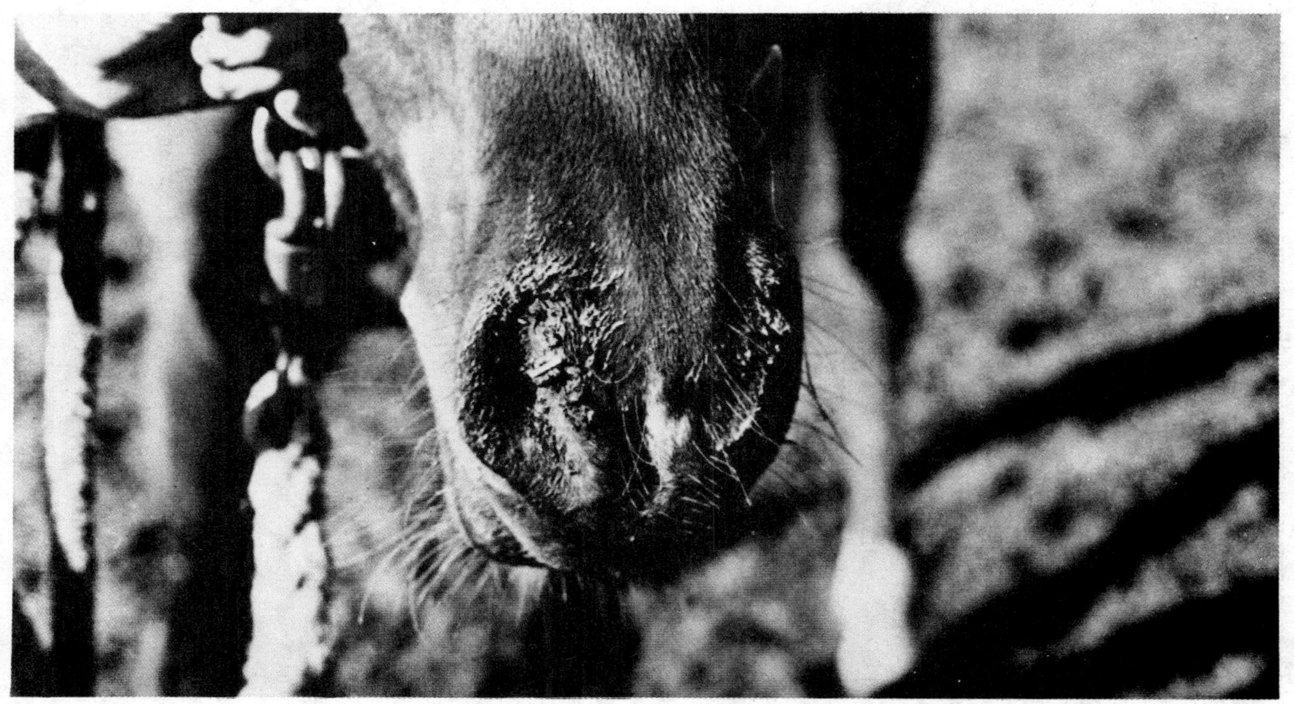

Fig. 8
Catarrh. Dirty nose resulting from dried nasal discharge in a horse with a cold.

eyes. These discharges later become thicker and of a yellowish-white colour if secondary infection with bacteria occurs. The animal has a slight fever, is dull, sneezes or snorts, but does not cough unless the throat is affected. In uncomplicated cases, the trouble clears up in 7 to 14 days. When there is a persistent cough and the animal has difficulty in eating and drinking, pharyngitis may be present. This may be followed in some cases by bronchitis and pneumonia.

Treatment The disease itself is not usually serious, but it should receive proper attention because it may lead to more serious disorders or become chronic. General attention to the comfort of the animal, isolation (because the disease is contagious), and good nursing are the main points to keep in mind. Soft feed including bran mashes, if adequate green feed is not available, and fresh water should be provided. If the horse is not stabled in cold weather, it should be rugged. A few days of rest, fresh air and good feeding will be of greater benefit than most medications. Antibiotics are not indicated in the treatment of most colds.

CHOKING

Choking is not as common in horses as it is in cattle, probably because horses chew their food better than cattle and do not usually feed on root crops. An apple is sometimes fed to a horse and a sudden fright may cause an improperly chewed piece of fruit to be swallowed. Choking sometimes occurs in horses that eat greedily and bolt their food, which becomes lodged in and fills up a portion of the gullet.

Symptoms The symptoms vary according to the position of the material causing the choke. The obstruction may be in the upper part of the oesophagus (gullet), at the middle portion, or close to the stomach.

In high choke the head is poked out, there is great distress and the horse has an anxious expression. There is hurried breathing, frequent cough, excessive flow of saliva, sweating, stamping and the horse runs backwards. The lump can usually be seen or felt in the upper part of the neck. The abdomen rapidly distends with gas.

In middle choke the symptoms are not so severe. The chin is drawn in to the chest, the horse hiccoughs and makes retching movements as though it wishes to vomit. The lump caused by the object can be seen and felt. The abdomen may be distended.

In thoracic choke the symptoms are less severe. Feed or water may be ejected through the nose or mouth after the animal has taken a few swallows. There are some symptoms of distress, fullness of the abdomen, cough, and sometimes retching movements. The obstruction will be encountered if a stomach tube is passed down the oesophagus.

Treatment Professional assistance should be obtained as soon as possible. In high choke it may be possible, if a mouth-gag is available, and with the aid of an assistant pressing the object forward from the outside, to pass the hand into the pharynx, grasp the obstruction and to gradually and steadily withdraw it. Frequently, the oesophagus goes into spasm around the object and the use of tranquillisers, under veterinary guidance, often results in the obstruction being passed into the stomach.

COLIC

The term "colic" is widely used to designate any form of severe abdominal pain in the horse. Through common usage, it usually refers to pain arising in the digestive organs. Whilst most cases of so called colic do arise from derangements of the digestive system and are usually amenable to treatment, pain in the abdomen may arise from diseases of the uterus, bladder and kidneys.

Cause It will be seen from the above that colic is a symptom rather than a disease. In this section, however, colic will be discussed as a disturbance of the digestive system.

It has been estimated, however, that up to 90 per cent of colic cases are associated with damage from worm infestations, particularly red worm, which damages the blood supply to the intestines. Owing to its relatively small stomach and the bulk of intestines, especially the large intestines which have many changes in diameter, the horse is particularly susceptible to digestive upsets. Most cases of digestive colic are caused by errors in feeding, faulty mastication or by factors which interfere with the process of digestion. To this, however, must be added the effects of overwork as a factor in the causation of colic. A sudden change in the manner of feeding; giving a large feed to an over-hungry horse; lush green feed producing rapid fermentation and gas formation; eating coarse indigestible material or mouldy, sour or fermented feed, are all prone to cause an attack of digestive colic in a horse.

Faulty mastication in young horses may be due to imperfect shedding of the temporary teeth. In older animals, the edges of the molar teeth often become so sharp that proper mastication is difficult. Indications of this may be shown by the horse dropping small balls of partly-chewed food out of the mouth, often referred to as "quidding". Horses so affected will often bolt their food without proper mastication, and this is likely to cause digestive upset through fermentation in the stomach. Removal of the sharp edges of the teeth with a tooth rasp will frequently result in the food being properly chewed. When a horse has developed a habit of bolting his food, a few big stones in the manger will prevent him getting too big a mouthful at a time.

Fatigue, exhaustion, and general weakness and debility will result in impaired digestion. Hard and exhausting work will have the same effect. Other factors which interfere with the process of digestion include heavy work on an overloaded stomach (especially in horses which do irregular work and are "soft"); severe worm infection; chilling due to exposure to cold when the animal is wet with sweat, and sometimes the drinking of a large quantity of very cold water.

The above remarks apply to the causes of colic in general. It is now proposed to describe briefly the main types of digestive colic, together with symptoms and treatment.

Spasmodic Colic This is a common form of colic which obtains its name from the fact that there are intervals of ease between the spasms of pain. It is commonly known among some horse owners as "water gripes", although it has nothing to do with the inability of the horse to pass urine. The pain is caused by sudden severe contractions of the muscular wall of the bowel. It might be termed a cramp colic. It may arise from chilling after heavy work or simply from overwork, from indigestible food, from a large drink of cold water or from exposure to severe cold and rain.

Symptoms

The pain begins suddenly and, although not continuous, is usually severe. During the attacks of pain, the horse paws the ground, stamps the hind feet, kicks at the belly, and crouches as if to lie down, looking around anxiously at the flank. The horse may straddle as though trying to pass urine. This last symptom gives rise to the common but erroneous deduction that the animal is suffering from an affection of the kidneys or the bladder. As the attack progresses, the pains get more frequent and last longer. The animal may throw itself down, roll and jump up again, paw the ground, kick at the belly, and become generally violent. "Rumbling of the bowel" may be heard by putting the ear to the flank of the horse.

Treatment

A veterinary surgeon has at his disposal a variety of drugs which will speedily deal with this condition. In the absence of professional assistance, quite good results are often obtained by comparatively simple treatment. Walk the horse around slowly, and, if possible, prevent it from rolling and injuring itself. Frequently horses convert a relatively simple condition into a severe one by rolling about. This can give rise to a twist in the intestines which can be fatal.

If the spasmodic colic recurs every 2 or 3 weeks, the most likely cause is damage to the intestinal blood supply by red worms. In these cases a cure is sometimes effected by having a veterinarian administer a large dose of a deworming mixture (for example, *Thiabendazole*) by stomach tube.

Flatulent Colic This is a form of digestive disorder which is sometimes referred to as tympanitic colic, wind colic or bloat, and is associated with the formation of gas, mainly in the large bowel. It usually follows the eating of lush green pasture, clover or other legumes. Feeding a large quanitity of green vegetables such as cabbages will cause the condition. It may arise from obstruction of the bowel. Feeding new oats or mouldy hay, or a heavy feed after a long day's work are other causes.

Symptoms

The pain is not as severe as in spasmodic colic, but is more continuous. The horse is dull, paws the ground, makes frequent attempts to urinate and may or may not lie down. The abdomen enlarges, being most noticeable in the upper right flank. Breathing may be interfered with and the animal may attempt to lie down carefully but seems afraid to do so. Dung may be passed in small quantities and is usually accompanied by flatus (gas).

If the condition is not relieved, more serious symptoms may follow, due to a twist or rupture of the intestines, and the horse may suffer respiratory distress due to pressure of the distended bowels on the diaphragm making breathing difficult.

Treatment

In the case of very severe distension, it may be necessary to puncture the bowel and a veterinary surgeon should therefore be called in. It is inadvisable for a layman to attempt to do this operation, which requires skill and care greater than that required to puncture the paunch of cattle or sheep. A small trocar and canula is inserted in the right flank, and the canula is not left in.

Frequently the condition resolves upon the administration of 2 to 4 litres of paraffin. This is best given by a veterinarian, using a stomach tube. A few days' rest and careful feeding on small feeds are advisable after recovery from a mild attack of flatulent colic.

Obstruction Colic This form of digestive disorder is usually more serious than those already described. It includes impaction of either the small or large intestine, and chronic constipation.

The common causes are overloading of the bowels, especially when food is hurriedly eaten, or after prolonged feeding on harsh dry feed and eating of straw bedding. Other causes include intestinal calculi, displacement of the bowel and tumour growths.

Symptoms

The symptoms of this disorder usually develop slowly. There is abdominal pain which may disappear for a day or 2 and reappear with more violence. The horse appears dull and the dung is passed in small quantities and is drier and harder than usual. The abdomen appears full, but is not distended, and the horse continually looks round at the flanks. Later the animal gets restless, lies down and assumes a characteristic attitude flat on its side with head and legs extended, occasionally raising its head to look at the flank. The horse may remain on its side for 5 to 15 minutes, then rise and may press its hindquarters against the stall or a fence and then go down again. On applying the ear to the horse's flank, no intestinal movement is heard. Pressure of the impacted bowel on the bladder may cause straining and frequent efforts to pass urine. When symptoms become more acute, the animal may break out into a sweat, the extremities are found to be cold, the mouth dry and the breath foul smelling.

Symptoms of obstruction colic may last for a week or longer and, provided auto-intoxication, enteritis (inflammation of the bowel) or rupture does not occur, the animal eventually recovers under suitable treatment.

Treatment

The aim of treatment is to soften the impacted mass, thus allowing it to be passed. This is usually done by a veterinary surgeon who administers medications such as paraffin and *dioctyl sodium sulfosuccinate* by stomach tube. Usually 1 to 2 treatments are sufficient to enable resolution of the condition.

Sand Obstruction

When there is reason to believe that the obstruction is due to sand, which may be indicated by sand in the scanty droppings, the horse should be given up to 5 litres of liquid paraffin for a large animal, preferably by stomach tube. The paraffin should be repeated in a day or 2, in smaller doses. However, sand colics are notoriously difficult to resolve completely.

Wheat Engorgement Colic Before farm mechanisation, many cases of digestive upset occurred when working horses gained access to wheat grain. Cases still occur in light horses on farms.

Symptoms

In mild cases there may be only dullness, lack of appetite and sluggishness at work. In severe cases there is violent pain, the horse becomes restless, paws the ground, looks around at the flank and kicks at the abdomen. As the pain increases, the horse throws itself on the ground and rolls about. The respirations are hurried, the mucous membranes of the eye and mouth become brick red in colour and the horse breaks out in a heavy sweat and may become violent. In some cases rupture of the stomach may occur. Following recovery from the acute effects of the condition, laminitis ("founder") frequently occurs.

Treatment

A veterinary surgeon would inject certain tranquillising and pain relieving drugs to quieten the horse and also pass a stomach tube to relieve any possible distension, and to administer paraffin and possibly other drugs. In the absence of a veterinarian, between 2 to 4 litres of paraffin could be given. Veterinary assistance should be obtained as soon as possible as injections of antihistamine and corticosteroid drugs may be necessary to prevent laminitis.

Worm Colic The common large roundworm (*Ascaris equorum*) is sometimes responsible for digestive upset and symptoms of colic. The worms may be so numerous that they become impacted in the small intestine, and the obstruction may be so severe that intussusception (telescoping of the bowel) and even rupture of the bowel may occur. Young horses up to 2 years of age suffer most from these worms.

Symptoms

The symptoms are similar to other forms of colic and may be accompanied by tympany (gas formation).

Treatment

If symptoms of constipation are shown, care is necessary in the treatment of the large roundworm when conventional methods, such as carbon bisulphide, are used. Under such circumstances it would be preferable to treat the horse as for obstruction colic and, when bowel movement has been obtained, to treat for the parasites.
See *Parasites — Internal*

Volvulus, Torsion and Intussusception These terms all refer to twisting and inversion of the bowel, causing severe colic.

Symptoms

Similar symptoms as shown in spasmodic colic, but horses show a much greater pain response with frequent rolling, profuse sweating and a greatly elevated heart rate.

Treatment

Early diagnosis is important as surgery to correct these conditions is now feasible. However, even with surgery the chances of survival are quite poor.

CORNS

The term "corn" is applied to a bruise of the sensitive sole of the hoof at a point between the bar and the wall. Usually corns occur in the fore feet, and more often in the inner rather than the outer heel. A bruise elsewhere on the foot is referred to as a bruised sole or frog. Depending on the site and the extent of the corn the horse will show varying degrees of lameness. If the corn becomes infected this is known as a suppurating corn.

Causes Corns are mainly attributable to faults in conformation, such as wide flat feet with low heels; long feet; weak feet with excessively thin horn; excessively flat soles and feet with high, contracted heels. Bad shoeing is also a common cause of corns which follow excessive paring of the sole, bars or frog. The type of shoe fitted may cause a corn. For example, calkins fitted too high destroy the counter pressure of the frog with the ground and cause undue pressure upon surrounding tissues, leading to the production of corns. Badly seated shoes have a similar effect. Direct injury from stones which may become wedged between the heel of the shoe and the seat of corn may lead to bruising.

Symptoms The main symptoms are lameness of varying degrees, sometimes very slight but increasing with work, and at other times very severe. Tapping with a light hammer or firm pressure over the area causes great discomfort. In the case of a suppurating corn, the foot will be hot to the touch and the animal will flinch when that portion of the wall adjoining the corn is slightly struck. If not properly treated, pus may burrow through to the coronet to produce a quittor or suppurating sinus.

Treatment The treatment of corns is not always satisfactory, especially in the cases of very long standing. The normal procedure when a diagnosis of corn has been made is to remove the shoe, and then to lightly pare the seat of the corn to see if there is any suppuration. Excessive paring should not be undertaken, as this deprives the sensitive sole of its natural protection. Only in the case of a suppurating corn should the sole be excessively pared, and then only sufficiently to allow exit of pus. The important thing to keep in mind when treating an ordinary corn in a horse's foot, is to remove pressure. This may be conveniently done by applying a three-quarter shoe, which is an ordinary shoe with about 4 cm of the side of the shoe, adjoining the corn, cut off. If there is a corn on both the inside and outside of the foot, a so called bar shoe may be used. The use of these shoes allows a horse to walk without pain and prevents further injury.

Anti-inflammatory drugs, such as *phenylbutazone,* when prescribed by a veterinarian, can hasten resolution of the condition.

Suppurating corns require special treatment. The main aim is to provide drainage and this is best performed by a veterinary surgeon, who knows how deep to cut into the sole with a hoof knife. Once the site of infection is reached irrigation of the area with a mild antiseptic is performed. This should be done once or twice daily until the infection resolves, and an Ezy-Boot applied to protect the sole. Tetanus is sometimes a sequel to suppurating corns and, therefore, tetanus vaccination and tetanus antitoxin administration is essential.

CORYNEBACTERIUM INFECTION IN FOALS

Corynebacterium infections in foals are a major cause of foal deaths on studs in Australia. Foals with this infection have been called "rattlers" due to the rattling cough they have.

Causes A particular bacteria, *Rhodococcus equi* (formerly *Corynebacterium equi*) causes this condition. These bacteria can live in soil and it is thought that foals either ingest or inhale the bacteria when in infected paddocks.

Symptoms The disease tends to develop insidiously with the foal becoming lethargic, not sucking and developing a rattling cough. There is usually a high temperature (up to 41 °C) and a rapid respiratory rate.

Treatment It is important that a correct diagnosis be established early in the course of this disease as once abscesses develop it is difficult to obtain successful treatment. Only a few of the more expensive antibiotics are effective against the bacteria and these include *neomycin, erythromycin*, *gentamycin* and *streptomycin.*

CRACKED HEELS

The term "cracked heel" is applied to an inflammation of the skin in the hollow of the heel at the back of the pastern, and appears as painful transverse fissures having thickened edges.

Causes The result of washing the horse and not thoroughly drying the heels, or any situation which results in the heels being continually kept wet. It was formerly a common condition in army horses picketed with heel straps on lines in the open.

Symptoms The skin of the heel is reddened, fissured and tender. The cracks may become infected and suppuration occur, but more commonly they become covered at the edges by firm encrustations resulting from inflammatory exudations. As a result of this, the skin becomes increasingly thick and rigid. Lameness is present.

Treatment Clip the area and wash the lesion thoroughly with warm water and good quality soap. Dry thoroughly. Dab on white lotion as recommended in treatment of corns and then apply zinc oxide ointment or zinc cream repeatedly.

CRIB-BITING AND WIND-SUCKING

Crib-biting and wind-sucking are acquired vices, both of which result in the swallowing of air by the animal. A crib-biter rests the chin on, or with his teeth grasps the edge of the manger or another object at convenient height, in order to get a firm purchase; he arches and sets the muscles of the neck, draws in air and gulps it down giving a characteristic "grunt" at the moment he swallows. The animal may even use a knee or other part of a limb as the point of support for the chin. A wind-sucker arches its neck, draws its head towards the chest, and swallows a gulp of air. It does not require any object to seize or support the chin.

Causes Varied are the reasons given as to why horses acquire these vices. It has been suggested that young horses acquire the habit of crib-biting from the irritation caused by teething. Idleness and boredom are also held to be predisposing causes. Horses are certainly prone to learn these two vices by imitation, and idle horses, particularly young horses, quickly acquire the habits if they are associated with confirmed crib-biters or wind-suckers.

Ill-effects The ill-effects caused by these vices are loss of condition, indigestion and colic. Crib-biters wear down the front portions of the incisor teeth so that they do not meet properly when the mouth is shut and this interferes with grazing.

Treatment Once the habits of crib-biting or wind-sucking are acquired they are never forgotten. In long established cases, there is no satisfactory treatment other than by the operation of myectomy (excision of a portion of muscle), quite an intricate operation which is effective in a large percentage of cases. Many corrective measures are adopted to prevent horses indulging in these habits, which may be effective for a time, until the horse learns to outwit the preventive. For both crib-biters and wind-suckers, a broad strap fitting tightly around the top of the neck,

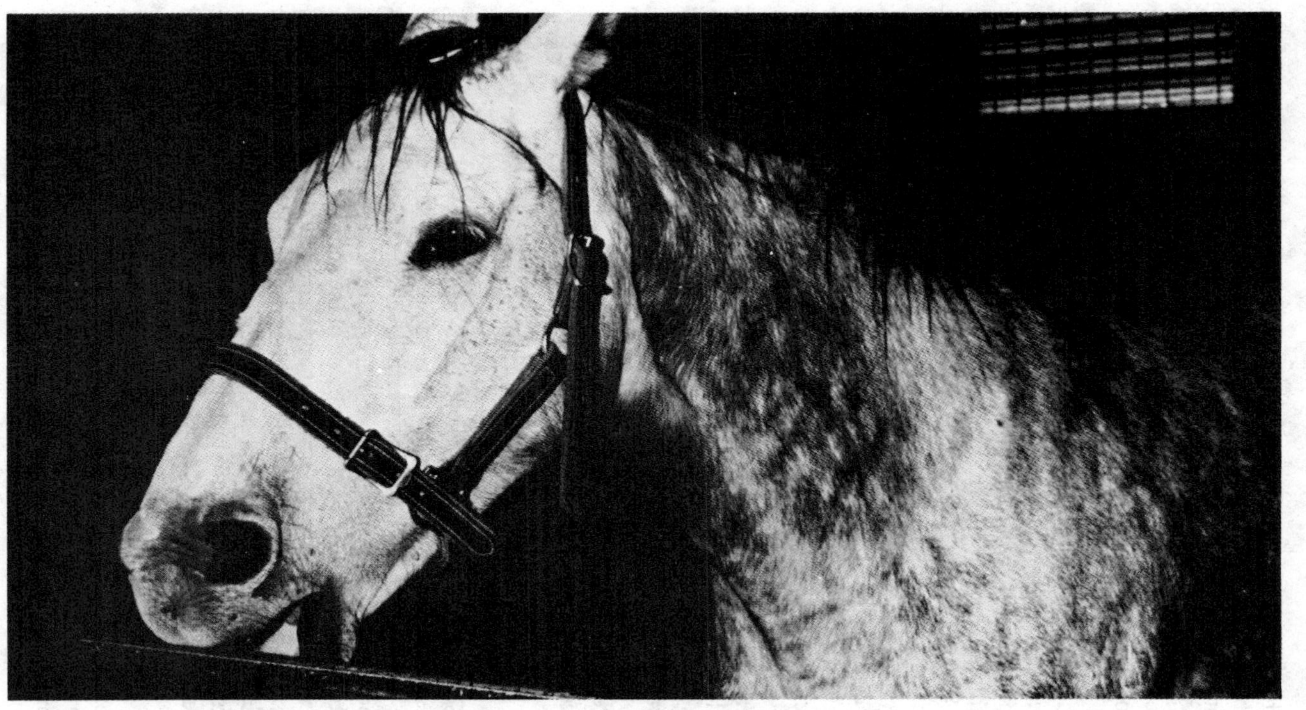

Fig. 9
Crib-biting

with a small wooden or metal gullet plate stitched on so that it projects on each side and sticks into the throat when the head is bent, may be used to control the habits. There are various types of commercial cribbing straps, one of which has recessed metal prongs which press into the throat region when the neck is arched. Even a plain leather strap fastened around the throat sufficiently tight to make arching of the neck uncomfortable, but not tight enough to interfere with breathing, will sometimes be effective. A hollow tube bit, perforated with holes throughout its length may be fitted so that when it is adjusted suction cannot be exerted owing to the impossibility of completely closing the mouth. Another device is a piece of thick rubber tubing with a strap passing through it, fastened around the lower jaw just behind the tushes. It is not always effective. Care must be taken, when these devices are removed during work or feeding, that they are immediately replaced, otherwise the horse will take full opportunity to indulge in the vices. A crib-biter may be put into a loose-box with four blank walls and fed from a removable trough, which is taken away as soon as the feed is finished. This can be effective until the horse learns to use its knee or other part of a limb to rest its chin on, or learns the vice of wind-sucking. Muzzles of various types have been tried in the past in an effort to prevent the teeth grasping or leaning against the manger or other object, but they were not sufficiently successful to warrant their adoption.

Irrespective of what preventive measure is adopted, there is every possibility that the vice will recur as soon as such measures are discontinued.

CURB

The condition known as "curb" is the sprain of a ligament at the back of the hock, shown by a swelling which is soft in the early stage, about a hand's-breadth below the point of the hock towards the inner side. It may be best observed by standing at the side of the animal. Another condition referred to as "false curb" occurs in approximately the same area and is due to an enlargement of the head of the small metatarsal or splint bone, which may be congenital or be caused by a bony deposit. It can be differentiated from true curb by being bone-hard and situated towards the outer side of the leg.

Cause Although curb may be caused when any undue strain is placed upon the hocks, such as by slipping forward with the hind legs, jumping and so on, hocks of a certain conformation seem to be more prone to curb than others. Faulty conformation, as when the hocks are too bent ("sickle hocks"), or too narrow from front to back across the lower portion,

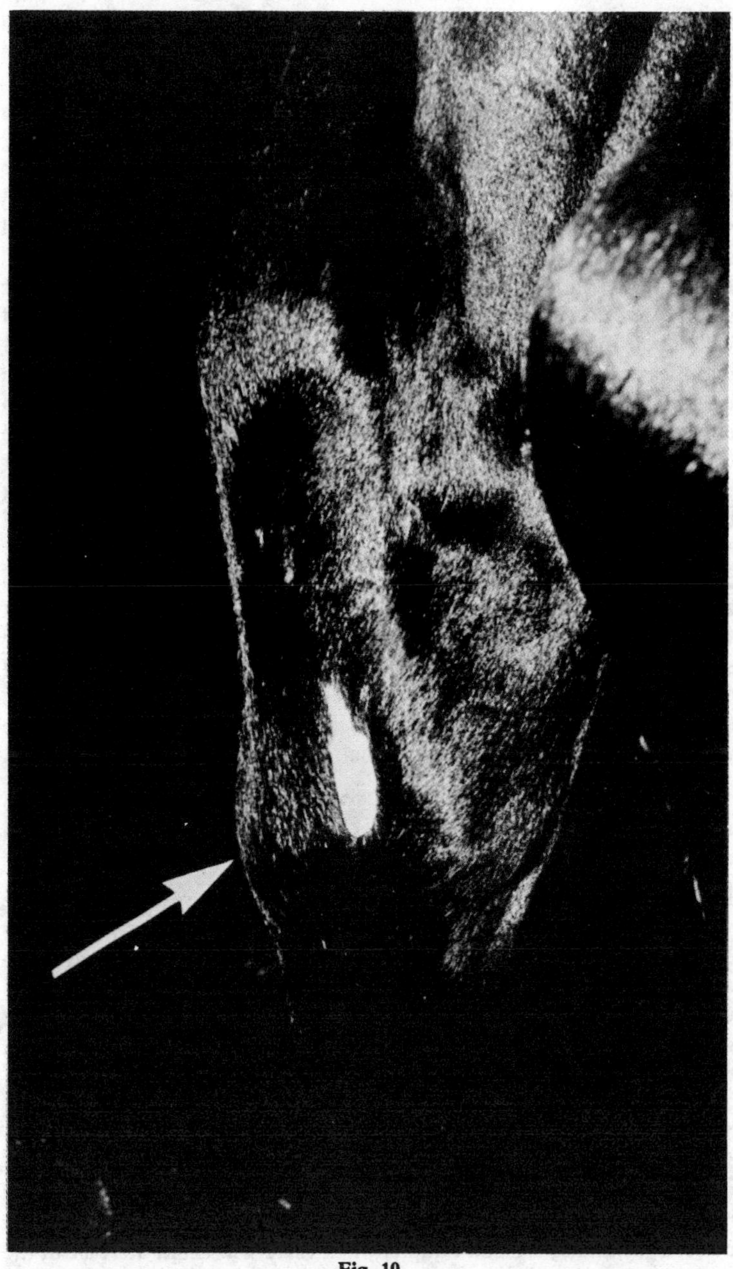

Fig. 10
Curb. Swelling due to sprain of plantar ligament (arrow).

appears to predispose horses to curb. A good hock should be large, and from its point the tendons of the hind limb should drop straight to the fetlock.

Standardbred trotters and pacers seem to be more prone to this disorder than other breeds.

Symptoms Lameness usually accompanies the formation of a curb, when the swelling is more or less diffuse with varying degrees of heat and soreness. The horse stands with the leg at rest and the heel elevated. Later, the swelling becomes better defined, the prominent curved line is readily detected and the thickness of the infiltrated tissue is easily felt with the fingers. The lameness may then become intermittent or disappear completely, but the enlargement remains. A hock thus affected is less able to endure severe work and is more likely to give way with effort; nevertheless many horses with pronounced curb work well and no further trouble is experienced. There is a tendency in young horses for the curb to disappear, but in older horses it remains as a permanent blemish and thus reduces the value of the animal

Treatment In the acute stage rest is essential and repeated cold applications should be applied to the curb in the form of ice packs or water from a hose. When the inflammation has been reduced and the swelling has assumed better defined boundaries, a period of rest extending over 3 or 4 months is necessary. Veterinary surgeons have certain injectable drugs which may be helpful. Special shoes, which have wedge-shaped heels, may be beneficial in the early stages of curb.

DEHYDRATION

Dehydration, which means loss of fluid from the body, is seen in a wide variety of disorders, and may be associated with either excessive fluid loss or inadequate fluid intake. Common conditions associated with dehydration are severe types of colic, diarrhoea and prolonged exercise where there has been excessive sweating. Endurance horses have been found to lose up to 50 litres of fluid via the sweat during the course of an 80 to 160 kilometre endurance ride.

Symptoms The main symptoms of dehydration are a dull coat, sunken eye-balls and a decrease in skin elasticity, so that when the skin on the neck is pulled up it will tend to stay elevated. There is usually an increase in heart rate and respiratory rate. Milder forms of dehydration can be detected by taking a blood sample, when there will be an increase in the number of red blood cells and an increase in the total plasma protein.

Treatment Treatment is aimed at establishing the cause of dehydration. If there has been inadequate water intake then fluid may have to be given by stomach tube. This should contain a balanced electrolyte (body salt) mixture, which should be prescribed by a veterinarian. Where there has been excessive fluid loss, if severe, then the horse's life may be in danger. This may necessitate the use of various fluid and electrolyte solutions given intravenously. Usually large volumes of these solutions are required (10 to 20 litres) due to the large blood and fluid volume of the horse.

DENTITION AND AGEING

The age of a horse may be determined fairly accurately by the appearance of the incisor teeth. If any real doubt arises, an examination of the molar teeth is necessary. Nevertheless, even the best of judges may be deceived unless they have some knowledge of the conditions under which the horse was raised. For example, horses pastured on sandy soil will wear their teeth much more rapidly than those raised on loamy soil with better pasture, or those that are entirely stable-fed. Even the water horses drink affects the development and appearance of the teeth. When some doubt exists as to the normal wearing of the teeth, some idea of the age of the horse can be determined by its general appearance. In the case of an old horse, there are certain pronounced indications of age apart from the appearance of the teeth. For example, in an old horse the bones on each side of the nose "fall-in" on account of the descent of the back teeth as it gets older. With grey or roan horses, there is a whitening of the coat, and in the case of almost all horses some white hairs are shown, especially about the temples, as the horse advances in years. The depth of the hollows above the eyes is, to a certain extent, a guide to the age of the animal.

There are 2 complete sets of incisor teeth, temporary or milk teeth, and permanent teeth. The temporary incisor tooth is small and white, has a distinct neck and a short root which practically disappears as the tooth gets older from the pressure of the growing permanent tooth beneath, until its remnant is pushed out of the jaw. The permanent incisor tooth is, by contrast, broad, thick and yellowish or brownish in colour. It has no marked neck but has a long stout root or fang stoutly implanted in the alveolus (socket) in the bone.

The parts of a permanent incisor tooth The surface which bites on the food or on the opposing tooth is the table or wearing surface. Each permanent incisor has on its table a blackened depressed ring known as the infundibulum, surrounded by a distinct narrow light-coloured ring of

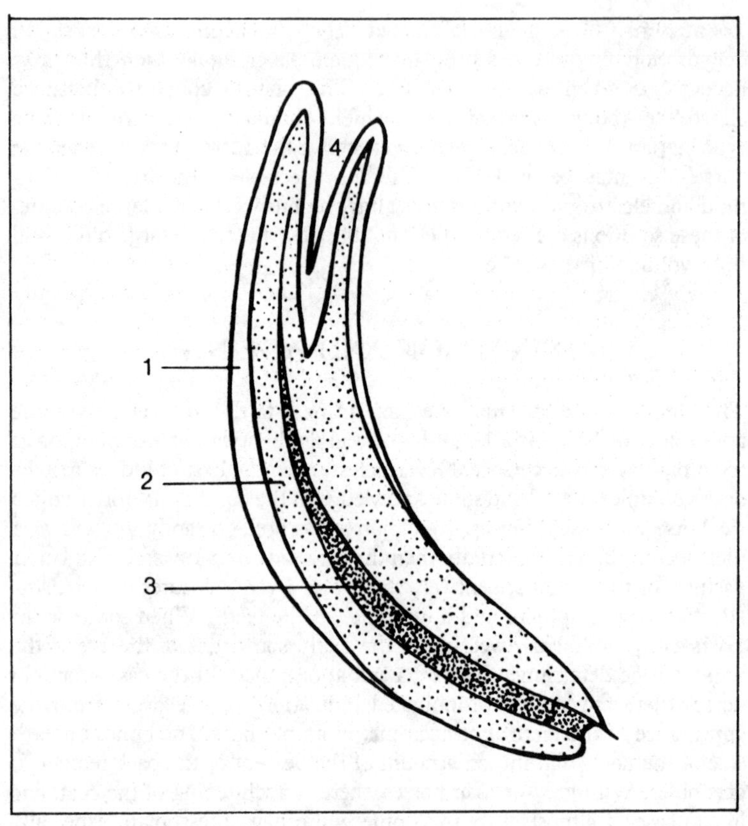

Fig. 11
Diagram to show the different parts of a lower incisor tooth and their relative positions. **1.** Enamel **2.** Dentine **3.** Pulp Cavity **4.** Infundibulum

(after "Animal Management" with permission of Her Majesty's Stationery Office, London)

enamel. This latter is easily seen and felt as it stands up a little above the rest of the surface. In the new tooth the infundibulum is very broad and deep, but with wear of the table it becomes shallower and smaller and gradually disappears. It some teeth, however, it persists for much longer periods than in others, the variation being due to the depth of the depression and the thickness of its enamel lining and also the manner in which the upper and lower teeth make contact with each other (uneven jaws). The blackening of the depressed area is due to discoloration from the food during mastication. As the teeth become worn away and continue to erupt, a central transverse darkish line appears on the tables in front of the disappearing infundibulum, due to exposure of the pulp cavity. The time of its appearance is variable depending on the method of feeding and quality of the tooth. The foregoing factors have to be taken into account when attention is paid to the so called "marks" on the table surfaces of a horse's teeth as an indication of the animal's age. The shape of the teeth, angle of projection and several other factors are more important than the "marks" in determining the age of a horse.

The *crown* of the tooth is that part which is above the gum and the point where the gum and tooth meet is the *neck*. The *root* or *fang* is the part within the bone which carries it. It is hollow and its cavity contains the blood vessels and nerves which nourish and sensitise the tooth (the pulp). Later the cavity becomes filled with a bone-like material known as dentine. All the permanent teeth in the horse are continually erupting, that is they are constantly being pushed out of the sockets by the slow proliferation of bone beneath their roots. (They do not actually grow longer.) This process is continuous throughout the life of the animal and compensates for the natural wear of the teeth. Thus, at first the crown, then the neck and finally the fang comes into wear. The "pushing-out" process continues in the absence of wear, and teeth which have none opposing them (as may occur when a horse loses a tooth in the upper or lower jaw) project beyond those in use.

Number of teeth There are 6 incisors, at first temporary and later replaced by permanent teeth, in each jaw. The 2 in the centre of the jaw are called "centrals", the next tooth on either side is referred to as a "lateral" and the outermost on each side of the jaw is the "corner" tooth. In the male, a tush or canine tooth appears behind the corner tooth on each side of each jaw when the horse is reaching maturity. This is a permanent tooth. Occasionally mares have rudimentary tushes.

There are 6 molar teeth on each side of each jaw, and they are numbered 1 to 6 in each jaw, top and bottom. The first, second and third are at first temporary and then permanent, but the fourth, fifth and sixth only appear as permanent teeth. Four other partially developed teeth, popularly called "wolf teeth" may be present, one in front of each first molar, but more commonly in the upper jaw only. They are vestigial teeth which were well developed in the early ancestors of the horse. They usually appear at the age of 5 or 6 months and generally fall out when the temporary molar behind is shed, and are not replaced. Occasionally they remain permanently in the jaw. Only the incisor teeth and the tushes will be referred to when discussing the age of the horse by the teeth.

FORMULA OF TEMPORARY TEETH

	Molars	*Incisors*	*Molars*	
Upper jaw	3	6	3	} = 24
Lower jaw	3	6	3	

FORMULA OF PERMANENT TEETH

	Molars	*Tushes*	*Incisors*	*Tushes*	*Molars*	
Upper jaw	6	1	6	1	6	= 40
Lower jaw	6	1	6	1	6	

If the four wolf teeth are included in the permanent formula, the number of permanent teeth is increased to 44.

Tushes are usually absent in the mare.

Order of appearance of incisor teeth *At birth* the foal usually has two central temporary incisors in each jaw. Their appearance may be delayed for 7 to 10 days.

At about 4 to 6 weeks the lateral temporary teeth are cut and the outermost or corner teeth come through *at 6 to 9 months.*

At 1 year all 6 temporary incisors in each jaw are in wear, the inner side of the corner teeth not yet grown up level with the front.

At 2 years the corner temporary incisors are well in wear, and all the teeth have well formed tables. Some care is necessary at this age in distinguishing between these well developed temporary teeth and permanent incisors.

At 2 years and 3 months there may be some evidence of the centrals giving way to the permanent teeth which erupt in pairs in both the lower and upper jaws. The gums may be red and swollen and the temporary teeth loose.

At 2 years and 6 months the central permanent incisors appear and at *3 years* they are in wear.

At 3 years and 6 months the lateral permanent incisors are cut and at *4 years* are in wear.

At 4 years and 6 months the corner permanent teeth come through and at *5 years* are in wear, but not fully (a typical 5 year-old mouth).

The horse has now 12 permanent incisor teeth (6 lower and 6 upper) and is referred to as having a "full mouth". The tushes or canine teeth usually start to appear when the horse is 4 years old. When present, there are 2 in each jaw, with the ones in the lower jaw closer to the incisors than the ones in the upper jaw. At first the tushes have sharp points and edges but these gradually become rounded with age.

At 6 years the corner teeth are in full wear over their entire surface, and such wear has caused the infundibula (depressions in the teeth) to become more shallow, especially in the central teeth where they may have disappeared. Reference has already been made to the cause of this variation. The wearing surfaces of the teeth are broad ones, the centrals showing perhaps a tendency to become triangular.

At 7 years the infundibulum has disappeared from the centrals and laterals but a trace of enamel may remain. There is a distinct notch on the upper corner incisor, where it overlaps the corresponding tooth on the bottom jaw. This is sometimes referred to as the "7-year hook".

At 8 years the infundibulum has disappeared from all incisors. Usually at this age, but sometimes earlier, a transverse darkish line appears on the wearing surface of the central teeth in front of the disappearing infundibulum. This is commonly referred to as the "dental star", and indicates that the teeth have worn down to the fang exposing the pulp cavity now filled with dentine. The shape of the table surfaces of the central teeth have become more triangular. The 7-year hook on the upper corner incisor has worn away somewhat or may have broken off. The "hook" completely disappears at 8½ to 9 years and the surface of the tooth is again level.

At 11 years the hook reappears and the notch becomes sucessively deeper, so that by 13 years it is very noticeable and usually persists throughout the life of the horse.

From 9 years onwards it becomes much more difficult to tell the age with any degree of accuracy. The wearing surfaces of all incisors have become changed from the broad oval to triangular, the back of the tooth forming the apex of the triangle. As the horse becomes still older, the table surfaces become round. The teeth project increasingly forward and appear to be longer on account of the receding gums. With increasing age, the dental star, which has gradually appeared on the wearing surfaces of all the incisors, becomes a "spot" rather than a line and occupies the centre of the table surfaces. At 10 years, sometimes a little earlier, a well-marked longitudinal groove known as "Galvayne's Groove" appears on the outer side of each upper corner incisor. It is first seen as a groove just protruding from under the gum and travels down the tooth as the horse ages. It reaches halfway down the tooth at 15 years, to the bottom at 20 years, is half grown out at 25 years and disappears at 30 years.

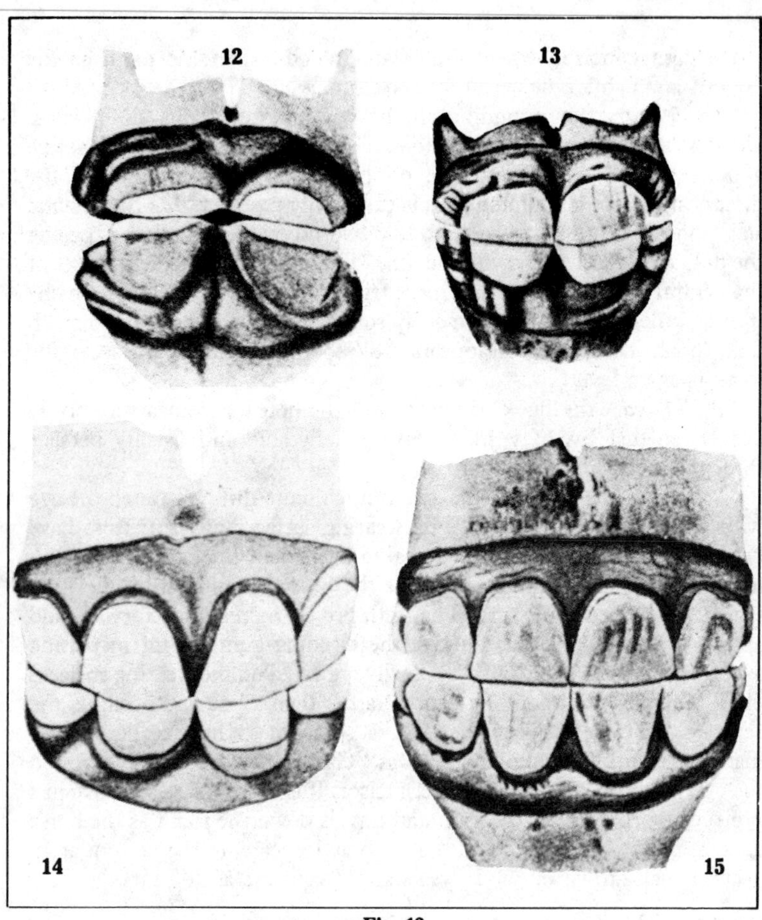

Fig. 12
Mouth at about 1 week. The 4 central milk incisors are cut. The 1st, 2nd and 3rd temporary molars also appear about this time.

Fig. 13
Mouth at 4 to 6 weeks. The 4 lateral milk incisors are through. The foal has now 20 milk teeth.

Fig. 14
Mouth at 5 to 6 months. The front edges of the central and lateral teeth are worn level.

Fig. 15
Mouth at 1 year. The corner milk incisors are well up and shell-like in appearance.The 4th permanent molars, 4 in number, are cut. The colt now has 28 teeth, 24 milk and 4 permanent.

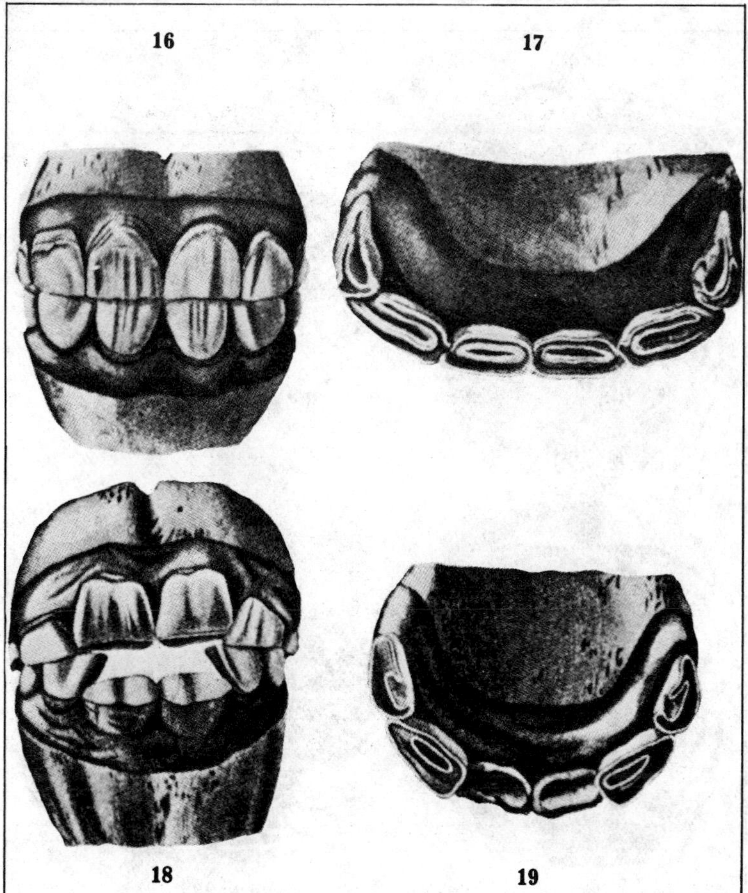

Fig. 16
2 years.

Fig. 17
Tables of lower incisors at 2 years. The tables of all the milk incisors are worn, the corner incisors have lost their shell-like appearance, and the 5th permanent molars are well up.

Fig. 18
Rising 3 years.

Fig. 19
Tables of lower incisors rising 3 years. The 4 central permanent incisors have replaced the corresponding milk teeth, and the 1st and 2nd permanent molars have replaced their temporary forerunners.

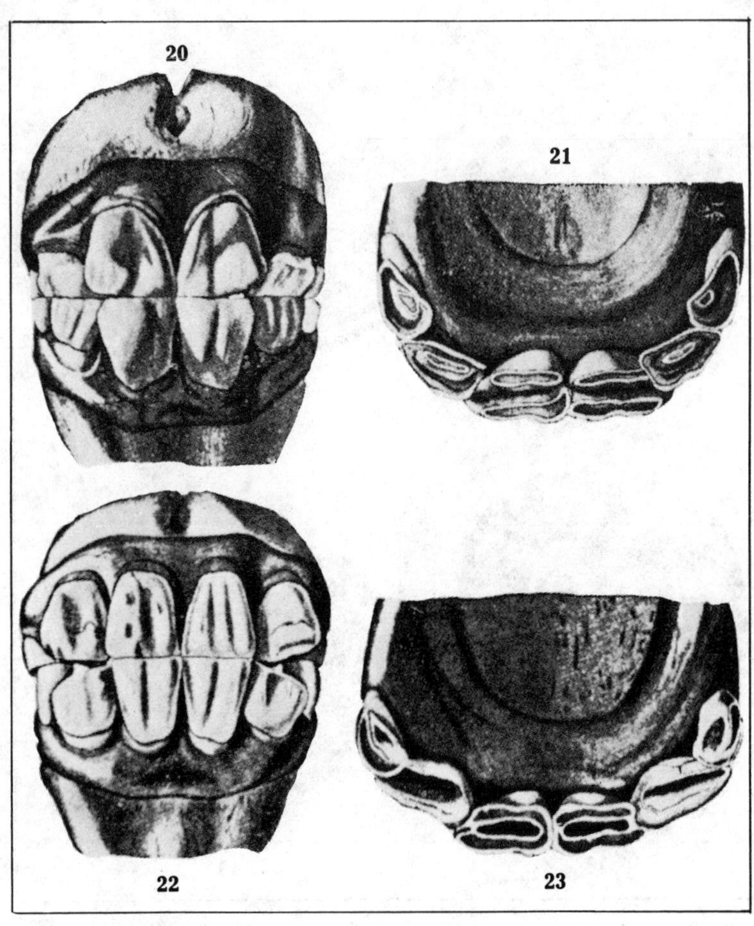

Fig. 20
3 years past.

Fig. 21
Tables of lower incisors 3 years past. The central permanent incisors are in wear, and the 1st and 2nd permanent molars are well up.

Fig. 22
Rising 4 years.

Fig. 23
Tables of lower incisors rising 4 years. The 4 lateral permanent incisors have replaced the milk teeth, as have the 3rd permanent molars, 4 in number. The colt has 32 teeth of which 28 are permanent.

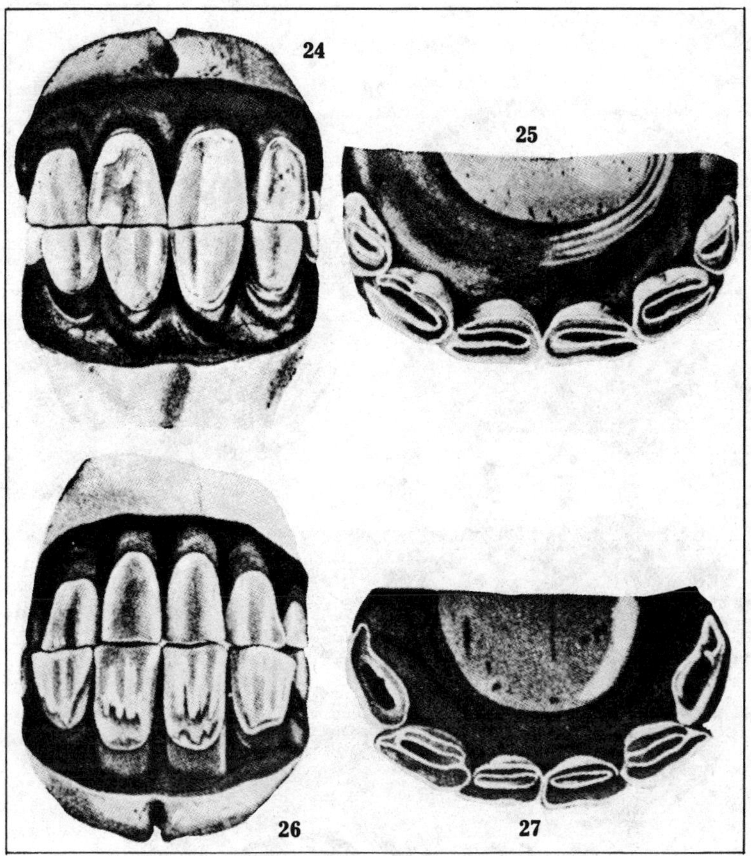

Fig. 24
4 years.

Fig. 25
Tables of lower incisors at 4 years. The 4 lateral permanent incisors are in wear, the 6th permanent molars are up, and sometimes the tushes are breaking through.

Fig. 26
Rising 5 years.

Fig. 27
Tables of lower incisors rising 5 years. The 4 milk corners have fallen out and are replaced by the permanent teeth. They are not on a level yet with the lateral incisors. The tables of the other teeth show more wear than at the preceding age.

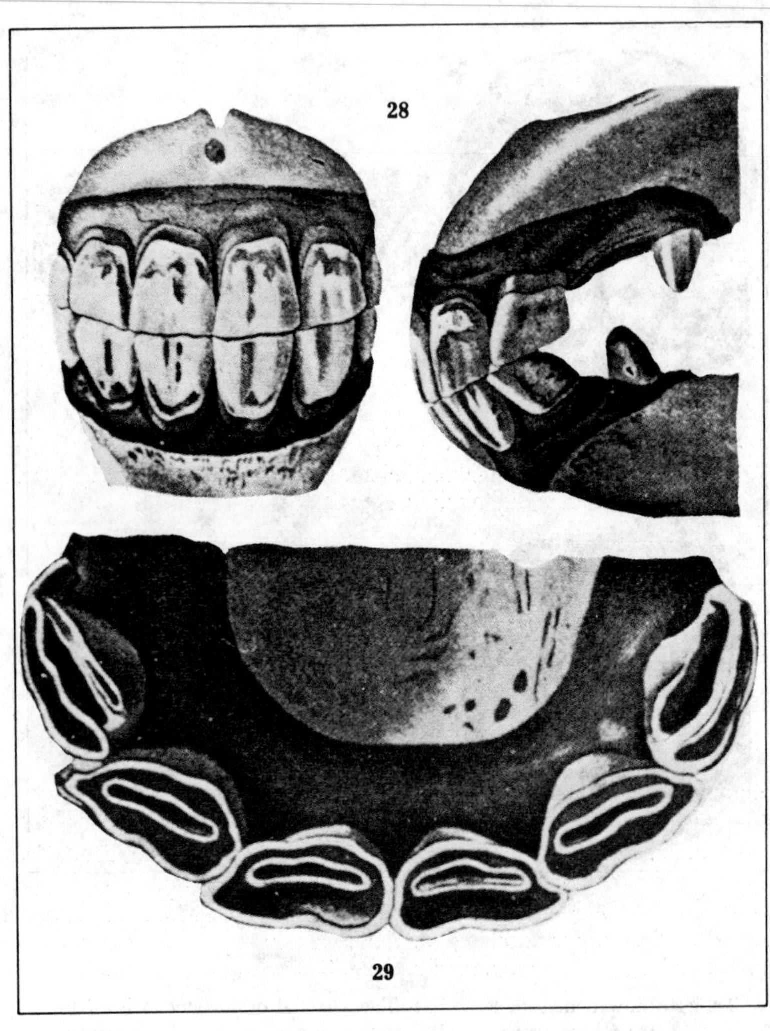

Fig. 28
5 years.

Fig. 29
Tables of lower incisors at 5 years. At 5 years the mouth is entirely made. All the permanent teeth are on the same level in the respective jaws, although the inner edges of the corner incisors have not yet come into use. The tushes are now well developed.

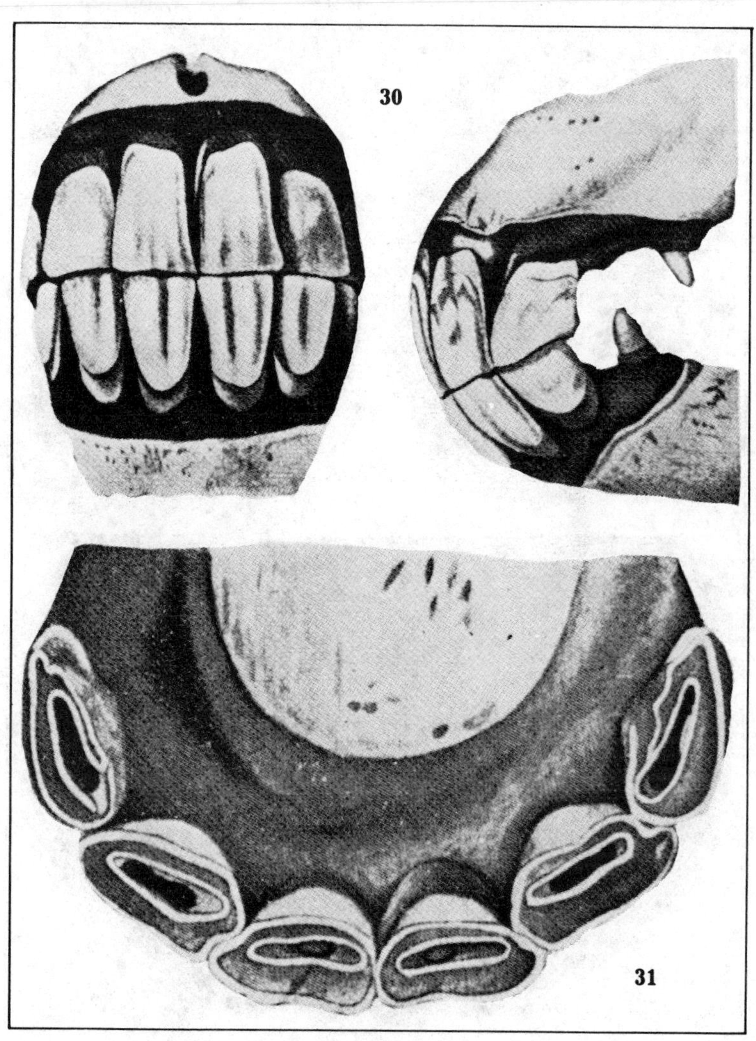

Fig. 30
6 years.

Fig. 31
Tables of lower incisors at 6 years. At 6 years the inner edge of the corner incisors is worn level with the outer edge. Wear has caused the infundibula of all incisor teeth to become more shallow, especially in the central incisors.

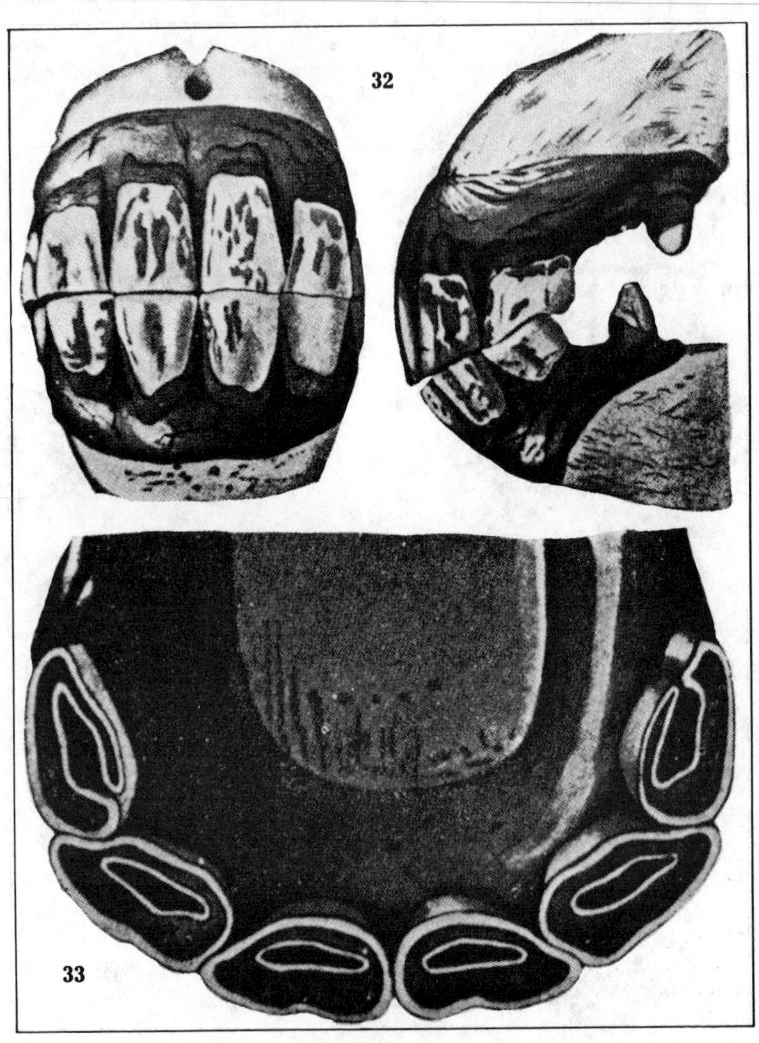

Fig. 32
7 years.

Fig. 33
Tables of lower incisors at 7 years. The infundibula have disappeared from the centrals and laterals but a trace of enamel may remain. There is a distinct notch on the upper corner incisor.

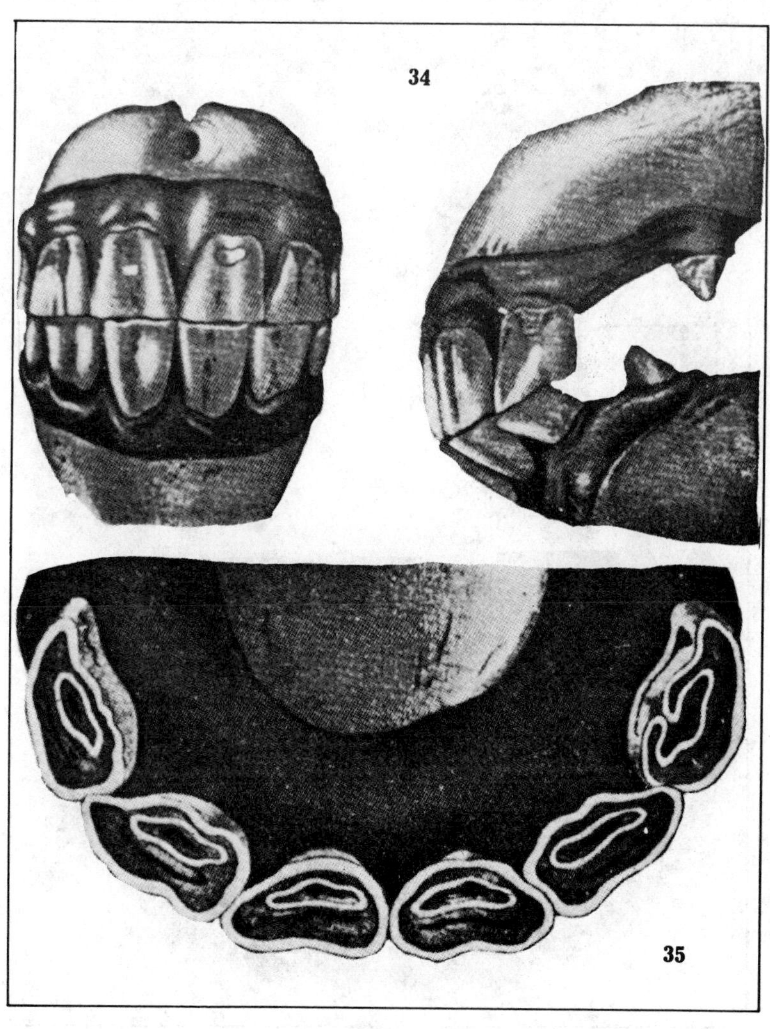

Fig. 34
8 years.

Fig. 35
Tables of lower incisors at 8 years. The infundibula have disappeared from all incisors. A transverse darkish line ("dental star") is present on the wearing surface of the central incisors in front of the disappearing infundibula. The directive of the incisors is notably changed in both upper and lower jaws, and they are opposed obliquely.

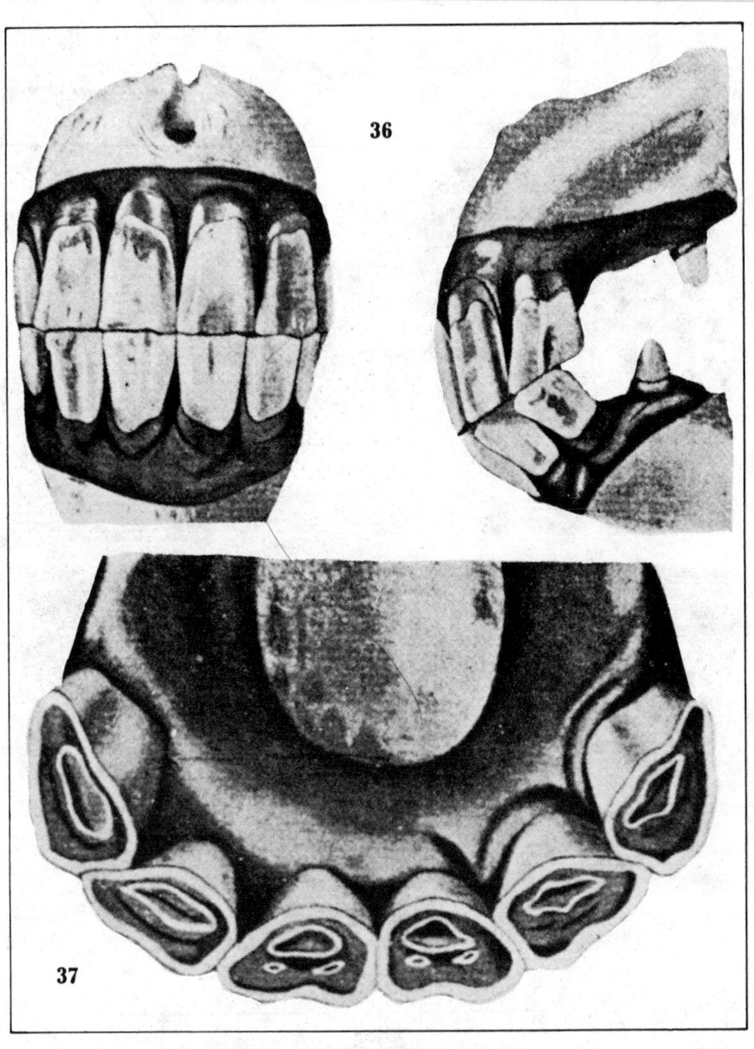

Fig. 36
9 years.

Fig. 37
Tables of lower incisors at 9 years. The incisor teeth are more oblique and appear to be longer than at the previous age. A slight groove may have begun to show at the neck of the upper corner incisor. The dental star is more prominent. Upon the table the central incisors are round, the laterals becoming round and the corner teeth are still broad ovals.

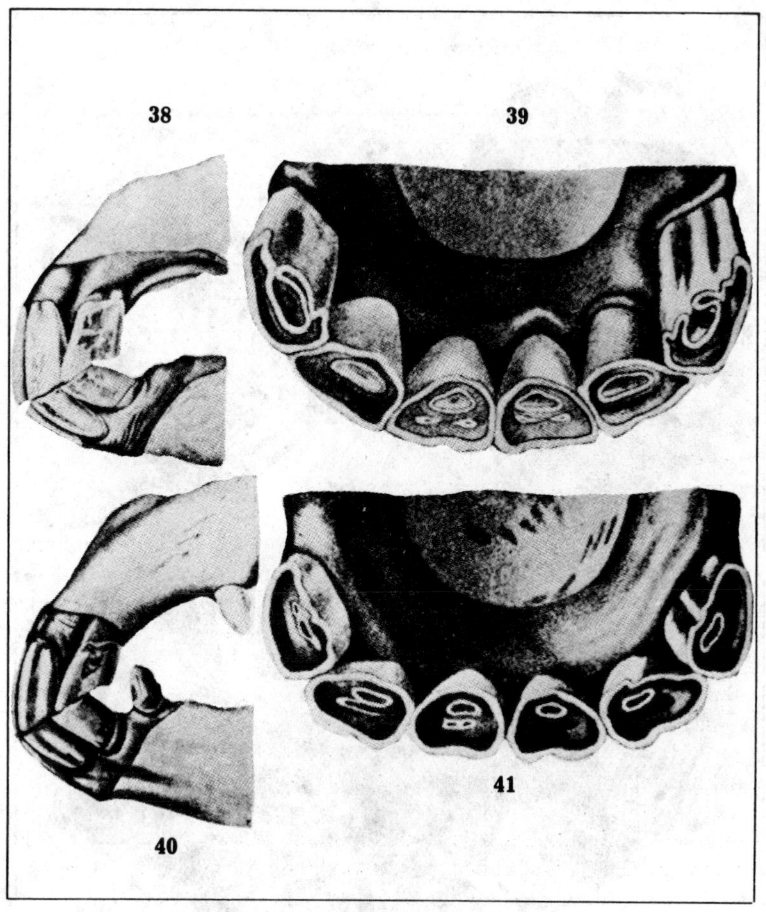

Fig. 38
10 years.

Fig. 39
Tables of lower incisors at 10 years. The incisor teeth have projected increasingly forward. The groove on the outer side of the upper corner incisors ("Galvayne's Groove") is more distinct, the tables of the laterals are round and the corners are tending to assume this form.

Fig. 40
11 years.

Fig. 41
Tables of lower incisors at 11 years.

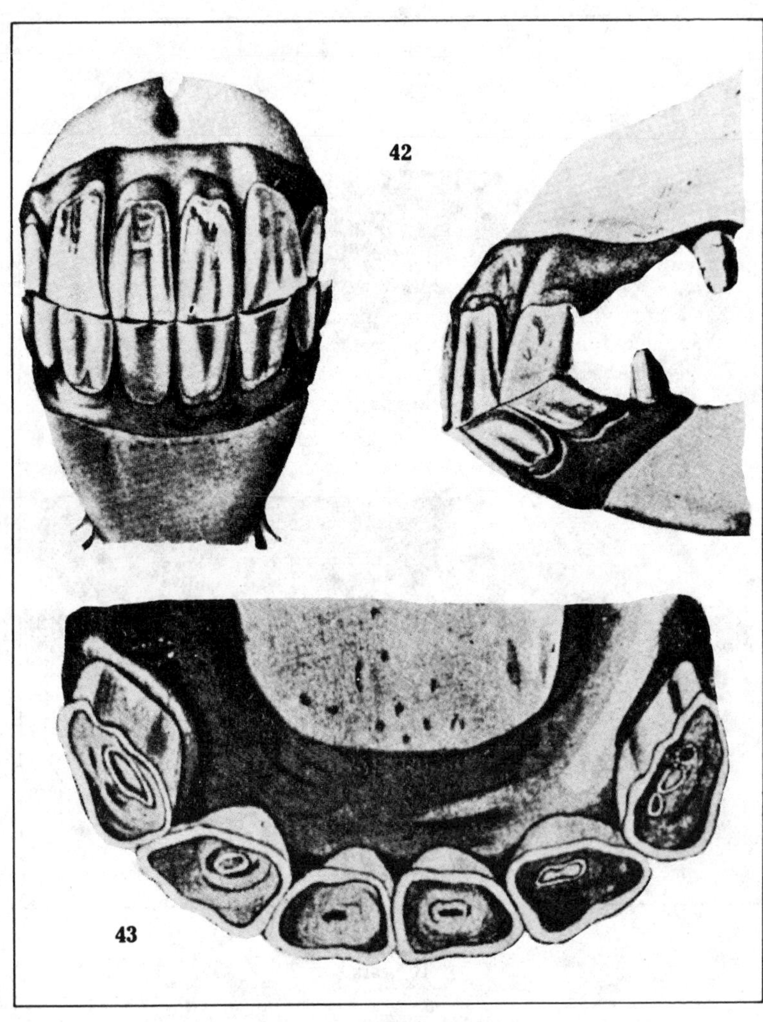

Fig. 42
12 years.

Fig. 43
Tables of lower incisors at 12 years. In profile, the upper corner shows a greater obliquity than the intermediates. It carries a notch behind, and the interspace which separates it from the lateral incisor is more marked. The tables of all the lower incisors are now round, tending to be triangular.

The foregoing figures of the teeth at various ages are from Goubaux and Barrier as reproduced by the New South Wales Department of Agriculture in Farmer's Bulletin No. 87 "The Teeth of the Horse and its Age".

DERMATITIS

See *Eczema, Mange, Leg Mange, Lice, Queensland Itch, Photosensitisation* and *Ringworm*

DESTRUCTION OF A HORSE

When it is necessary to destroy a horse, the most convenient and humane method is by shooting, provided it is done in the right place. A pistol or small bore rifle may be used, standing close with the gun almost touching the forehead, and held at a right angle to the head. The head can be brought into a convenient position by offering a handful of hay or grass. Aim at the centre of the forehead, about 10 or 12 cm above the level of the eyes, which is commonly in the centre of the "star". This site lies at the intersection of lines drawn between one ear and the opposite eye. The animal will not fall forward but will collapse exactly where it stands, death being instantaneous, the bullet having passed through the brain. Care should be taken that nobody is standing within sight behind the horse.

DIARRHOEA

Diarrhoea, usually referred to in animals as "scours", is a symptom rather than a disease and arises from damage to the bowel, from either infection or irritants.

Causes Diarrhoea can be caused by infection, sudden changes of feed, irritation of the bowels from eating mouldy or musty food, irritant plants, chemicals and so on. Many racehorses develop persistent diarrhoea as a result of the stresses of training. Diarrhoea may also exist as a symptom of a number of serious diseases, including worm infections. Persistent diarrhoea can be resistant to most forms of treatment.

Symptoms Frequent evacuation of loose stools, with or without pronounced abdominal pain, rumbling of the bowels, loss of appetite, weakness and staggering. Founder of the feet sometimes supervenes on persistent scouring. Increased thirst is usually apparent.

Treatment As diarrhoea is associated with a number of different disorders, the cause should be ascertained wherever possible before treatment is instituted. This may mean having a veterinarian carry out diagnostic tests, which could include blood counts, culture of droppings and tests of the intestines' absorptive capacity. Whenever diarrhoea lasts more than 1 to 2 days, professional assistance should be obtained, because large amounts of fluid and electrolytes (body salts) are lost. This may necessitate the injection of large volumes of electrolyte-containing solutions into a vein.

Horses with diarrhoea will usually drink an increased amount of water and so water should be made available at all times. Small tempting dry feeds, such as crushed oats and good quality chaff, should be given to keep up the horse's strength.

Other treatment, such as drugs to slow down the activity of the intestines, or antibiotics may be prescribed in specific situations by a veterinarian.

DIARRHOEA IN FOALS

Diarrhoea is commonly shown by foals during the first heat period of the mare, which is 6 to 9 days after foaling. This is a simple diarrhoea which usually passes off without any treatment being necessary. On the other hand, foals not infrequently are affected by a condition similar to that known as "white scours" in calves, which is due to bacterial infection. Foals may also show symptoms of diarrhoea from other causes.

Causes Foals are prone to eat dung and may also ingest genital discharges from the mare which have contaminated the udder and teats. The intestines of the very young foal are not ready to handle any solid material, so that eating dung and genital discharges causes irritation to the bowels, and resultant diarrhoea. Another cause of simple diarrhoea, apart from changes in the mare's milk, is over-engorgement of milk by the foal which has been separated from its mother for a prolonged period.

Diarrhoea caused by infection with various types of bacteria is more commonly seen on horse studs where large numbers of mares foal, and infection occurs from contaminated foaling paddocks, loose boxes or yards. It seldom occurs when an isolated mare foals in a clean paddock. The condition is also seen associated with other diseases of foals, such as joint-ill or navel-ill.

Symptoms The symptoms of simple diarrhoea, unassociated with bacterial infection, are the appearance of offensive-smelling liquid stools and a reduced appetite. When caused by bacterial infection, the scour is usually yellow, offensive and may contain blood. The foal is dull, disinclined to suck its mother, the temperature is usually raised and the foal may show colicky pains. Some foals quickly become debilitated and dehydrated, have a characteristic smell, and die within a week. Pneumonia may be a complication and be responsible for death.

Treatment Simple diarrhoea in foals requires little treatment other than keeping the foal warm and making sure that it is continuing to suck. *Kaomagma* with peptin (Wyeth), which is readily available from chemists, can be given with good effect to foals in volumes of 20 to 30 ml every 6 to 8 hours orally using a syringe.

If the foal stops drinking then attention from a veterinarian should be sought as soon as possible. Extensive fluid losses can take place in foals with severe diarrhoea, with resulting dehydration and death within 24 hours. In these cases prompt treatment with electrolyte solutions and plasma can replace the fluid disturbances and save the life of the foal.

DISLOCATIONS

Dislocations are the result of rupture of supporting structures such as ligaments and tendons around joints. This results in loss of stability of the bones so that malalignment results. Dislocations of bones in the horse are rare and when they occur usually involve the fetlock, pastern or coffin joints.

Symptoms of a dislocation There is an alteration in the shape of the joint and in the normal relationship of the articulating surfaces of the bones. The horse will generally not bear weight on the affected leg if a limb dislocation occurs. If there is a dislocation of the neck then the horse will usually show signs of paralysis or unsteadiness on the feet.

Treatment The main difficulty in treating dislocations is that although joints may be reapposed, the damage to ligaments and supporting structures is so severe that the joint may be unable to be retained in apposition. Therefore, surgery may be required to stabilise dislocated joints, or in less severe cases, plaster casting. Following dislocation of a joint, the damage to cartilage and ligaments may be so severe that the horse may not become sound on the limb.

When dislocation of vertebrae occurs in the neck, the resulting pressure on the spinal cord causes a paralysis of the legs or unsteadiness. In these cases no treatment is successful. (*See Fig. 44 on p. 66*)

DRENCHING HORSES

Drenching horses is frequently necessary to administer various medications, in particular deworming preparations. The current availability of many drugs in a paste form has reduced the need for administration of medications by stomach tube. These pastes allow

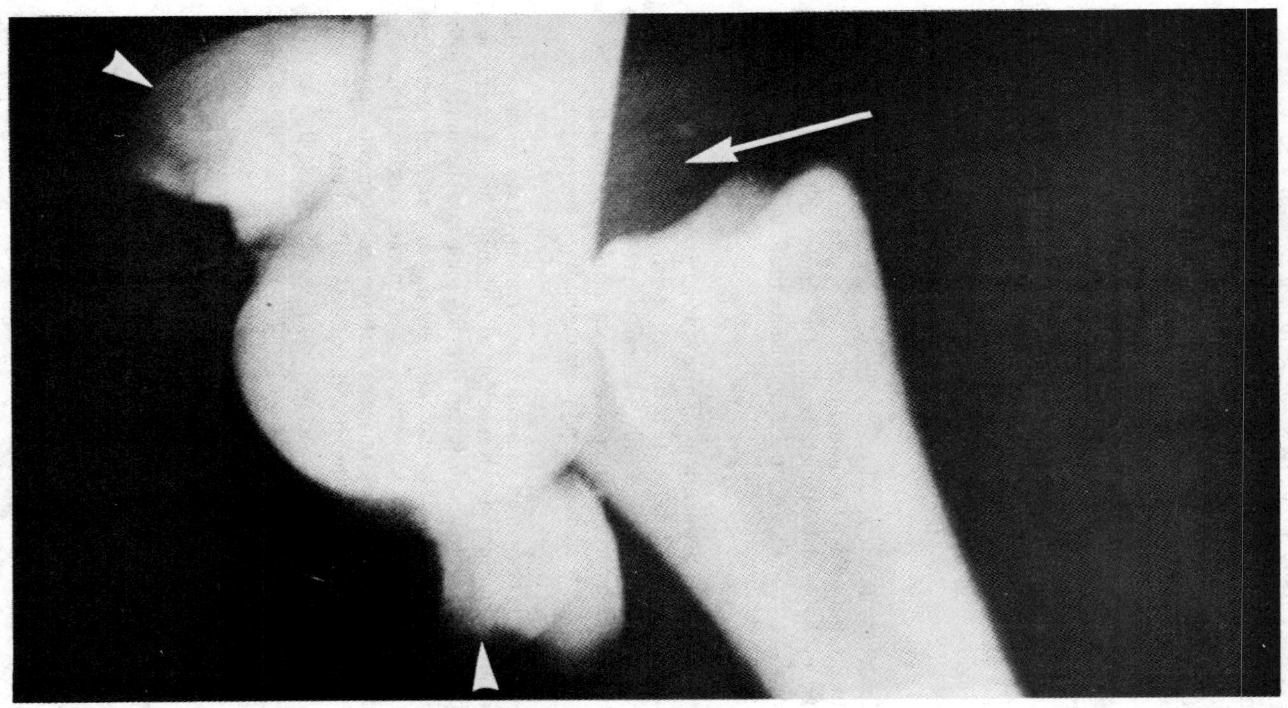

Fig. 44
X-ray showing dislocation of the fetlock joint and fracture of both sesamoid bones (small arrows).

simple administration of drugs which are deposited on the back of the tongue with a syringe. Preparations available in paste form include deworming mixtures, vitamins, anti-inflammatory drugs, antibiotics, cough mixtures and anabolic steroid hormones.

Passage of a stomach tube by a veterinarian is sometimes necessary to allow administration of preparations such as paraffin and other medications. This is performed by passing a rubber or plastic tube, approximately 3 metres long and 15 mm in diameter, into the stomach via the nose. This procedure should not be attempted by laymen as the tube may be inadvertently passed into the windpipe. Damage to the fine bones in the nose may also result from improper placement of a stomach tube.

Drenching has also been carried out in the past using a smooth-necked beer bottle passed into the side of the mouth and the medication poured into the back of the throat. Most horses resent this, and additionally, fluid may be poured into the windpipe.

ECZEMA

Eczema is a term usually confined to humans where there is an inherited sensitivity of the skin to inflammation. This term is sometimes used in horses to describe dermatitis (inflammation of the skin), which may occur in association with various diseases and infections.

Symptoms Irritation, rubbing of the skin, formation of scabs, pustules and raw areas in the skin may be seen at various stages of this disorder. It is important to establish the cause of the eczema or dermatitis by having a veterinarian examine the horse and take samples of hair and skin for a laboratory analysis.

Treatment In some cases of eczema, topical washes may be the most suitable form of treatment. Antihistamine and cortisone injections may also be given to reduce inflammation and irritation of the skin. Specific treatment will vary depending on the particular cause of the condition.

ELECTROLYTES

Electrolytes are the various body salts which are important in maintaining fluid balance and normal circulation. The most important electrolytes are sodium, potassium, chloride and bicarbonate, and these can be measured in the blood. In recent years it has become apparent that electrolyte imbalances in the body can result in impairment of the performance of racehorses, trotters and endurance horses. Losses of electrolytes are particularly common in horses that sweat heavily and in horses with diarrhoea.

Treatment Various commercial electrolyte replacement mixtures are available to correct electrolyte losses. Of these, *Humidimix* and *Stressalyte* (Medical Research Pty Ltd) have been formulated for horses with different electrolyte abnormalities. *Humidimix* is used for horses with very heavy sweat conditions, whereas *Stressalyte* is used in those with normal sweat losses.

ENCEPHALOMYELITIS — VIRAL

Equine encephalomyelitis ("sleeping sickness") is a serious infectious disease which at the time this book goes to press has not occurred in Australia, but against which every precaution is being taken to prevent its introduction. It is a specific viral disease of the brain and spinal cord which has affected millions of horses in the Americas and elsewhere, and has caused great mortality. There are 3 distinct types of virus involved, namely the Eastern, Western, and Venezuelan strains, named for the geographical regions in which they were originally recognised.

In recent years (1969-71) a serious outbreak of the disease caused by the Venezuelan strain of virus occurred in Central America and Texas (U.S.), when American authorities mounted a large scale control campaign. Viral encephalomyelitis is spread by various biting insects, chiefly the mosquito, and, particularly in the case of the Eastern and Western strains of virus, is transmitted from infected mosquitoes to birds. The virus multiplies in the bird host and the birds then serve as sources of infection for other mosquitoes which feed on them. Infected mosquitoes transmit the virus to the horse or man when feeding on them. In the case of Venezuelan equine encephalomyelitis it appears that the virus multiplies mainly in the horse and that spread of the disease occurs mainly from horse to horse. Birds may also be infected. Viral encephalomyelitis is a seasonal disease, occurring mainly in mid and late summer when the insect population is highest.

Symptoms In general the symptoms of infectious viral encephalomyelitis in the horse caused by the 3 strains mentioned are similar but the prognosis varies. The following are some of the symptoms. Sluggishness and drowsiness are early symptoms in the developing stage of the disease. The temperature varies from 39 °C to 41 °C and may remain for 24 to 48 hours, then drops to near normal. Groups of muscles about the head, shoulders, or flank may be seen to twitch spasmodically.

With the progress of the disease thc animal stands dejectedly and moves with an awkward staggering gait. Some animals may blunder blindly into obstructions in their path. In some cases there is extreme sensitiveness as shown by flinching at the slightest touch or by jerking muscular contractions when disturbed. The dejectedly sleepy horse may show a momentary interest in feed or water, only soon to lapse into a stupor with unchewed food in the mouth, or water trickling from the mouth or nostrils.

Treatment This is difficult and is essentially a matter for a veterinarian.

Control Very little can be done to control insect vectors such as mosquitoes, and because of this method of spread of the disease and the high incidence in wild birds, especially in relation to the Eastern and Western types, complete eradication of the disease once it has been introduced into an area appears to be impossible. Annual immunisation of horses, using vaccines prepared from the appropriate strains of the virus, is the most satisfactory way of controlling the disease. Because man is susceptible to the causative virus the possible introduction of the disease is also of considerable public health significance.

EQUINE INFECTIOUS ANAEMIA (Swamp Fever)

Equine infectious anaemia or swamp fever, as it is commonly called, is an acute or chronic contagious disease of the horse, ass and mule, characterised principally by intermittent fever, marked depression, loss of condition, oedema and anaemia. The disease is found in most countries, including Australia, where it was first diagnosed in 1959, but it would appear to have been present and fairly widely distributed before then. The disease occurs most commonly in low lying and swampy country, particularly during the summer months, although chronic cases persist throughout the year.

Cause The disease is caused by a specific virus which persists in the body of an affected animal for many years and is eliminated in the milk, semen, nasal and eye secretions, and in the urine and dung. Although essentially a disease of members of the horse family, possible experimental transmission to pigs and sheep has been recorded, and cases have been reported in humans with anaemia as the main symptom.

Methods of Transmission Biting flies, mosquitoes and other blood sucking parasites mechanically transmit the virus from a "carrier" animal to healthy horses. This would appear to be the reason why the disease spreads more readily in spring and summer and in swampy areas. Contaminated food and water may be a source of spread of the disease, but relatively large amounts of virus must be ingested to cause infection. Stabling of a "carrier" animal with healthy horses, especially over a period, will spread the infection. Foals sucking infected mothers can contract the disease through the milk, and a stallion could transmit the disease to mares at service. Infection can also be spread by contaminated surgical or tattoo instruments or the use of unsterilised hypodermic needles, when horses are being inoculated against some other disease.

Symptoms The incubation period of the disease in natural outbreaks is generally considered to be 2 to 4 weeks. The symptoms vary greatly depending largely on the form of the disease. Ordinarily the disease appears to spread slowly, occurring in isolated cases, but it may occur as an epidemic in a large group of susceptible horses following the introduction of "carriers", when circumstances are favourable for its transmission. The disease may occur either as an acute rapidly fatal disease with continuous or intermittent high fever, the temperature ranging to 38 °C, with great prostration and death within a few days, or the attacks of fever may gradually decrease in intensity and frequency, and the disease becomes sub-acute or chronic. Usually the disease begins in the sub-acute form and the symptoms come on more gradually, being less severe intermittent fever attacks; depression; lack of appetite; progressive weakness; loss of condition; dropsical swellings of the lower portions of the body and legs; jaundice; pin-point haemorrhages on the mucous membranes of the eyes, nose and mouth, and later signs of anaemia. There may be a slight watery discharge from the eyes and nose and, if the weather is warm, profuse sweating occurs. Frequent urination may be noted and a foetid, watery diarrhoea is sometimes seen. It is common for animals to recover from this sub-acute form of the disease over a period of about 3 weeks and then to suffer a relapse. The symptoms shown, however, are usually less severe, although an animal may die during such a relapse. Subsequent attacks become less frequent, the animal finally developing into a chronic case or a recovered "carrier".

During the attacks of fever and immediately afterwards, there is destruction of red blood corpuscles which causes the anaemia, as shown by paleness of the visible mucous membranes, for example, the eyes and inside the nose. There is also considerable enlargement of the spleen, which at post-mortem examination is seen to be very dark in colour.

In general, the chronic form of the disease is manifested by unthriftiness, rough coat, loss of weight, sluggishness and general weakness. Symptoms of anaemia may be evident as shown by pallor of the visible mucous membranes. Horses affected with this form of the disease eat well, but in spite of this do not put on weight, and are subject to recurrent febrile attacks. Death may occur during one of these attacks, or the animal may subsequently die from exhaustion.

The disease may exist in a form in which no clinical symptoms are shown, yet the affected animal carries virulent virus in the bloodstream and is a constant source of infection to other horses through the insect vector.

The mortality rate from this disease is high and pregnant mares may abort.

Diagnosis Definite diagnosis of the disease is difficult as it may be confused with a number of other diseases, especially in acute cases. The only reliable way is by transmission tests at a laboratory, thus calling for veterinary attention. The disease may be suspected when a number of horses in a horse establishment or on a property suddenly become sick for no apparent reason and develop symptoms as described. A test for the presence of antibodies in the blood, called the Coggins test, is available to test for the presence of equine infectious anaemia.

Treatment No specific treatment or vaccination procedure has been developed for the disease. Many chemicals, drugs and antibiotics have been tried, but with poor results and no lasting value. Supportive therapy, including blood transfusions, may help.

Control Equine infectious anaemia is a notifiable disease in all States of the Commonwealth of Australia, and suspected cases should be reported to the nearest official veterinary officer in order that suitable control measures can be carried out. Attempts should be made to control flies and mosquitoes and care taken that any surgical instruments, including tattooing outfits and hypodermic syringes and needles, are properly sterilised. The introduction of horses from known infected areas should be avoided.

EYE — CONJUNCTIVITIS

Conjunctivitis, or inflammation of the conjunctiva, is a common condition amongst animals and is probably the most common condition affecting the eye of the horse. As a rule, it is not in itself a serious disease, but it may give rise to serious complications such as ulceration of the cornea, which may be incurable and lead to loss of sight. Conjunctivitis, with accompanying eye discharges, occurs in association with a number of febrile infectious diseases such as strangles and influenza.

Cause Apart from conjunctivitis associated with febrile infectious diseases, which usually clears up if the disease is overcome, inflammation of the conjunctiva occurs from blows or other injuries to the eye; from the presence of foreign bodies in the eye, such as sand, pollen, seeds, oat husks, chaff, lime and irritant gases. All these agents act as exciting causes, the direct cause of the inflammation being the activity of organisms which are already present on the moist surface of the conjunctiva or which are blown on to it from the air. Flies may also carry infection to the eyes.

Specific bacteria and viral infections of the eyes, and allergies, also cause conjunctivitis.

Symptoms The first symptoms of conjunctivitis are redness and swelling of the lining membrane of the eyelids, a watery discharge and a tendency for the animal to keep the eyelids closed and to seek the shade. Later the watery discharge thickens and may become purulent, blister the surrounding skin and mat the hair together. The eye may be kept completely closed or only slightly opened, or the discharge may glue the eyelids together. An inflammation of the conjunctival membrane, or of the cornea beneath it, may result in an opacity of a part or the whole of the front of the eye. This may partially blind the animal for a time.

Treatment It is important to allay inflammation and control infection quickly to avoid structural alterations to the eye. Discharges should be cleaned away with warm water to which a little boracic acid has been added and a search then made for any foreign body which may have become lodged in the eye. If found, action should be taken along the lines indicated below under *Foreign Bodies in the Eye*. Frequent irrigation of the eye is desirable, using normal saline solution (1 teaspoonful of salt to 600 ml of boiled water), either by means of a small syringe, or a piece of cotton wool soaked in the solution and squeezed into the corner of the eye. Irritant eye lotions should not be used. A range of antibiotic preparations is available as eye drops and ointments which can be used to advantage, but preferably under veterinary supervision. The horse should have access to shade or be kept in a loose box. A piece of cloth attached to a headstall and hung over the affected eye will shade it from light.

EYE — DERMOID CYSTS

A so called dermoid "cyst" may develop in various situations in the body. The growth is a piece of skin which has become misplaced during the formation of the embryo before birth. This piece of embryonic skin continues to grow and produce hair wherever it is located in the body. In the eye, a dermoid "cyst", which should more correctly be referred to as a tumour, is commonly attached to the margin of the white tough outer membrane of the eyeball where it joins the cornea, and looks like a smooth wart. From its free surface grow hairs of variable length which cause irritation and excessive flow of tears, and may cause interference with vision and even ulceration of the cornea. The tumour can be removed under an anaesthetic by delicate surgery.

EYE — FOREIGN BODIES IN

Foreign bodies, such as oat husks, chaff and other material of plant origin occasionally enter the horse's eye, and not uncommonly mud or grit enters the eyes during racing. Usually the foreign bodies become lodged on the internal surface of the eyelids or in the conjunctival sacs, but sometimes they penetrate more deeply. The irritation causes an acute conjunctivitis, the eye is half closed and it weeps. The third eyelid or haw may protrude across the eye and the animal avoids bright light. Complications due to ulceration or infection may occur if the foreign body is not speedily removed.

Treatment Because the eye is so extremely sensitive and the animal resists examination, it is often a difficult task to remove a foreign body. It is, therefore, advisable to obtain professional assistance and have the foreign body removed under a local anaesthetic. If a veterinarian is not available, it may be possible with the aid of a twitch, to syringe out the eye with normal saline solution, 30 g of salt to 600 ml of boiled water. This may in itself dislodge the foreign body but, if not, and the object can be seen, it may often be removed with the corner of a clean handkerchief or the little finger covered with the handkerchief or a piece of fine linen. After the foreign body has been removed antibiotic ophthalmic ointments can be used to help to prevent infection. It is very important that the foreign body be removed as soon as possible otherwise ulceration of the cornea may occur and lead to loss of sight. To prevent this, veterinary attention should be sought as quickly as possible.

Occlusion of the lacrimal duct, through which tears escape from the conjunctival sac into the nasal chambers, may also occur as a result of obstruction by a foreign body or other material. Such an obstruction will make itself apparent by overflow of tears down the face and can be remedied by having a veterinarian examine the horse and syringe out the blocked duct.

EYE—HABRONEMIC CONJUNCTIVITIS

House flies, bush flies and stable flies act as intermediate hosts of certain species of stomach worms of horses of the genus *Habronema.* Infected flies feeding on the borders of the horse's eyelids, especially at the inner corner of the eye, may deposit *Habronema* larvae, which penetrate the mucous membrane. This causes considerable irritation, followed by a persistent conjunctivitis and frequently the development of a nodular ulcer. On the third eyelid the nodule may be as big as 6 mm in diameter. A profuse, watery and sometimes purulent discharge from the eye attracts more flies, thus aggravating the condition. These *Habronema* nodules are frequently mistaken for cancer of the eye (see *Tumours*) and indeed may develop into the malignant condition.

Treatment Habronemic conjunctivitis does not respond to the usual treatments and it may be necessary to remove the nodules surgically. Repellants applied around the eyes are not very satisfactory in keeping the flies away. Heavy fly veils should be fitted to headstalls on the horse, and attention paid to disposal of manure to destroy the worm eggs and so prevent hatching of the flies.

EYE — PERIODIC OPHTHALMIA (Recurrent uveitis)

Periodic ophthalmia has been recognised as a disease of horses and mules since ancient times and, although much study has been carried out, the cause of the disease has not yet been definitely determined. The latest theory is that it is associated with a hypersensitivity reaction to bacteria or parasites which cause a recurrence of the symptoms seen.

Equine periodic ophthalmia is characterised by periodic attacks of general inflammation of the eyeball, subsequent shrinking of same and finally blindness. It occurs under a variety of circumstances, usually in mature horses, and has in the past been more commonly seen when large numbers of horses have been congregated together, such as in the army. Odd sporadic cases do occur.

It had been observed that the disease was prone to occur in damp surroundings, on low-lying country and in dark ill-ventilated stables, and such conditions were held to be predisposing causes. The disease is much less common now throughout the world than it was formerly, due no doubt to decrease in the number of horses and improved sanitation. It is still, however, reasonably common in Australia.

Symptoms The onset of the disease is sudden, and the first indication of the disease occurs when the horse is seen with half closed eyelids on one side, tears trickling down the face and evasion of bright light. The horse objects to handling of the eye and, when this is attempted, will keep the lids tightly closed. Careful examination will reveal inflammation of the conjunctiva and deeper parts of the eye, contraction of the pupil and perhaps some opacity of the cornea. This is usually associated with a slight rise in temperature and general depression. Other changes, including lack of lustre of the iris also occur in the eye. This initial period of inflammation may last from between 2 to 10 days. This is followed by a gradual decline of all symptoms over a period of about 3 weeks, when, to a casual observer, the eye appears to be normal. Only very close examination and use of an ophthalmoscope will reveal remaining abnormalities. The characteristic recurrence of the disease occurs from 3 weeks to 3 months after the first attack. It may be in the same eye or in the other one. In the second attack, the symptoms are much the same as in the first but it takes longer for the eye to clear again. Each succeeding attack leaves its additional damage to the vital structures of the eye. After several attacks, the lens will show a number of fleecy lines running in towards the centre and soon the whole lens will become a white and opaque mass and the animal will be blind. After an animal has had 1 or more attacks, the eyeball becomes perceptibly smaller than normal and the upper eyelid is wrinkled. The attacks vary greatly in severity in different cases, but the recurrence is quite distinctive and will lead to permanent blindness.

Treatment This is essentially a matter for a veterinarian. Excellent results have been obtained by the injection of a cortisone-type preparation under the conjunctiva. A darkened stable or shed or even an eye-shade contributes to the animal's comfort during the period when it is very sensitive to light.

EYE — ULCER

Keratitis means inflammation and ulceration of the cornea, the clear part of the front of the eye. It not infrequently supervenes on neglected cases of conjunctivitis, the basic causes being the same.

Symptoms The early symptoms are similar to those of conjunctivitis, but as the pain is more intense than in the latter condition, the horse is inclined to keep the eye permanently closed and examination is carried out with some difficulty. A close inspection shows the surface of the cornea to be duller than usual, the dullness varying from a slight haze to a bluish appearance. Later the blood

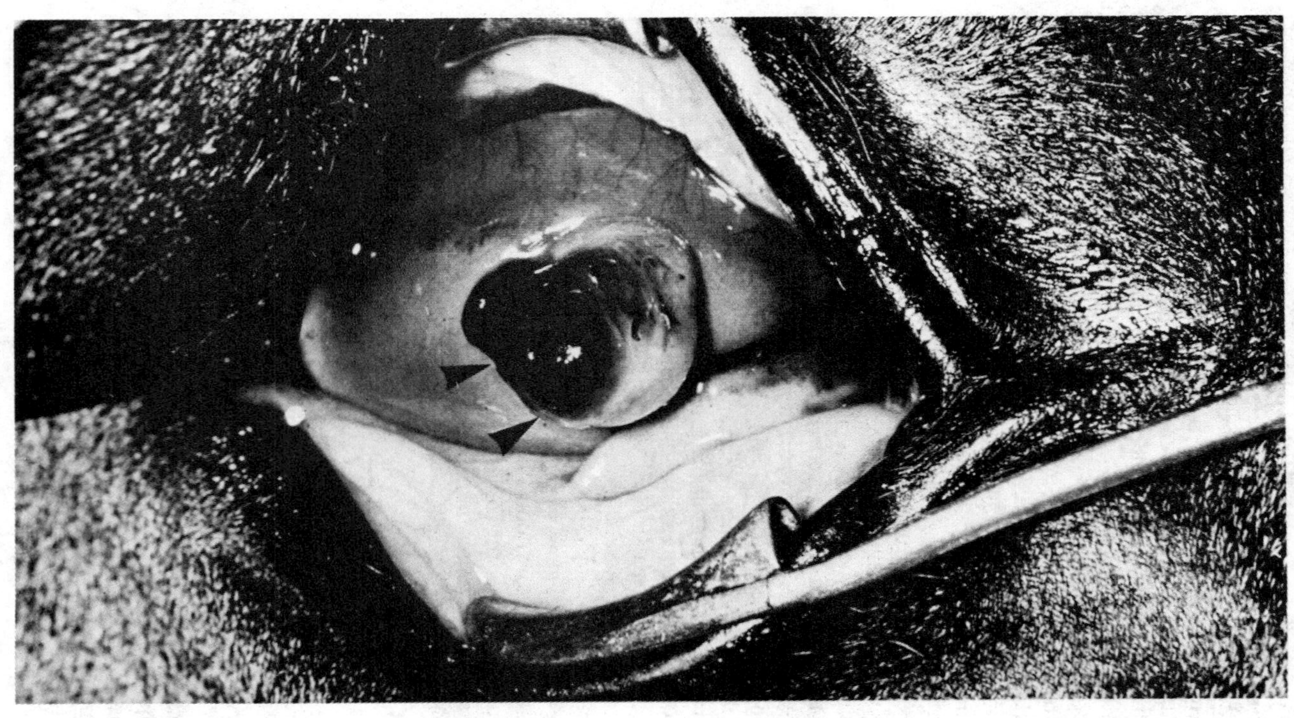

Fig. 45
Severe ulcer of the eye, resulting in rupture of the cornea and prolapse of the iris (arrows).

vessels around the margins of the eye are congested and begin to spread over the eye when the white of the eye appears blood-shot. This condition is usually associated with a discharge of pus from the eye. Still later, irregularities occur on the cornea and commonly a small projection may be seen on the surface of the cornea, usually greyish in colour or tinged with pink. This indicates that ulceration has destroyed the wall of the cornea and the pressure of the contents of the eyeball has pressed outwards the membrane which lines it on the inside. Recovery may occur at this stage, and the eye revert to normal, although a slight film may remain. In severe cases, continued ulceration causes the membrane to rupture, the fluid content escapes through the hole in the cornea, and the front of the eyeball collapses, causing permanent loss of sight in the affected eye.

Keratitis is frequently accompanied by fever and constitutional disturbance, probably occasioned by pain and fear.

Treatment To prevent permanent loss of sight it is important for a veterinarian to carry out prompt treatment. This may involve antibiotic ointments and/or local medications in simple cases, or surgery to close the eyelids in more severe cases. Local treatment with antibiotic ointments should be performed at least 6 to 8 times a day to achieve rapid resolution of the infection.

EYELIDS — ENTROPION

Entropion means a turning-in of the eyelid, usually the lower, in such a way that the lashes rub against the globe of the eye and cause irritation. The condition is more commonly seen in foals, when not infrequently the lids of both eyes are affected. In adult animals the condition may follow laceration and faulty healing of the eyelid. It may also occur as a sequel to severe conjunctivitis or an attack of periodic ophthalmia.

Symptoms The irritation caused by the inverted lashes rubbing against the cornea may result in keratitis and loss of sight. The condition of entropion is recognised by a continuous closure of the eyelids with some suppuration and matting of the lashes.

Treatment In most cases foals will recover without surgical intervention and will respond simply to pulling out the lower lid and repeating the procedure from time to time during the first few days of the foal's life. On some studs this is carried out with adhesive tape.

In more severe cases quite a minor operation will cure the condition, but this should be left to a veterinarian to perform under local or general anaesthesia. It may only be necessary to suture the lid back into place, or remove an elliptical piece of skin from below the offending lid and suture the edges of the cut together. Either of these procedures, but particularly the latter, will cause sufficient contraction of the skin to pull back the lid and prevent it from curling inwards.

FALSE QUARTER

False quarter is the term applied to that condition of the horn of the quarter of the foot in which, owing to disease or injury of the coronet, the wall has grown in a manner that is incomplete. It is seen more commonly on the fore feet and usually on the inner side, but does occur on the hind feet.

Causes As already mentioned, false quarter can result from any disease of the foot that involves destruction of a portion of the coronary cushion, because it is from the papillae of this body that the horn tubules of the wall are secreted. Destruction of any part of it results in a corresponding loss of horn in that position. Therefore, wire cuts to the coronet frequently result in this condition. It may also result from a suppurating corn or from a severe tread or overreach.

Symptoms The condition appears as a gap or shallow indentation, narrow or wide, in the thickness of the wall, with its length in the direction of the horn fibres. The condition is aggravated should there be a sandcrack in the quarter. On either side of the indentation an abnormal growth of horn occurs, which protrudes and stands above the level of the horn surrounding it. This might be regarded as a form of hypertrophy—abnormal increase in the size of a part—brought about by the increased stress imposed by the loss of substance in the region of the false quarter. So long as the sensitive structures of the foot are not exposed, the horse does not go lame. Sometimes, however, as a result of concussion, a fissure appears in the narrow veneer of horn that covers the sensitive structures in the indentation, aided perhaps by a sandcrack in the quarter. Infection then takes place, leading to inflammatory changes and pus formation, and the horse becomes lame. Many horses are not adversely affected for work by a false quarter which has not become infected, but the latter is always possible.

Treatment The treatment of false quarter is exceedingly difficult because of destruction of the horn-secreting substance of the coronary cushion. The fissure in the wall usually remains, rendering the horse liable to occasional lameness and making that side of the hoof weak.

Attention should be given to the coronary cushion injury and the hose appropriately shod to keep weight off the affected quarter.

FISTULA

A fistula is a passage of scar tissue which provides an abnormal communication between 2 body surfaces. In horses, the term "fistula" has come to be commonly accepted as applicable only to such lesions when found on the withers. Poll evil is a fistula or sinus in the region of the poll and in no sense differs from *fistulous withers* other than in location. Fistulous passages may also be developed upon the sides of the face, through which saliva is discharged instead of flowing into the mouth, and they are called salivary fistulas. A dental fistula may arise from necrosis of the root of a tooth, providing a discharge of pus to the exterior of the upper or lower jaw.

A fistula is sometimes noted at the umbilicus (navel) associated with hernia, and recto-vaginal fistula have been developed in mares, following difficult parturition. A fistula of the oesophagus may occur as a result of misuse of a probang or stomach tube for the relief of choke.

Fistulous tracts persist whilst irritation occurs from some foreign body, necrotic bone, cartilage or other cartilage or other infective material, particularly when there is poor drainage from the part.

FISTULOUS WITHERS AND POLL EVIL

Fistulas are particularly prone to develop at the withers or poll because the exposed position of these parts renders them liable to injury, but trauma or mechanical injury is not always necessary for infection to occur. Once infection is located in these areas it is inclined to extend further downwards, because of the fan-shaped way the muscles and tendons are arranged in these situations, thus allowing it to gravitate to the deeper-lying structures. It will be readily appreciated how quickly the bursa (the protective sheath covering the bones and even the bones themselves) together with the main ligament of the neck become involved, leading to *necrosis.* One of the most significant features of fistulous withers is that there are so many variations of the arrangement, size, location, and anatomical relations of these lesions. A knowledge of anatomy is necessary to fully appreciate why this is so.

Cause Because the organisms of *Brucella abortus* and *Brucella suis,* the germs responsible for brucellosis in cattle and pigs, have been cultured from cases of fistulous withers and poll evil, the possibility of infection of the horse with these germs has to be kept in mind as a cause of these conditions. Further, a microfilarial parasite (small thread-like worm) *Onchocerca reticulata* is not uncommonly found in the neck ligament of horses and has been held responsible for some cases. On the other hand, injury to the parts and subsequent infection with pus-producing and other organisms is a more common cause. Among the more common predisposing causes of fistulous withers are ill fitting collars or saddles; direct injury from blows or stallion bites, and rolling upon rough or sharp stones. Saddle horses that are very low in the withers permit the saddle to ride forward and bruise the parts, and are prone to be affected with fistulous withers. *Poll evil* may follow chafing by a halter, headstall or heavy bridle, blows from the butt end of a whip, the horse striking its head against a beam, low stable doors and so on.

Following the initial injury, infection occurs, leading to inflammatory swelling and often to abscess formation below the skin, which, if not quickly and properly treated, may become fistulous. This results from pus seeping between the muscles and escaping only when pressure forces it to the surface, and it bursts through the skin.

Should the fistulous wither or poll evil be caused by *Brucella abortus* infection, the discharges can contaminate the pasture, so that a horse affected with these conditions can be the means of transmitting brucellosis to cattle or other horses grazing over such pasture.

Symptoms The symptoms vary according to the progress of the fistula. When the wither is affected, the horse may at first show some soreness or stiffness of the front legs. In a day or 2 a swelling commonly occurs on 1 or both sides of the wither, which is usually hot and painful. The stiffness of the limbs may disappear at this time and the heat and soreness of the swelling may become less noticeable, although it continues to enlarge. Several months may elapse before the swelling bursts at some point and discharges. The discharge may cease and the opening may apparently heal, only to break out again later.

Poll evil may be first indicated by the animal becoming sensitive to the application of the bridle or to a grooming brush. The disease in its early stages may be recognised as a soft fluctuating swelling on 1 or both sides of the mid-line of the poll surrounded by inflammatory swelling, and stiffness of the neck. Later the inflammation of the surrounding tissues may disappear, leaving a prominent tumour-like swelling. Subsequently this swelling bursts and discharges and, as in the case of fistulous withers, heals up temporarily and discharges again.

Treatment The treatment of fistula of the withers or fistula of the poll (poll evil) is determined by the changes that have occurred in the affected structures. It is essentially a matter for a qualified veterinary surgeon. In the earliest stages of the diseases, when there is soreness, perhaps enlarged lymphatic vessels, and only slight swelling, the trouble might be checked by hot fomentations, massage and antibiotic treatment. In other cases, where the swelling is simply due to a sterile distension of the synovial sac covering the bones, the condition may respond to local injections of cortisone. Once the swelling has burst and is discharging pus, treatment is outside the province of the horse owner. Home treatments with strong caustic drugs and arsenic, and the use of setons, are seldom successful and usually involve much suffering to the horse. From the foregoing description of the 2 disease conditions, it will be appreciated that surgical intervention is the only way of arranging for proper drainage and the removal of necrotic material which is causing the trouble. Combined with surgery, the veterinarian will adopt antibiotic and other forms of treatment in an attempt to cure these very troublesome conditions. Sometimes an extended daily course of antibiotic treatment given by or under the supervision of a veterinarian will effect a cure, and then only if there is not extensive involvement of the bone and ligaments.

FLIES

The common house-fly (*Musca domestica*), the bush-fly (*Musca vetustissima*) and the stable-fly (*Stomoxys calcitrans*) are the main flies which worry horses in Australia. March-flies (*Tabanus spp.*) also worry horses and inflict a severe bite. All these flies can carry disease. Reference has already been made (see *Eye—Habronemic Conjunctivitis*) to the fact that house-flies, bush-flies and stable-flies act as intermediate hosts of certain species of stomach worms of the genus *Habronema.* The larvae of these worms are carried by flies into the eyes and on to abrasions on the body of the horse and give rise to *habronemic conjunctivitis* and a skin condition known as "summer sores". It is suggested that swamp cancer of horses may have a similar origin.

Bush-flies, when feeding on the secretions of the mouth, eyes, ears, nose and around the vulva, as they commonly do in great numbers, cause considerable irritation to the animal. The flesh around these areas is indented and the skin raised, due, it is presumed, to the secretion of digestive juices by the flies.

Stable- and March-flies annoy horses and the females of certain species of the latter suck blood.

The buffalo-fly, which is normally associated with cattle and buffaloes, will attack horses but only when they are with cattle. This fly can only live where its bovine host exists, as it breeds in the freshly dropped dung.

Control The most effective method of controlling house-flies and stable-flies is by the regular and thorough collection of manure, and its treatment or disposal so that flies cannot breed in it. Manure is most attractive to flies during the first 3 to 5 days. Flies will not breed in dry dung and desiccation kills the eggs. If practicable, dung should be collected and spread as soon as possible over pasture where it will quickly dry out. Alternatively, dung should be tightly packed, and every 4 days the heap should be raked and the old dung placed on top of the fresh dung. This raises the temperature of the dung heap and the fly eggs are destroyed. Fly-proof pits can be used, or the dung heap sprayed with one of the organic phosphorus preparations to destroy the emerging flies. It is much more difficult to control bush- and March-flies by the above methods as their breeding places are very extensive. Various sprays may be used to kill the adult flies on the horse, which will at least afford temporary relief to the animal. The hair on the tail, mane and forelock should not be interfered with, and a leather fly veil attached to a headstall will assist in protecting the eyes. When severe waves of bush-flies occur, it is a common practice in the country to light smudge fires around which horses will congregate to get smoke protection from the flies.

FOAL — REARING OF ORPHAN

When a mare dies or has no milk, it becomes necessary to raise the foal by hand. If the foal has not had a suck from its mother it is essential to give 200 to 400 ml of colostrum (first milk of the mare) before the foal is 24 hours old. This milk is rich in antibodies which protect the foal from infection. Colostrum can be collected from recently-foaled mares and frozen for later use. Sometimes it is possible to arrange for another recently-foaled mare to take the foal in addition to her own, or to put the foal on to a recently-calved cow of a large breed, such as a Friesian or Shorthorn. Usually it is necessary to rear the foal on fresh cow's or goat's milk diluted with one-third the quantity of warm, boiled water and sweetened with 30 g of glucose or lactose to the litre of milk mixture. This milk mixture is similar to the milk of the mare which has low butter fat and high sugar content. One to 2 teaspoonfuls of vitamin A standardised cod liver oil should be added to each litre of milk and water mixture for the first 10 days. Lactose or milk sugar is the best kind of sugar to use and is available from any chemist. Glucose can also be used. The milk mixture should be warmed to blood heat and the foal given 300 to 400 ml every 2 hours at the beginning.

After a few days, if the foal is doing well, the quantities of milk and the intervals between feeds can be increased until the foal is getting 2 to

4 litres of milk 3 times a day when a month old. More milk may be given if the foal seems to need it, but overfeeding should be avoided. The sugar may be reduced at 3 weeks of age and discontinued at 1 month. At 6 to 8 weeks, skim milk may be gradually substituted for whole milk. By 3 months, the foal may be given all the milk it can drink, which may be up to 20 litres a day. It should, of course, have access to clean drinking water. A bottle with a large rubber teat can be used to feed the very young foal but it should be encouraged to drink from an open vessel as soon as possible. Scrupulous cleanliness must be observed with the bottle and teat, which should be sterilised after use and kept covered with a clean cloth until used again. All vessels used to hold milk must be rinsed with cold water immediately after use and then scalded and kept covered.

The foal will begin to nibble grass or concentrates at 2 to 3 weeks of age. Feeding of a dry meal or crushed oats may be commenced at 4 weeks. Three parts of crushed oats to 1 part of bran makes a suitable concentrate mixture. Some prime quality lucerne hay should be available to the foal and, if there is a shortage of green grass, some greenstuff should be fed. At about 2 months the foal will be eating a considerable quantity of crushed oats and hay, especially if the grazing is poor. Lucerne hay is a valuable source of calcium (lime) and it is recommended that some be fed, even if the foal is running on good grass pasture. If lucerne hay is not fed regularly 1 per cent of finely ground limestone should be added to the concentrate mixture. Skim milk feeding should continue until the foal is 5 to 6 months old or even a little longer if the milk is available, when the foal may be weaned. At least 1 feed of crushed oats should be given daily until the end of the first year.

An orphan foal should be suitably housed and protected from cold winds and rain. The shed should be kept clean and any bedding, such as straw, frequently changed. If possible, a companion animal should be kept with the foal. A quiet old pony is best, but a quiet calf, sheep or goat will help. This prevents the foal from being lonely, and it learns to eat, seek shelter, and fend for itself more rapidly.

Young foals are subject to a number of diseases which are discussed elsewhere. Within the first 12 hours of life, a foal is likely to be constipated, especially if it has not sucked the mother and obtained the colostrum. The constipated condition is due to retention of the meconium (the first dung discharges of the newborn). A home method of correcting this is to give the foal an enema of 1 part glycerine in 5 parts of warm water, using an ordinary human enema syringe, after lubricating the nozzle with white petroleum jelly. A human prepackaged enema mixture caled *Microlax* (Pharmacia) is also useful to have on hand for the treatment of foals with constipation.

FOALING

See *Parturition*

FOALS — LIMB DEFORMITIES

In newborn foals, a number of limb deformities are of common occurrence. Many of these deformities are only temporary in nature and result from weakness of muscles, tendons and ligaments in the post-natal adaptive period. However, some of the more severe limb deformities require treatment.

Contracted tendons Contracted tendons are most commonly found in the forelimbs of foals, but occasionally develop in weanlings and yearlings.

Cause

This is largely unknown, but is thought to be associated with malpositioning of the limbs *in utero.* In weanlings and yearlings, the condition usually develops when horses are placed on high protein diets and have a rapid growth rate.

Symptoms

Excessive pull of the flexor muscles and tendons results in the foals standing on "tiptoes", or in severe cases, to knuckle over on to the front of their fetlocks.

Treatment

In most young foals restriction of movement within a loose box will result in correction of the deformity in mild cases of the disorder. In more severe cases surgery is necessary to decrease the pull of the flexor tendon by cutting the inferior check ligament. When the condition develops in older horses, strict control of their diet is necessary.

Weak flexor tendons Weak flexor tendons may be found in the fore limbs and/or hind limbs of newborn foals. The condition tends to affect the hind limbs more commonly.

Cause

The cause is unknown, but may be associated with the maturity of the foal as it is seen in most premature foals.

Symptoms

Affected foals are unable to stand upright on their pasterns and when walking the back of the fetlock sometimes touches the ground. In

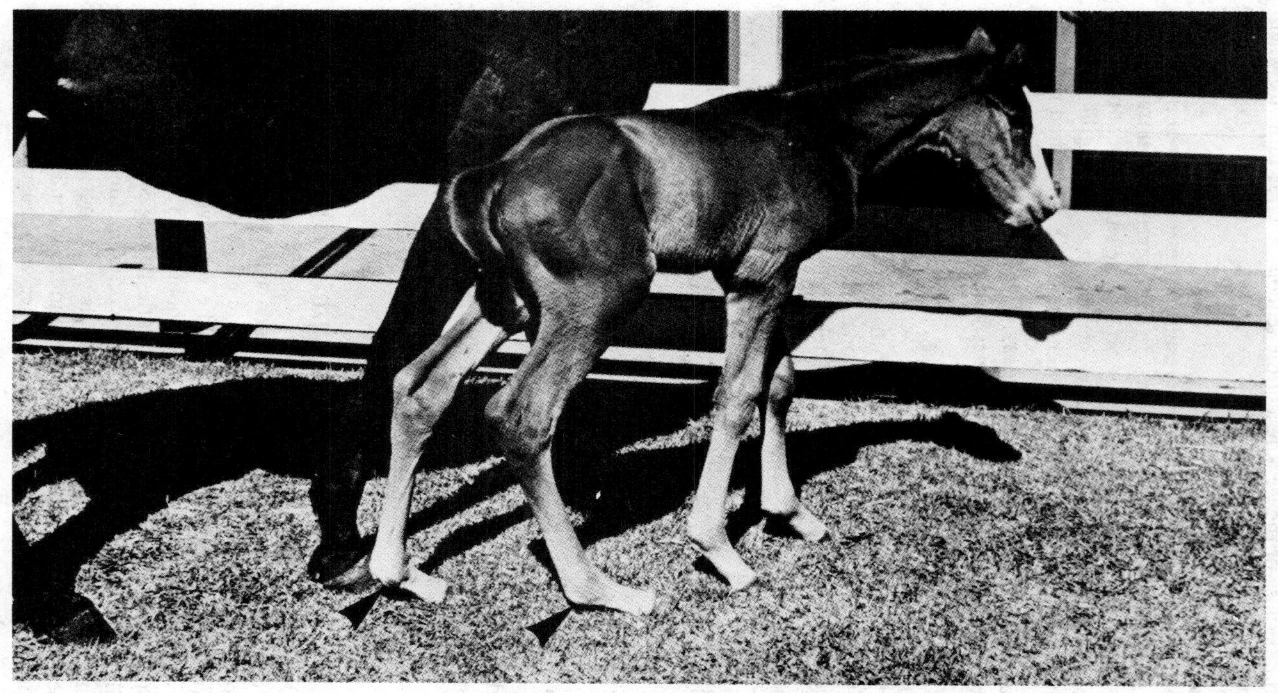

Fig. 46
Five-day-old foal demonstrating weakness of the flexor tendons (arrows).

addition, because of the weakness of the tendons, the toe turns up when weight is placed on the foot.

Treatment

Confinement to a loose box will result in strengthening of the flexor muscles and tendons over 7 to 10 days. In some severe cases a trailer-type device can be fitted to the affected feet, so that the fetlock does not sink to the ground. This can be achieved by bandaging something like a steel door hinge to the foot, so that it projects out 5 to 8 cm behind the foot.

Deviation of the knees (knock knees) This condition may be found in newborn foals, but generally becomes accentuated as the foal grows.

Cause

Damage to the growth plate just above the knee results in faster growth of the inside of the leg. The initiating cause for this differential growth may be due to conformational abnormalities, resulting in differential pressure on the growth plate.

Symptoms

The foal will appear "knock-kneed" in the fore limbs, although the same condition can affect the hind limbs. In some cases only one fore limb may be affected. As the foal grows the limb deviation becomes more severe.

Treatment

Supportive bandaging or plaster casting of the legs in the early stage of the disorder will usually prevent the disorder from progressing.

Foot trimming to pare down the outside of the hoof wall also serves to reduce the pressure on the leg. In more severe cases surgery may be necessary to staple or fix the inside of the growth plate to prevent it from growing while the outside catches up. This is best performed before the foal is 6 months old.

FOUNDER (Laminitis)

The correct name for founder is laminitis and this gives a clue to the nature of the disease. It is an inflammation of the sensitive laminae and other vascular structures of the foot. The sensitive laminae form the junction between the hard insensitive hoof and the underlying soft sensitive structures. They consist of thin fleshy ridges or plates running parallel with each other, which fit into corresponding depressions on the inner surface of the horny wall and sole of the foot. Inflammation of the sensitive laminae leads to an increase in the volume of blood within the horny box of the hoof which, together with stagnation of venous

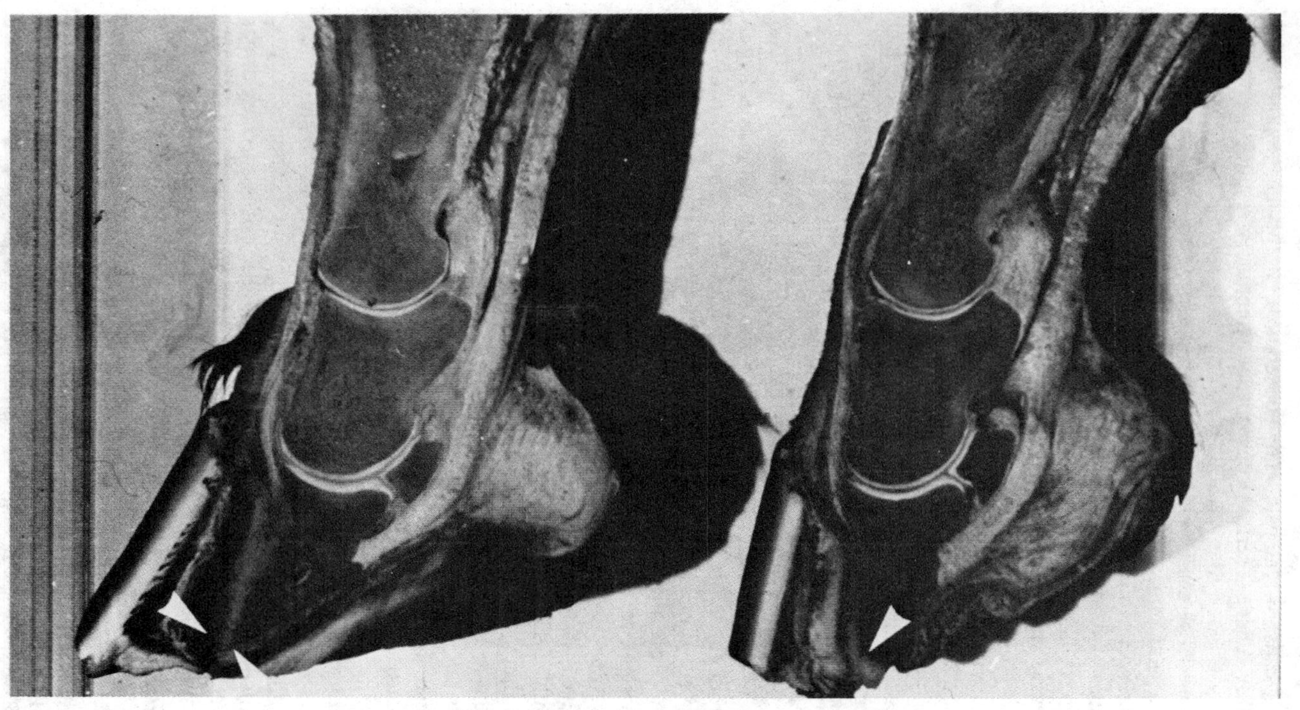

Fig. 47

Founder (laminitis). Cross-section of the front feet of a horse with severe founder where the pedal bones have rotated through the soles of the feet.

blood, causes great pain and foot-soreness. If this congestion is not speedily relieved, serious consequences commonly result.

Causes The causes and predisposing causes of the disease are of great variety and some horses are more prone to contract the disease than others. The following are some of the causes of laminitis: sudden changes of food, especially engorgement on wheat and other grains to which the horse is unaccustomed; severe work after a period of idleness, or severe work at fast pace on hard ground; lack of exercise, as when horses are sent on long sea voyages, or when they are kept in stalls for long periods and do not lie down; overweight, especially if associated with lack of exercise, and commonly seen in fat ponies at grass; metritis (inflammation of the womb) after foaling; exhaustion; flat-footedness, and as a complication of pneumonia. Horses which are lame in one foot or leg and favour this limb, may develop laminitis in the foot of the opposite leg.

Symptoms Laminitis more frequently affects the fore than the hind feet. The symptoms, which usually occur suddenly, vary according to whether the animal is affected in one or more feet. The most marked symptom is lameness, the animal being unwilling to move. When the fore feet are affected, the body is thrown backwards, the horse putting the weight on the hind legs, which are placed well forward under the belly. The fore legs are extended well in front. If the hind feet only are involved, all four legs are held under the body to relieve the hind feet of as much weight as possible. When all feet are affected, the horse stands with the back arched and the hind legs drawn forward under the body to take most of the weight on the heels. If forced to move, the animal walks on its heels, lifting the feet quickly in a characteristic crouching manner. In acute cases, the temperature is raised, the breathing is heavy and hurried, the pulse rate is increased and the animal may break out in a sweat.

Examination of the feet at this stage will reveal nothing abnormal except that the hooves of the affected feet will feel hotter than normal, and pressure with the thumbs, or light tapping with a hammer, may be resented because of pain. The artery at the back of the fetlock throbs beneath the finger. In most cases of laminitis the horse remains standing, but in some cases it lies down on its side with the legs extended. In severe laminitis the pedal bone may rotate to move down towards or even through the sole of the foot.

Treatment Recovery from this disease depends on early diagnosis and prompt treatment before permanent injury takes place. Professional assistance should be sought if possible. Relief of pain and inflammation with anti-inflammatory drugs such as *phenylbutazone* are indicated. A very important part of treatment which should be commenced without delay, and even before arrival of the veterinarian, is cold applications to the feet after removal of the shoes. It may be carried out by standing the horse in a dam or creek, or in a foot-bath dug in the yard or paddock and filled with water. The horse should be tied to a rail or held in such a way as to compel him to keep the affected feet in the water. Alternatively, the feet may be placed in buckets of very cold water, using ice if available, for an hour at a time 3 or 4 times a day. Forced exercise by a short slow walk for 10 minutes every hour for the first 48 hours is also recommended, provided the pain is not too severe. If the pain is extremely severe, nerves to the foot can be blocked with local anaesthetic to enable the horse to be walked.

Bleeding from the jugular vein may be beneficial but this is a matter which should be decided by the veterinarian. The horse should be given a laxative diet of bran mashes and green grass, if available.

If treatment as outlined above is begun early, the acute cases usually subside within 5 or 6 days. The animals should not be returned to work for at least 3 weeks after recovery. In cases where the pedal bone rotates to move through the sole of the foot, the horse may have to be destroyed.

Chronic laminitis

Chronic laminitis results when the acute disease progresses to produce deformity of the foot. The sole drops, rings develop on the hoof running parallel with the coronet, the hoof may become misshapen and the pedal bone rotates.

A cure of this condition is extremely difficult, and the horse is usually rendered unfit for ordinary work. By judicious paring of the foot and with special shoeing, a horse may have some degree of usefulness.

X-rays are useful in showing the degree of rotation of the pedal bone which allows the amount of foot trimming to be assessed.

FRACTURES

All the bones of the body are subject to fractures but in the horse most fractures are of the bones of the limbs. Other fractures which are not so common involve the face, the lower jaw, the ribs, cervical vertebrae and the pelvic bones. Different terms are given to the various types of fractures, the more common ones being *greenstick* or *incomplete fracture,* where only part of the bone is broken or the bone cracks or splits; *simple fracture,* when the bone is broken right through but the soft parts have

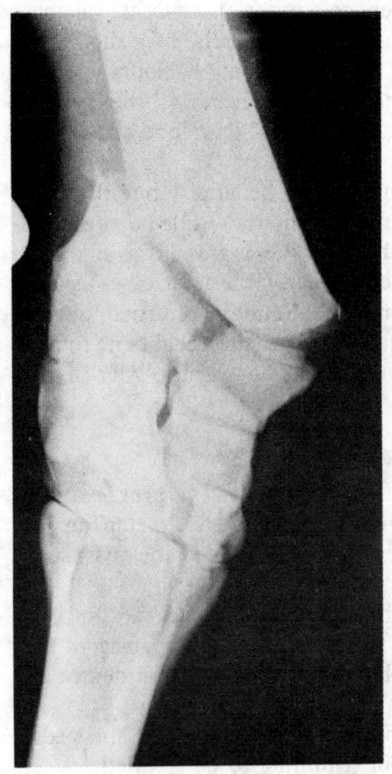

Fig. 48
Fracture of the radius.

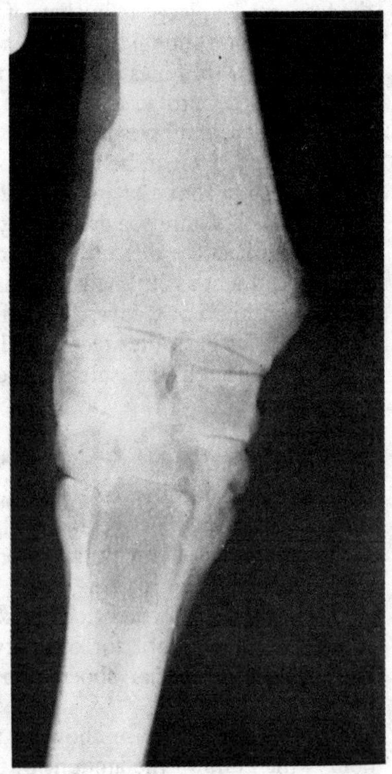

Fig. 49
Fracture of the radius showing healing after 9 weeks in a plaster cast.

received no injury and there is no external wound; *compound fracture,* when one broken end of bone causes a skin wound; *comminuted fracture,* when the bone has broken in several places and shattered; *impacted fracture,* when one broken end of a bone is driven in to the other broken end.

Causes Apart from certain predisposing causes such as age, fragility of the bones due to disease, slippery conditions of roads and tracks, most fractures in horses are caused by direct violence, such as kicks, falls, errors in judgement during jumping, collisions, casting for operations, or from sudden or excessive muscular contractions as may occur in galloping or jumping, or by struggling when cast for operation.

Symptoms Usually fractures are easily diagnosed because the part is rendered useless, crepitation—grating of fractured bones—can be heard or felt when manipulated, and there is unnatural mobility and deformity. Sometimes, however, such as in the case of a fractured pelvis or split pastern bone, these symptoms are not observed, and, although they may be revealed by careful manipulation, an x-ray is often necessary.

Treatment Skilled veterinary attention is required for the treatment of most fractures in the horse but the type of animal, the use to which it is put, the nature of the fracture and economic considerations influence the decision as to whether treatment is justified. In recent years the availability of larger stainless steel plates and screws has allowed bones to be repaired where formerly the horse would be destroyed. However there are still some fractures that are untreatable and necessitate destruction of the horse.

In young horses the bones heal quite well if broken parts can be kept immobilised—a much more difficult matter than in the case of small animals. After reduction of the fracture, splints, plaster of paris bandages and other supports may be used for this purpose and bones may be plated or pinned surgically. The difficulty is to keep the patient in a state of rest and quietness, hence the difficulty of getting complete recoveries. As long bones have a tendency to shorten when uniting, a break of the leg commonly leaves a horse slightly lame.

In the case of incomplete or greenstick fractures in foals where there is no displacement, complete recovery may occur if the foal can be kept quiet in a loose box or shed.

FROG — DISEASES OF

The frog is intended to act as a cushion to take the first weight of the limb. A healthy frog does not bruise, and the best way of bringing a diseased one back to health is to lower the heels and give it ground pressure. Ragged edges of the frog which harbour dirt may be trimmed off, but no cutting away of the healthy frog should be allowed. Attention to stable hygiene and cleanliness of the part are essential in preventing disease of the frog. This entails cleaning out accumulated straw and moist material in the deep crevices either side of the frog twice daily.

See *Canker, Thrush*

GASTRO-ENTERITIS

See *Diarrhoea*

GIRTH GALLS

A gall is an excoriation (erosion) of the skin and commonly results from excessive pressure or friction imposed on a horse's body by the saddle, the girth and harness generally, and is frequently associated with the condition or shape of the animal. Condition certainly plays an important part in the causation of girth galls, as horses in soft condition gall much more readily than horses in hard condition. Hard, dirty girths contribute to galling, but under ordinary conditions it is not so much the hardness of the girth that causes the gall, but rather its movement forward so that the edge of the girth is dragged forward behind the elbow. The shape of the brisket around which the girth fits, and the general conformation of the chest contribute to this. It can sometimes be overcome by using a split leather girth (not generally recommended) which catches not only the edge of the brisket, but also the skin. A girth should be kept fairly tight to ensure that it moves as little as possible. In this connection it should be remembered that a saddle is never girthed to a back as tightly as it seems, because when the rider's weight is in the saddle, the girth at once becomes slacker. Some horses learn the trick of keeping their chests distended with air when they are being girthed up. If necessary, such horses should have their girths tightened again by someone after the rider is in the saddle.

When, owing to malformation of the horse, the girth persists in slipping forward, it can be held back by means of a surcingle and a strap. The surcingle is placed under the seat towards the rear arch of the saddle, and passed obliquely under the belly and buckled. A strap is then applied along the underline from girth to surcingle which should be about 30 cm to the rear of the girth. If the horse already has a girth gall, the saddle girth can be drawn back as far as is considered necessary to avoid the injured surface, and then drawn tight. The strap is adjusted and then the surcingle tightened, but only sufficiently to prevent it from being drawn forward. With such a contrivance, the girth does not slip forward, galling is prevented and it is possible to work a horse with a simple girth gall.

When girth galls occur because of soft condition, a piece of sheepskin or soft rubber tubing placed around the girth will prevent galling until the horse improves in condition.

Treatment for simple girth gall Wash the excoriated skin with warm water and soap; allow to dry; dab on white lotion (zinc sulphate 30 g, lead acetate 15 g, water 500 ml) several times a day, or apply a solution of triple dyes, obtainable from any chemist. Neglected galls which have become infected will require veterinary attention.

GREASY HEEL

The scientific name for grease or greasy heel is *seborrhoea*, which means an abnormal secretion of the sebaceous or oil glands. It is accompanied by deep-seated inflammation of the skin at the rear surfaces of the pastern and fetlock and is really a chronic dermatitis. The specific cause is unknown, but the condition is usually seen in heavy horses with coarse thick legs, when such horses are kept in damp, dirty stables or are long subjected to mud and filth without proper grooming. It can, however, occur in any type of horse and is sometimes seen in horses with clean legs kept under hygienic conditions.

Symptoms The early symptoms are swelling and redness of the skin, with some itching. Later there is increased secretion from the sebaceous glands in the affected area, over which the hair stands erect, the individual hairs being glued together by the oily secretion. The skin, which is at first moist and sensitive, tends to become thickened and later fungoid masses commonly referred to as "grapes" may be found, and the part enlarges considerably. Secondary bacterial infection occurs, leading to *necrosis* and ulceration. There is an offensive odour. The infection may spread to the frog and even undermine the sole of the foot. The hind legs are more commonly affected but the condition is seen in the fore legs. Lameness may or may not be present.

Treatment Early cases of the disease, when only the superficial layers

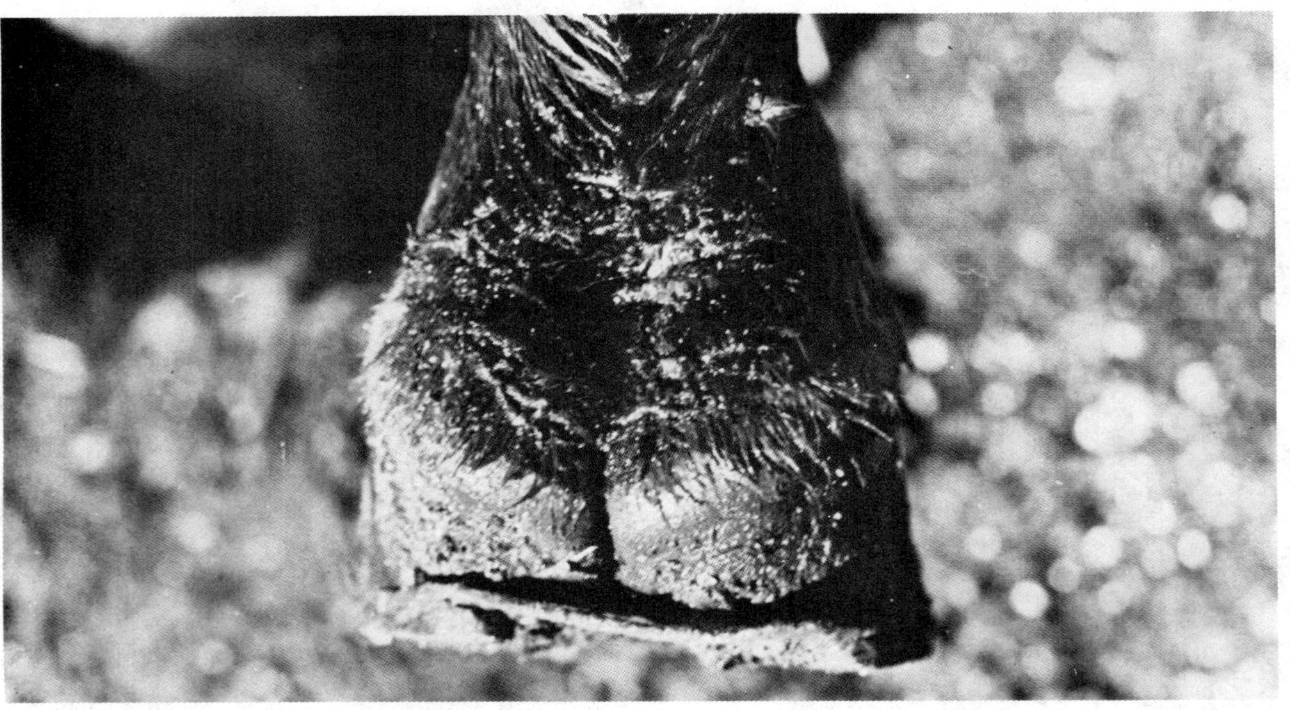

Fig. 50
Greasy heel at the back of the pastern region.

of the skin are involved, will respond to local treatment. When the condition is advanced, the prognosis is not so hopeful. The hair should be clipped closely over the affected areas, and the part then cleansed with good quality soap and water, rubbing the soap in gently for some time. Wipe off any fungoid or greasy material. When thoroughly dry, apply a mild astringent lotion, such as white lotion (see *Girth Galls*) repeatedly, but keep the part soft with benzoated zinc oxide ointment or zinc cream. Bluestone solution (30 g bluestone to 600 ml of water) may be used as an early application. Good results have been reported following repeated dusting of the affected areas, after thorough washing and drying, with a sulphonamide dusting powder. Advanced cases of the disease will require attention by a veterinarian.

Preventive measures for greasy heel include refraining from unnecessary washing of the legs and feet and, when this is unavoidable, thorough drying of the legs. Clipping the legs for appearances' sake should be avoided. Oiling behind the pastern and fetlock in prolonged wet weather, and attention to hygiene are the most effective ways to prevent occurrence of the condition.

HEART DISEASES

Heart diseases similar to those occurring in man are uncommon in the horse. However, abnormalities of the electrocardiogram (ECG) are common in racehorses and result in a significant reduction in racing performance. These abnormalities cannot be detected with a stethoscope and require recording of an ECG.

Symptoms Horses with myocarditis (heart strain), which is the most common condition found in racehorses, will usually stop or fail to run on over the terminal stages of a race. Horses with this condition often race erratically and will work well on the track and race poorly on race day. In more severe heart diseases, where there may be failure of the heart, a pronounced jugular pulse may be noticed. This will be seen as a pulse wave moving up the jugular groove with each heart beat.

Treatment In the case of heart strain all that can be done is a long rest period for the horse and often horses recover following a spell of 9 to 12 months. When there is severe damage to the heart and congestive heart failure sometimes drug treatment is successful in alleviating some of the symptoms associated with heart failure. However long-term drug treatment for heart disease is seldom practical in the horse.

(See Fig. 51 on p. 96)

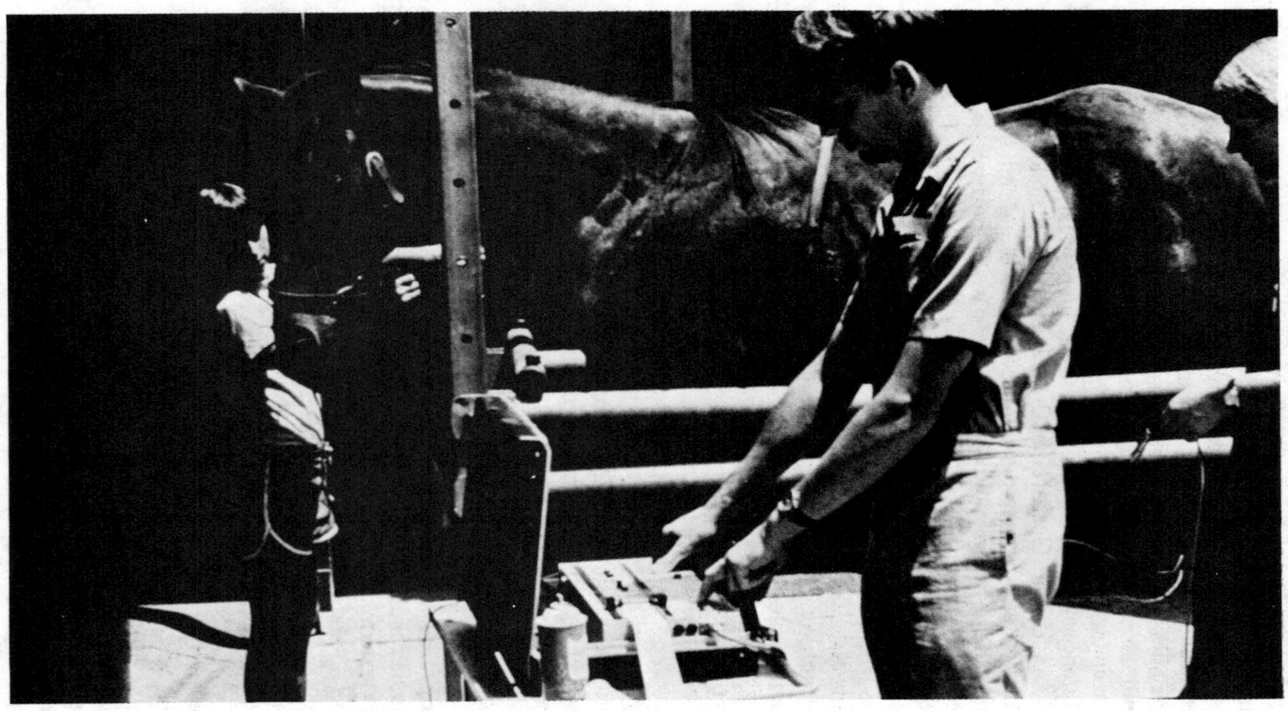

Fig. 51
Heart diseases. Recording the electrocardiogram from a horse.

HEATSTROKE — HEAT EXHAUSTION — SUNSTROKE

The conditions known as heatstroke, heat exhaustion and sunstroke are due to upset of the heat-regulating mechanism of the body. In general, they result from high environmental temperature, high humidity and sometimes inadequate ventilation. Heatstroke and heat exhaustion occur in excessively hot humid weather when horses are crowded together in yards or cattle trucks, or are forced to work hard in such weather. Sunstroke is caused when animals are unable to find shade and are exposed to direct rays of the sun, and more particularly, if they are worked continuously in the sun during very hot weather. Lack of water is an important contributing factor.

Symptoms The symptoms of heatstroke, heat exhaustion and sunstroke, which develop suddenly, are with minor variations, very similar. The horse is usually very distressed, the breathing is hurried, the temperature very high, the nostrils are dilated and highly reddened, the pulse is rapid and weak, usually sweating is checked, the pupils of the eyes are dilated, and the horse staggers and falls to the ground partially or totally unconscious. Whilst on the ground, if not fully unconscious, he may struggle and attempt to get up but be unable to do so. Muscular spasms or convulsions may be shown. Death occurs quickly in some cases but less severe ones recover, especially if treatment can be carried out promptly.

Treatment The horse should be moved to a cool and shady spot and the whole body hosed with cold water. Ice packs should be applied to the top and sides of the head and along the jugular furrow. It is important to reduce the body temperature and so hosing should be repeated at regular intervals so that the temperature drops gradually. Cold water should be available to the animal to drink immediately he is able to do so. Good nursing, a light diet and a lengthy spell from work are necessary for full recovery. Veterinary surgeons administer various drugs and supplement the cold applications by intravenous injections of saline and other solutions.

HEAVES — CHRONIC OBSTRUCTIVE PULMONARY DISEASE (COPD)

Heaves is a chronic condition of the lungs, commonly seen in horses in England, Europe and the United States. It appears to be due to horses spending a large proportion of their time in stalls where various substances in straw and hay cause an allergic condition within the lungs.

Although it is found in horses in Australia, it is quite uncommon.

Symptoms The symptoms usually develop gradually, there being a frequent dry wheezing cough, which becomes more pronounced with exercise. Due to the damage to the lungs, inadequate amounts of oxygen are transferred from the lungs to the bloodstream, and therefore horses often appear distressed during exercise. Horses with heaves or COPD have a characteristic respiration where there is a double lift of the flank during the expiration of air. This double movement of the flank is an attempt by the animal to remove air from its lungs. In the early stages of the condition the horse may appear normal at rest, but as the condition worsens a typical broken-winded breathing appears and is accompanied by a hollow cough. It will usually be noted that horses with broken-wind improve when they are turned out to pasture, the symptoms returning when they are put back into a stable.

Treatment The main aim of treatment is to improve the horse's environment for it is this environment that usually maintains the symptoms seen with this condition. If horses have to be stabled, then it is best that they are stabled on shavings or cut-up newspaper, which is now commerically available. Horses with COPD are allergic to various moulds and allergens within hay and straw, and therefore attempts should be made to exclude these materials from the horse's environment. Most horses will improve quickly when they are turned out in a paddock and this is probably the best form of treatment. If it is impossible for the horse to be turned out into a paddock then attempts must be made to improve the ventilation of the horse's stable, as well as the changes in management previously mentioned.

HEELS — DISEASES OF

See *Cracked Heels, Greasy Heel*

HERNIA (Rupture)

A hernia is a protrusion of any organ or part of an organ through the containing wall of its cavity, beyond its normal confines. The term is usually applied to the abdominal cavity, but hernias occur elsewhere in the body.

Abdominal hernias, or ruptures, may be classified as *reducible,* when the protruding structures can be readily pushed back into the abdominal

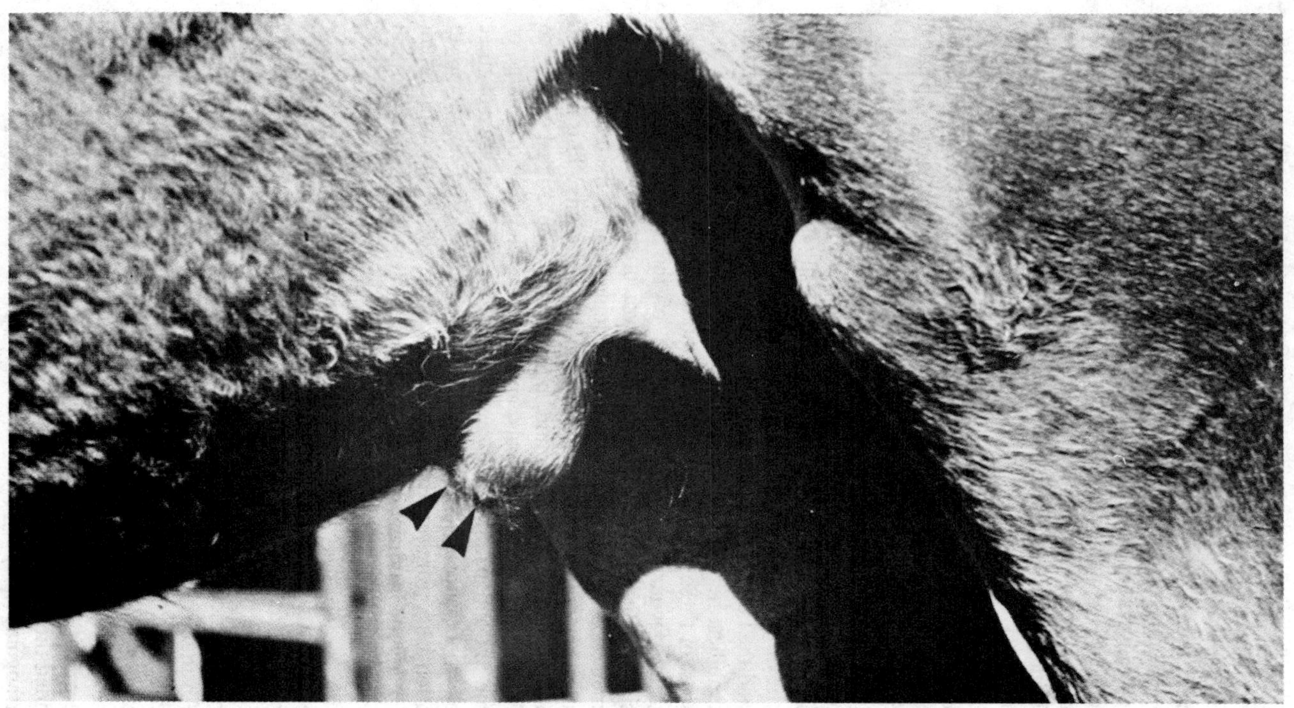

Fig. 52
Umbilical hernia (arrows) in a yearling.

cavity through the hernial ring; *irreducible,* when the structures have become adherent to the surroundings, or have become enlarged after emerging, or for other reasons cannot be pushed back; *strangulated,* when the circulation of the blood to the herniated bowel is cut off by the margin of the opening through which the loop of bowel has passed, thereby causing congestion, swelling and inflammation which, if not promptly relieved, leads to gangrene of the part and death of the animal.

According to their situation, abdominal hernias are described as umbilical, scrotal, inguinal, and ventral, and may be congenital or acquired.

Umbilical Hernia This form of hernia commonly occurs in foals and results from imperfect closure of the umbilicus, which is the opening through which the umbilical cord passes before birth. A loop of bowel or omentum (caul) passes through this opening, either at birth or subsequently, as a result of strain and weakness of the muscle, and lies just beneath the skin. The soft swelling can usually be pushed back easily with the fingers, especially if the animal is placed on its back. There is no pain and the health of the foal is not affected. It should be borne in mind that umbilical hernias may be hereditary.

Most of these hernias disappear spontaneously without any form of treatment, favoured by the small size of the rupture, absence of adhesions, youth of the animal and growth of the abdomen. As the abdomen expands in diameter, the protruding portion of the intestine and omentum are drawn gradually into the abdominal cavity. This may take 12 months. Bearing this in mind, hasty action should not be taken to rectify umbilical hernias in foals, and provided they do not enlarge or become hot and painful, they are best left alone. Should any of these complications appear, professional assistance should be sought, as an operation is then frequently necessary to correct the hernia and prevent strangulation. Umbilical hernias which occur later in life require surgical attention.

Scrotal and Inguinal Hernias These forms of hernia are also fairly common in foals as congenital conditions. The foal is born with an enlarged scrotum ("purse"), caused by a piece of omentum or bowel having descended through the inguinal canal into the scrotum.

An inguinal hernia is one in which the piece of omentum or bowel descends, but remains in the inguinal canal. It is not so evident as a scrotal hernia. Both these forms of hernia are due to the abdominal end of the canal being unusually large. Again, as in the case of umbilical hernia, these conditions rectify themselves over a period of 12 months or less provided there are no complications. In those cases where pain is shown or strangulation appears to be imminent, an immediate operation is necessary. Acquired scrotal and inguinal hernias in older animals, caused as a result of strain or over-exertion, can only be reduced by operation.

If the horse has had a scrotal hernia as a foal the veterinarian should be informed when a colt comes to be gelded. Colts with previous scrotal hernias are more likely to prolapse intestines through their castration wound at the time of gelding, and therefore the veterinarian can take steps to ensure that this does not happen at the time of surgery.

Ventral Hernia This is a hernia which mostly occurs as a result of some injury to the abdominal wall, which is weakened and allows portion of the bowel or omentum to pass through an artificial opening. Congenital perforations of the walls of the abdomen of the foal do sometimes occur, but are rare. An injury, such as a kick from another horse, a fall upon a stump or large stone, or even a kick from a man's boot, are common causative factors. These hernias vary greatly in size depending on the dimensions of the aperture, and may occur anywhere on the dependent parts of the abdomen. Treatment is by operation under a general anaesthetic. Ventral hernias are sometimes found in old mares in foal and are due to rupture of the supporting tendons of the abdominal muscles. This condition is very difficult to treat and may necessitate destruction of the mare.

HOCK — DISEASES OF

See *Capped Hock, Curb, Spavin, Thoroughpin*

HOOF — DISEASES OF

Whilst the hoof is the hard horny casing of the foot, it is so intimately related to the other structures of the foot that it is common to consider hoof disease and foot disease together. Books have been written on diseases of the horse's foot, including the hoof, and when one considers the importance of a horse having 4 good feet this is not surprising. The scope of this book does not permit a detailed desciption of the anatomy and physiology of the horse's foot, but the following brief discussion will help to explain a number of troubles attributable directly or indirectly to improper management or to faulty conformation.

The hoof of the horse and of other solipeds may well be compared with the human fingernail except that it completely encases the digit. The wall of the hoof consists of more or less dense, fibrous, horny material derived from the coronary band (the spongy tissue just above the hoof at its junction with the skin). Within this horny box are bones, tendons, ligaments, nerves and an intricate network of blood vessels. The hoof wall and sole are attached to the underlying structures by means of so called sensitive and insensitive laminae (see under *Founder*). These consist of small leaf-like structures which are closely united in dovetailed fashion. Although the hoof would appear to be unyielding, it expands and contracts in waves when the animal moves on it, particularly at the heels and coronary cushion. Even the sole of the foot, which is superimposed over a padlike structure known as the plantar cushion, flattens out when weight is borne. The so called lateral cartilages (referred to under *Sidebones*) play an important part in this normal expansion and contraction. The nutriment for the structures of the foot is received from the blood, the flow of which is largely controlled by the expansion and contraction of the parts referred to above. The hoof wall grows at the rate of about 6 mm a month, being pushed down from the coronet regularly all round the foot. Growth is favoured by moisture, good nutrition and general health, as well as by exercise. The unshod hoof grows more rapidly than one with shoes.

The white line at the junction of the wall with the sole marks the point of union between the horny leaves of the sole and those of the wall. In shoeing, the nails are driven through the hoof at a point just outside this line. The sole is marked by a deep V-shaped cleft, outlined on each side by the bars, which are a continuation of the wall. The triangular-shaped horny structure within the lines of the V formed by the bars is known as the frog. The entire sole of the hoof, as well as the walls, cover highly sensitive tissue richly supplied with nerves and blood vessels.

The conformation of the ideal foot, that is the general form, outline and arrangement of parts, varies somewhat with the type of animal and even with the breed. Broadly, the well-shaped hoof is roughly like a cone from above downward. The print made by the hoof is generally oval, being slightly greater in length than in width. The walls of the hoof slope gradually and evenly outward from above and are free from deep grooves or bulges. The substance of the normal hoof is dense and firm but not brittle, and it has a distinctive natural gloss, the result of a varnish-like substance called periople, which lessens the evaporation of the moisture normally present in the horn. The bars are well defined, strong and widely spaced. There is no compressed narrowing of the foot at the heel, and the frog is clean and well formed. The feet should be centred on a perpendicular line from the point of the buttocks through the hock and fetlock in the hind leg and from the shoulder through the knee and fetlock in the front leg. Viewed from the side, the axis through the fetlock, pastern, and hoof should consist of a straight, unbroken line forming an angle of about 34° with the base of the foot. The hoof at the heel should generally be approximately one-third as long as in front. The foot of the donkey or mule is considerably smaller and rounder than the foot of the horse.

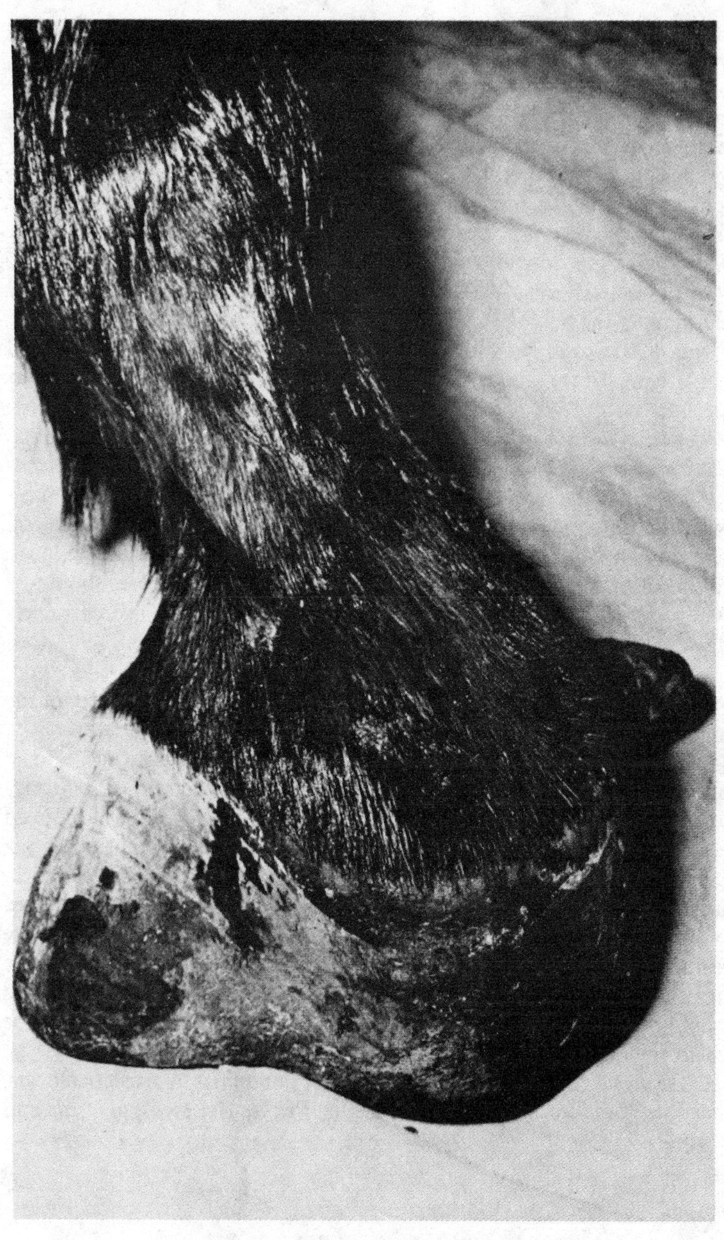

Fig. 53
Abnormalities in growth of the hoof wall due to poor hoof care.

Contracted Heels A condition not uncommonly seen affecting the heels and quarters, particularly of the feet of light horses, is that of contracted heels or "hoofbound". Horses which have been improperly shod so that the frog does not receive normal ground pressure are apt to be affected with contracted feet, particularly at the heels. Flat feet and low weak heels also predispose to this condition. Excessive use of the rasp from heel to toe, so that too much horn is removed from the heel and bars, may also be a factor in causing the condition. Lameness may occur especially at speed or after hard work.

Contracted heels of long standing may be difficult to rectify, and any treatment of the hoof is a slow process, extending over 6 months or more. If the animal can be allowed to go barefooted, this permits natural pressure on the frog, and spreading of the heels will follow. If shoeing is necessary, the toe of the foot should be kept short and the bars and frog left alone as much as possible. Several grooves, parallel to the coronet and 12 mm apart, may be cut into the quarters with a saw, starting 20 mm below the hairline and extending from the heel halfway to the toe. This operation must be repeated as the quarters grow out until the heels and quarters are normally expanded. Hoof ointments, containing such substances as turpentine, tar and wax in an oily or fatty base, should be used to assist in softening the horn. Special shoes, having as their object the spreading of the heels, are also useful.

Brittle Hooves As the name indicates, an abnormally dry state of the horn may develop as a result of which the hoof chips and cracks easily. Brittle hooves tend to predispose to toe and quarter cracks and lead to difficulties in shoeing. Long-continued dryness or stabling on hard dry floors is conducive to the trouble as is also the horse's diet (lack of green feed). Brittle hooves require very careful shoeing to ensure that the bearing surface is as level as possible. Only thin nails should be used, placed in the strongest parts of the hoof wall. A hoof ointment of the type referred to under *Contracted Heels* should be used. Castor oil and lanoline make useful hoof dressings for this condition. Attention should be paid to the diet of the horse and, if natural grazing is not available, cut green feed should be fed. Should this not be possible, stabilised vitamin A should be fed in the concentrate ration.
See *Canker, Corns, False Quarter, Founder (laminitis), Navicular Disease, Ringbone, Sandcrack, Seedy-toe, Shoeing Pricks, Sidebones, Thrush* and *Wounds*

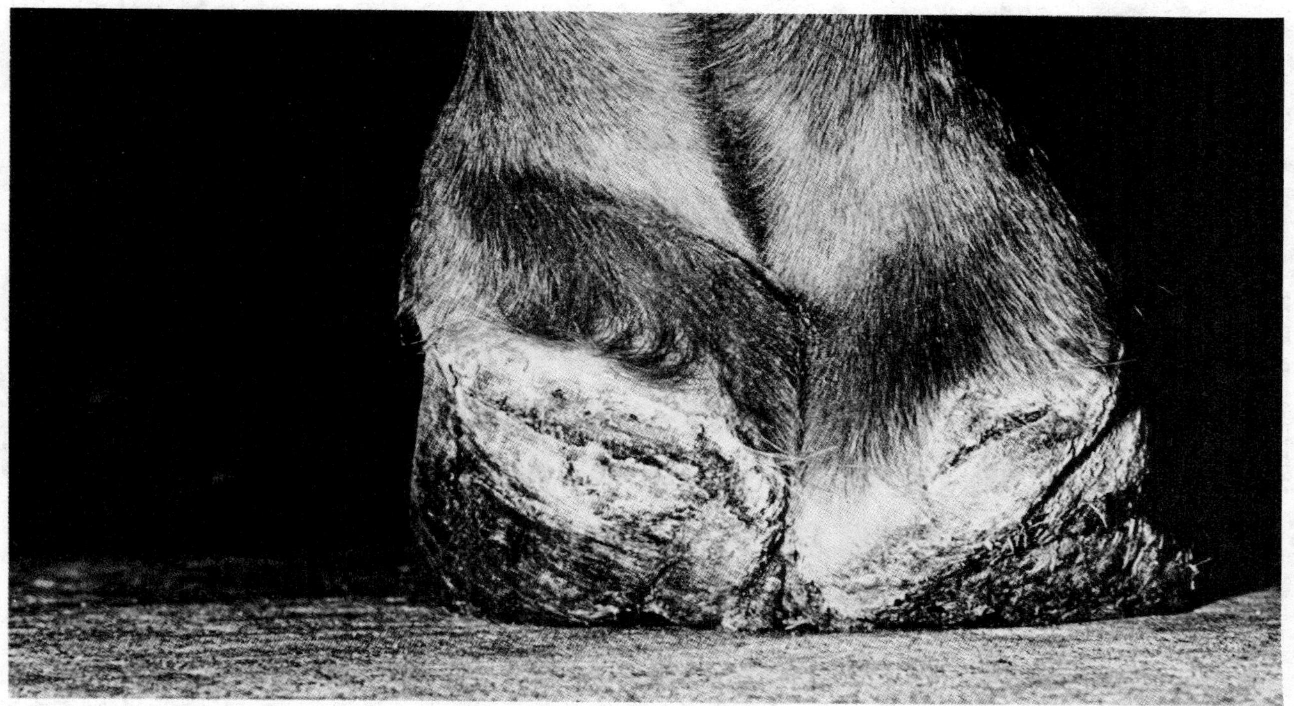

Fig. 54
Sheared heels in the foot of a horse due to uneven foot trimming.

INFERTILITY

The Stud Book figures testify to the significance of infertility as a major problem. Of all mares served approximately 65 per cent produce a live foal. This percentage has not altered perceptibly over the last 100 years, despite improvements in the understanding of reproductive physiology.

Cause The reasons for infertility are too numerous to discuss at length here. However, the most common ones are infection of the uterus (metritis), hormonal abnormalities and management problems.

Symptoms The most obvious symptom is failure of the mare to become pregnant. It is important to have information on cycle lengths, number of services, number of foals etcetera, so that a veterinarian is able to carry out effective treatment.

Treatment Before undertaking treatment a veterinary surgeon will perform various tests which can include a rectal examination of the reproductive tract, a swab to determine if bacteria are causing infection, and a uterine biopsy to determine if the uterus is capable of carrying a pregnancy. Treatment is then instituted on the basis of these findings.

INFLUENZA — EQUINE

Equine influenza is a specific viral infection not yet present in Australia. The virus is very similar to that causing human influenza. Equine influenza is widespread throughout the world and outbreaks occur where horses are congregated together.

Symptoms The horse will usually go off its feed, appear depressed, have a nasal discharge and a cough. Affected horses become severely ill for several weeks and may have a temperature up to 41 °C. Often several months are required for complete recovery.

Treatment Good general nursing is necessary and even then some horses are left with damage to the heart where the virus can sometimes localise. Vaccination is carried out in countries where the disease is endemic, and is successful in preventing infection.

INJECTIONS

It is sometimes necessary for horse owners to administer various medications, such as antibiotics, which have been prescribed by a veterinarian. When injections are required, it is important that these are performed carefully, using sterile needles (19 gauge, 3.75 cm long) and sterile syringes. The skin over the injection site should be disinfected using a 70 per cent solution of alcohol. This solution can be prepared by taking 815 ml of methylated spirits and making this up to 1 litre with water. For an intramuscular injection the needle should be inserted, after disconnection from the syringe, to its full depth. If blood emerges from the needle it should be inserted in a different site. The syringe is then connected to the needle and the plunger is withdrawn for 1 to 2 seconds to again check if the needle is in a blood vessel. If no blood emerges the material is injected. The sites for intramuscular injections are depicted in the illustrations and include the neck, chest and rump. When a series of injections are required over several days the injection sites should be alternated.

See Figs 55 to 59 on pp. 108–9

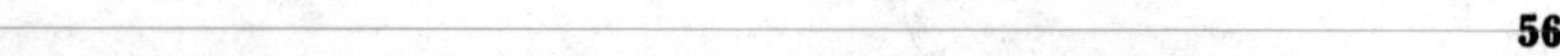

55

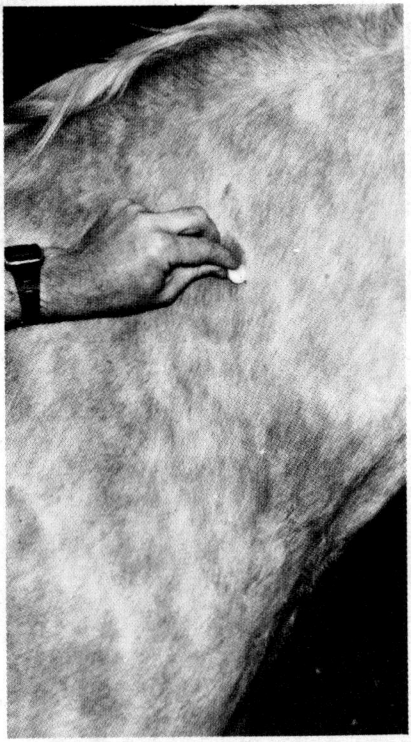

56

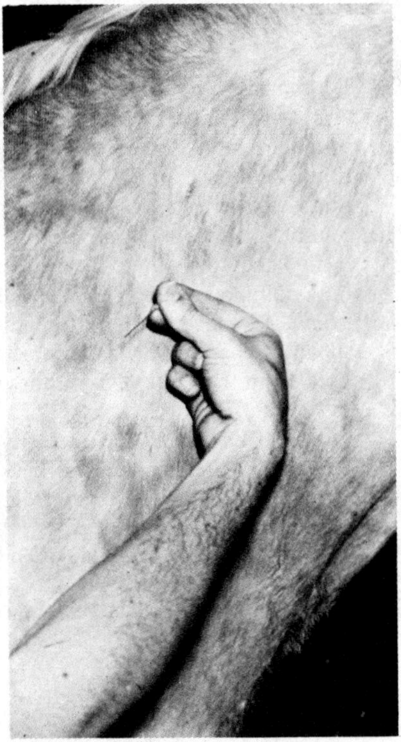

Fig. 55
Disinfection of skin with methylated spirits prior to injection in the neck.

Fig. 56
The needle is held by its hub and the area to be injected is hit a few times with the back of the hand. This has the effect of minimising the reaction of the horse.

Fig. 57
The needle is inserted up to the hub and the syringe connected. After drawing back on the plunger to make sure that the needle is not in a blood vessel, the material is injected. If blood is present, the needle should be removed and reinserted in a new site.

Fig. 58
Intramuscular injections may also be given in the pectoral muscles in the front of the chest.

Fig. 59
Another site for intramuscular injections is in the rump.

57

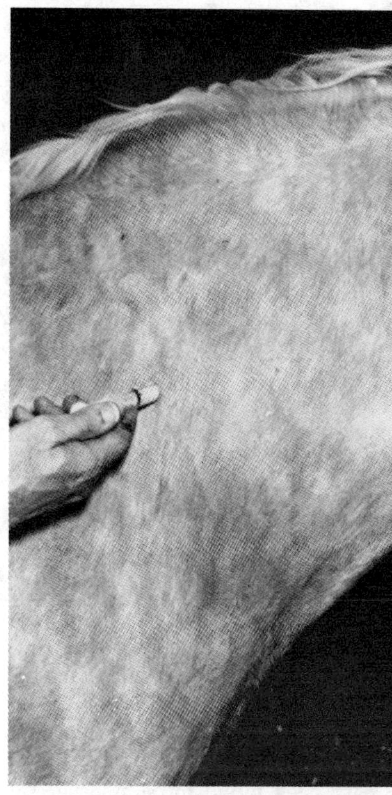

58

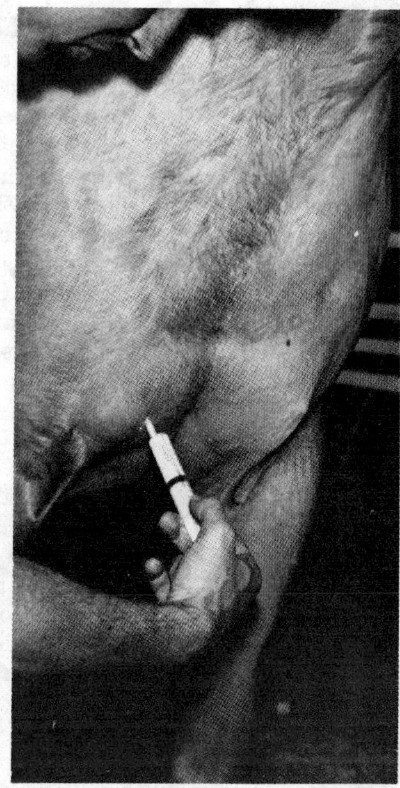

59

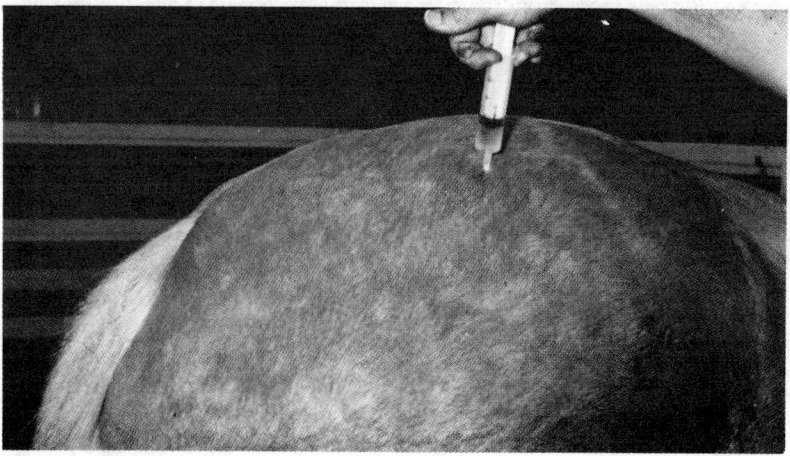

JAUNDICE (Icterus)

Jaundice, icterus or "yellows" is not a specific disease but is a clinical symptom which arises from disorders of the liver and biliary system and also in association with other diseases. There is a yellowish discoloration of the visible mucous membranes such as the eyes, nose, mouth and genital organs. In white or light-coloured horses even the skin may show this yellow tint. Although jaundice occurs as a common symptom of certain well-known diseases, it can occur as a symptom of almost any inflammatory disease accompanied by high fever. Obstructive jaundice, due to occlusion of the bile duct by calculi or from other causes—the horse has no gall bladder—is not common in the horse, but can occur. *Neonatal jaundice* is sometimes seen in foals. The treatment for jaundice depends entirely on the cause.

JOINT-ILL (Navel-ill)

Joint-ill (navel-ill or polyarthritis) is a serious disease of foals and, prior to the advent of antibiotic drugs, was responsible for many deaths. It arises from infection through the navel shortly after birth, and sometimes whilst the foal is still in the uterus. The infection spreads to various organs of the body causing a variety of disease conditions, and occasionally a fatal septicaemia. It commonly attacks various joints, leading to the term "*joint-ill*".

Cause A large number of bacteria have been found to be associated with the development of this disease complex. It is well recognised that the disease is more prone to occur when the mare foals in a foaling-box or stable, or when assistance is given to the mare when foaling. It is far less likely to occur when the mare foals in a well-grassed paddock and without human interference.

Symptoms In most cases symptoms appear within the first few weeks of life, depending on the mode and type of infection. If infection has occurred in the uterus, the foal may be born dead or in a weakened condition, is fevered, obviously sick and disinclined to suck its mother. Death commonly occurs in 2 to 3 days. When infection occurs shortly after birth, symptoms are generally shown in 7 to 8 days, sometimes longer, depending on the type of infection. There may be little or no evidence of infection at the navel with certain types of organisms. On the other hand, when the infection is due to pus-forming organisms, there is abscess formation at the navel. The foal is depressed and listless, has a temperature above normal and shows increased respiration and pulse rates. Swelling of the joints with accompanying lameness occurs, particularly of the stifle and hock, but also of other joints such as the knee, shoulder, elbow and fetlock. The joint swelling becomes hot, tense and painful and after a few days may burst and discharge a serous, blood-stained fluid and sometimes pus. Alternatively, the swelling may regress, the heat subside and the joint appear normal again, but such a joint may cause lameness later in life. In addition to fatal septicaemia, the disease is particularly serious when abscess formation occurs in the lungs, liver and other internal organs.

Treatment This disease in foals is far too serious for any attempt at treatment by the horse owner. Immediately any symptoms are shown which suggest navel infection, the services of a veterinary surgeon should be obtained in order that culture of joint fluid to determine the type of bacteria is performed. Following this, appropriate antibiotic therapy is instituted which will usually successfully overcome the infection. However, despite the infection being cured many foals are left permanent damage to the cartilage lining the joint and may be subject to arthritis and lameness as they become older.

Prevention It will be obvious that prevention lies mainly in good hygiene at foaling time. The best environment is that of a well-grassed, spelled paddock. In Australia, most mares do foal in the paddock and when they do so and the navel cord breaks naturally and no assistance is necessary at foaling, joint-ill is unlikely to occur. It is very important that the young foal should receive the colostrum in the first milk from the mother, as this contains antibodies which protect the foal against infection by various organisms. Should the foal be weak at birth, it should be assisted to the mare's teats and encouraged to suck, but the navel should not be interfered with. If it is necessary to render assistance at foaling, the strictest hygiene should be maintained. The fingernails of the attendant should be cut short and the hands and arms washed thoroughly in hot water and soap to which some antiseptic has been added. The external genitals and tail of the mare should be washed in antiseptic solution and other precautionary measures taken to prevent infection, particularly if the cord is broken in the course of the manipulations or has to be cut with sterile scissors. The application of strong antiseptics to the navel stump is likely to do more harm than good, as this retards healing and may encourage bacterial infection. Although it is the practice of some studs to give antibiotics to foals at birth, this is to be deplored. It seldom achieves the desired effect as few antibiotics will cover all likely bacteria and the use of antibiotics in this fashion leads to bacteria developing resistance to antibiotics.

KIDNEYS — INFLAMMATION OF (Nephritis)

Contrary to the general opinion of horse owners, it is comparatively rare for the horse's kidneys to be primarily diseased. Except in old horses, acute and chronic inflammations of the kidneys do not commonly occur. Horses excrete a lot of calcium carbonate in their urine, which gives the urine a characteristic whitish or thickened appearance on some occasions. This is entirely normal and not a sign of kidney disease as thought by many horse owners.

KIMBERLEY OR WALKABOUT DISEASE

A fatal disease of horses occurs in the Kimberley Division of Western Australia and in the Nothern Territory of Australia. It has been the subject of considerable research.

Cause A native plant *Crotalaria retusa,* which grows in the low-lying areas of the main river systems which are subject to flooding, has been found to be the poisonous plant which causes the disease.

Symptoms It is called walkabout disease because the affected animals walk in a straight line into fences and other obstructions and may stand for hours pushing at the obstacle. They also walk into creeks and rivers and stumble over logs. The earlier symptoms are those of sleepiness, irritability, depraved appetite and yawning. Affected animals also show inco-ordination of movement, and twitching of head and neck muscles. They are reluctant to lie down, and when down may be unable to rise without assistance. The urine is coffee-coloured or red and symptoms of jaundice may be shown.

The walkabout symptoms extend over a period of weeks or months with progressive and extreme emaciation. Eventually the horse goes down, is unable to rise, goes into a coma and death occurs. The main post-mortem finding is cirrhosis of the liver.

Treatment There is no known treatment.

Prevention The only preventive measure that can be adopted is to endeavour to prevent horses grazing over areas which are subject to flooding and where the plant grows.

Differential Diagnosis Kimberley horse disease must be differentiated from another horse disease known as "Birdsville disease", which occurs also in the Northern Territory of Australia and in western

Queensland and the north of South Australia. This disease is caused by a poisonous plant *Indigofera enneaphylla* and the symptoms are in some respects similar to Kimberley horse disease. Early symptoms are sleepiness and inco-ordination of gait in which the front feet are lifted high from the ground and there is some absence of control of the hind limbs. Horses affected with Birdsville disease are inclined to stand still rather than to wander, and if forced to move are inclined to drag the hind limbs. Chronically affected cases drag the hind limbs constantly and wear away the horn of the feet. Mildly affected cases may recover, but usually an affected horse, which does not die from starvation or thirst, is left with some chronic disability. There is no effective treatment and all that can be done is to deny horses access to the *Indigofera* plant, if possible.

KNEE — FRACTURES OF

The horse's knee is not actually the knee at all. It corresponds to the human wrist and is composed of 2 rows of bones, 3 in each row and a seventh one placed at the back of the upper row of bones. In racehorses, fractures of the bones of the knee are a common form of lameness and have ended many horses' racing careers.

Causes Bad conformation, particularly a calf knee or back of the knee conformation, can predispose to fractures of the knee bones. These fractures may vary from small chips, which are not so serious, to multiple fractures of the knee bones, which may necessitate destruction of the horses. Fractures of the knee bones occur much more commonly in thoroughbred racehorses than in horses used for other types of racing or sport.

Symptoms Varying degrees of lameness are usually apparent, together with distension or "bubbles" over the front of the knee. The horse usually shows pain on flexion of the knee. X-rays are necessary to determine if a fracture exists.

Treatment In some horses with small chip fractures, a rest period of 6 to 9 months may relieve the lameness. However, in the majority of cases surgery is necessary to remove the small fragments of bone, or, in the case of larger fragments, to screw these pieces back into place. After sustaining a knee chip horses have only 50 per cent chance of racing successfully again as damage to the joint surfaces frequently results in arthritis.

(See Fig. 60 on p. 114)

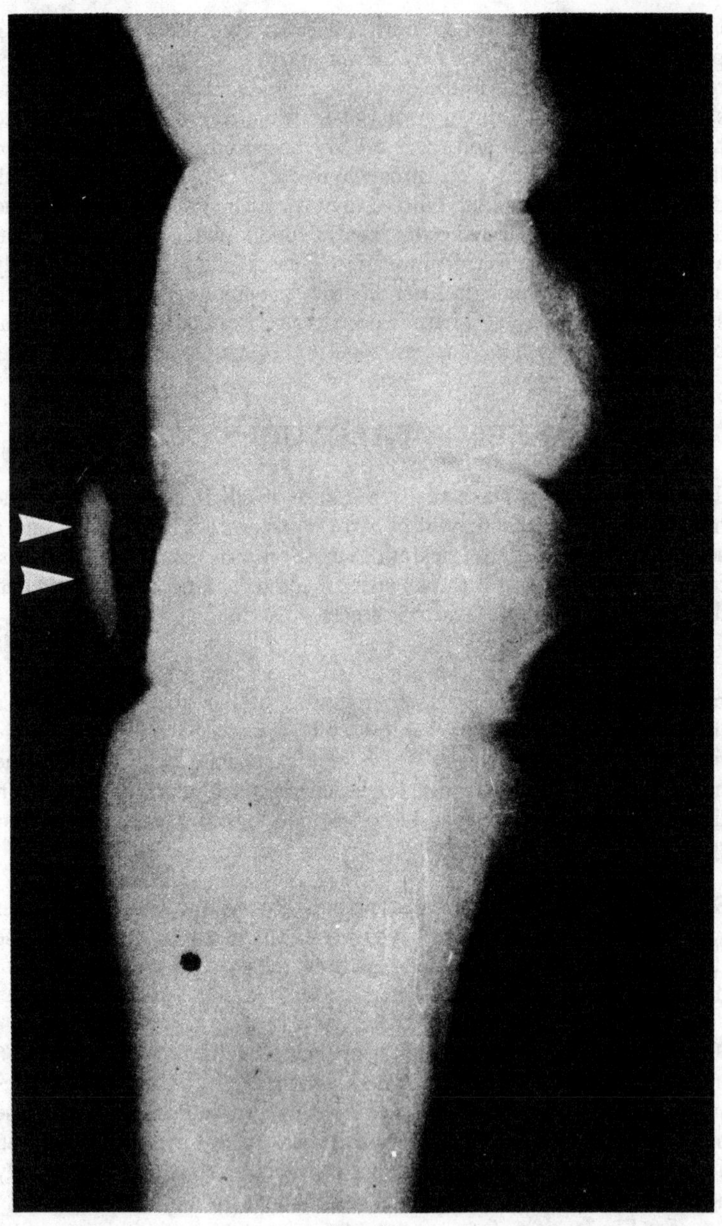

Fig. 60
X-ray of the knee showing a large slab fracture of the 3rd carpal bone (arrows).

LAMENESS

Books have been written on lameness and its diagnosis in the horse. Lameness may be defined as any irregularity or derangement of the function of locomotion, irrespective of its cause. Detection of the cause of the lameness is often very difficult, even for a veterinarian, who has the advantage of a knowledge of the anatomy of the horse. It is easy enough to detect the cause of lameness when some obvious injury, such as a wound or open joint, exists, but quite another matter when a horse just "goes lame". Slight lameness is more difficult to diagnose than more pronounced lameness. In horses, most causes of lameness occur at or below the knee and hock, whereas lameness in the shoulder and hip are comparatively rare. Where no apparent and sufficient cause of trouble can be detected and the affected limb has been recognised, the foot must be thoroughly examined and, if necessary, the shoe removed to further the examination.

Detection of the Seat of Lameness Close observation of a horse at rest or as he stands in a stable will often reveal the affected leg. If he "points" one fore limb, the trouble will probably be in this leg. If the trouble is in both fore feet, the horse is inclined to "point" each leg alternately. Watching a horse turn in a stable may show that he drops on one side, thus indicating lameness on the other side, either in front or behind.

Usually the best method of detecting the seat of lameness is to have the animal led away by a halter and then trotted slowly on hard ground. The horse should be observed from various points — in front, from behind and from each side. When an animal is lame, it takes as much weight as possible off the injured or painful limb and places it on the opposite one. The extra weight placed on the sound limb causes irregularity of action. In the case of fore leg lameness, it will be noted that when the horse is trotted towards the observer, the animal nods its head when the foot of the sound limb strikes the ground and the head rises when the foot of the lame leg is on the ground. If no abnormality of action is seen in the fore legs, the action of the hind legs should be observed as the horse is trotted away. In hind leg lameness, the hock of the sound leg rises higher and dips lower than that of the lame one, and the hip drops on the sound side.

Briefly then, when the horse nods its head as the foot of the right fore leg strikes the ground, the animal is lame in the fore leg, and if it dips the hock and drops the hip as the foot of the right hind leg strikes the ground, it is lame in the left hind leg. If the nodding of the head and drooping of the hip are on the near or left side, the lameness is on the off or right side. When the animal is lame in both fore legs, it takes short strides and walks in a rather stilted fashion with what is commonly referred to as a "proppy" gait. Double hind limb lameness may also be indicated by short strides and stiffness of movement suggestive of injury to the loins. Backing is difficult in these cases.

A horse which is very lame in one fore leg may appear to be lame in the diagonal hind leg also when trotting away. This can be very deceptive to the inexperienced observer.

When there is a combination of fore and hind limb lameness, the detection of the seat of lameness becomes much more difficult and usually requires the assistance of a veterinarian, both for detection and diagnosis of the cause of the lameness.

When a horse has been found to be lame in a given leg, it becomes necessary to decide what structure is involved and this is not always easy. It may be possible to localise the seat of the trouble by noting the way in which the lame leg is performing its functions; by observing the motions of the whole leg, especially of the various joints; by minutely examining every part of the leg; by observing the outlines and by feeling for heat and testing for sensitiveness. All these will be a guide to a correct localisation of the trouble, but a hasty conclusion should not be formed, and it must never be forgotten that all parts of the foot must be carefully examined. It is not at all uncommon for lameness to have an apparent location elsewhere when the foot is the true seat of the trouble.

It is possible for a veterinarian to desensitise various regions of the leg by using a local anaesthetic injection to block the appropriate nerve. This is extremely useful in differentiating various forms of lameness, as, if the horse goes sound after blocking the foot for example, then it can be definitively diagnosed that the problem exists in that area.

The various disease conditions which cause lameness are dealt with alphabetically throughout the book.

LAMINITIS

See *Founder*

LARYNGITIS AND PHARYNGITIS

Laryngitis (inflammation of the larynx) and pharyngitis (inflammation of the pharynx) are usually associated with some general infection of the upper respiratory tract, including tracheitis, rhinitis and sometimes bronchitis, or with certain infectious diseases such as strangles. Simple or acute catarrhal laryngitis commonly follows some predisposing factor, such as exposure to cold or dampness, inhalation of dust, smoke, gases, the lodging of foreign bodies such as grass seeds in the larynx, and careless use of the stomach tube. These factors bring about a catarrhal inflammation of the mucous membrane of the larynx, accompanied not infrequently by considerable oedematous swelling. Inflammation of the larynx is commonly complicated by pharyngitis, constituting what is popularly known as "sore throat".

Symptoms These depend on the severity of the inflammation of the mucous membranes of the area. The outstanding symptom is a frequent, short, dry and harsh cough, which later becomes more prolonged and is accompanied by a discharge from both nostrils.

Pressure over the laryngeal region with the fingers causes pain and attacks of coughing. The respiration is normal while the animal is at rest and the laryngitis remains localised. Not infrequently, however, it is complicated by bronchitis when there is an alteration in the normal respiratory rate. Fever is generally absent or slight, but the appetite is somewhat diminished. The horse may have difficulty in swallowing, and water and sometimes food is returned through the nostrils. There may be some swelling in the throat region and the head may be "poked out". Redness of the mucous membrane of the nose is commonly seen and there may be a harsh rasping snore. Diagnosis is based on the cough and the sensitiveness of the throat region. The prognosis is favourable in cases of simple laryngitis, the course of the disease being about 10 days, sometimes longer.

Treatment Simple laryngitis frequently responds to home treatment. The animal should be kept warm, but if stabled the ventilation should be adequate without draughts. If the weather is cold, Newmarket bandages might be applied to the legs for warmth and support. The horse should be given soft feed, such as bran mashes, scalded oats, linseed gruel and the like. Dry feed should be dampened to control dust. Steam inhalations by holding the horse's head over a bucket of hot water containing 2 tablespoons of Friar's Balsam afford relief to the animal. Drenching should be avoided. External treatment is of little value, and antibiotics are seldom useful as most pharyngitis and laryngitis is associated with virus infections. Frequently a rest period of up to 6 months may be necessary to achieve resolution of the condition.

LEG MANGE (Itchy Heel)

Leg Mange is a fairly common parasitic disease of the skin and in the days when draught horses were used on farms, was the cause of much damage to fences as a result of horses rubbing their heels on the wires. Although the condition is mainly confined to the legs below the hocks and knees, it occasionally reaches to the inner thighs and armpits. It may appear along the belly, and the muzzle and nose may be affected as a result of the horse biting at the legs.

Cause The disease is caused by a minute mange mite, *Chorioptes equi*, which is picked up by close contact with infested horses or from fences, posts, stumps and so on, recently contaminated by them. It is usual, therefore, for several horses on a farm or riding school to be affected in varying degree.

Under warm conditions eggs laid by the female hatch in about 3 days and burrow under the surface layer of the skin, feeding on skin scales and other debris. The young mites reach sexual maturity in about 6 days and begin to breed, so that the mite population increases rapidly in spite of the fact that the average life of the mite is only about 14 days. Since warmth favours the rapid multiplication of these parasites, the condition is more apparent during the summer months, becoming dormant during a cold dry winter, only to flare up again the following summer.

As already pointed out, infestation by the parasite of leg mange is mainly confined to the lower extremities of the legs and especially the hind legs. In this way it differs from other mange parasites of horses, not known to be present in Australia, which spread all over the body or affect the mane and tail.

Symptoms The activities of the mites cause a reddening of the skin around the affected areas from which moisture oozes to form hard crusts. Later the skin becomes thickened and thrown into ridges. Intense irritation occurs, which is shown by the affected horse stamping, pawing, kicking and rubbing the pastern with the opposite foot or biting at the affected area. The horse is inclined to back up against fences, stumps and logs and rub its heels or backs of the legs against these objects. This constant rubbing causes the hair on the legs to be worn and ragged in appearance. If the condition is not treated, serious complications may result, such as greasy heel or damage to the foot from stamping, and even fractures may occur.

Diagnosis of the disease may be confirmed by microscopic examination of skin scrapings from the affected areas for the presence of mange mites.

Treatment Clip the affected areas closely and wash with warm lime-sulphur (containing 1 per cent polysulphide). Lime-sulphur concentrates are prepared by a number of firms as orchard sprays and are guaranteed to contain 20 per cent polysulphide. If this concentrate is diluted 1 in 20, it makes a satisfactory wash. If large numbers of horses have to be treated, this 1 per cent solution can be used in a foot-bath. Re-treatment should be given in 1 week to 10 days and still further treatments may be necessary at the same intervals to clear up the condition. Various organophosphate preparations used to treat lice in cattle have also been used to treat leg lice in horses. Older treatments, such as 1 part sulphur to 4 parts lard, applied warm, are not as effective as the warm lime-sulphur wash.

Stables and other premises should be disinfected and attention given to rugs, brushes and harness which may remain infective for up to 3 weeks.

LICE

Horses are commonly infested by two species of lice, the horse sucking louse (*Haematopinus asim*) and the horse biting louse (*Damalinia equi*). These lice have similar life histories, the eggs hatching in 8 to 10 days or a little longer. The louse spends the whole of its life upon the host, which it does not leave unless to transfer to another horse, and which it can readily do when there is close contact between horses, or it is forcibly removed or reaches the ground with fallen hair. The sucking louse may remain alive off the host for 2 to 3 days and the biting louse for as long as 10 days. Eggs attached to fallen hair remain viable for 20 days away from the host, hatch under favourable conditions and the young lice survive for a further 2 to 3 days. Harness, saddles, rugs and grooming utensils may harbour the lice and eggs for similar periods. The parasites increase rapidly during the winter when the hair is long and decrease when the hair is shed in the spring. Sucking lice are more commonly found at the base of the mane and tail, while biting lice favour the lower parts of the body and jaws, but also congregate on the back and flanks. In heavy infestations lice extend all over the body.

Symptoms The irritation caused by lice causes the horse to stamp, kick and rub against objects. The hair is rubbed off in patches and the skin may be bruised and lacerated. Heavy infestation with sucking lice causes blood loss and weakens the animal, and is often one of the reasons for poor condition or "poverty".

Treatment Horses with heavy coats should be clipped and the clippings burnt. Dipping or spraying are the usual methods of applying insecticides for the control of lice infestation and, in the case of horses, owing to the lack of dipping facilities, spraying is mainly carried out. This must be done thoroughly, taking care that the horse is wetted all over. Because insecticides cannot be relied upon to kill the eggs or nits, or to remain toxic long enough to kill all the young lice which hatch from

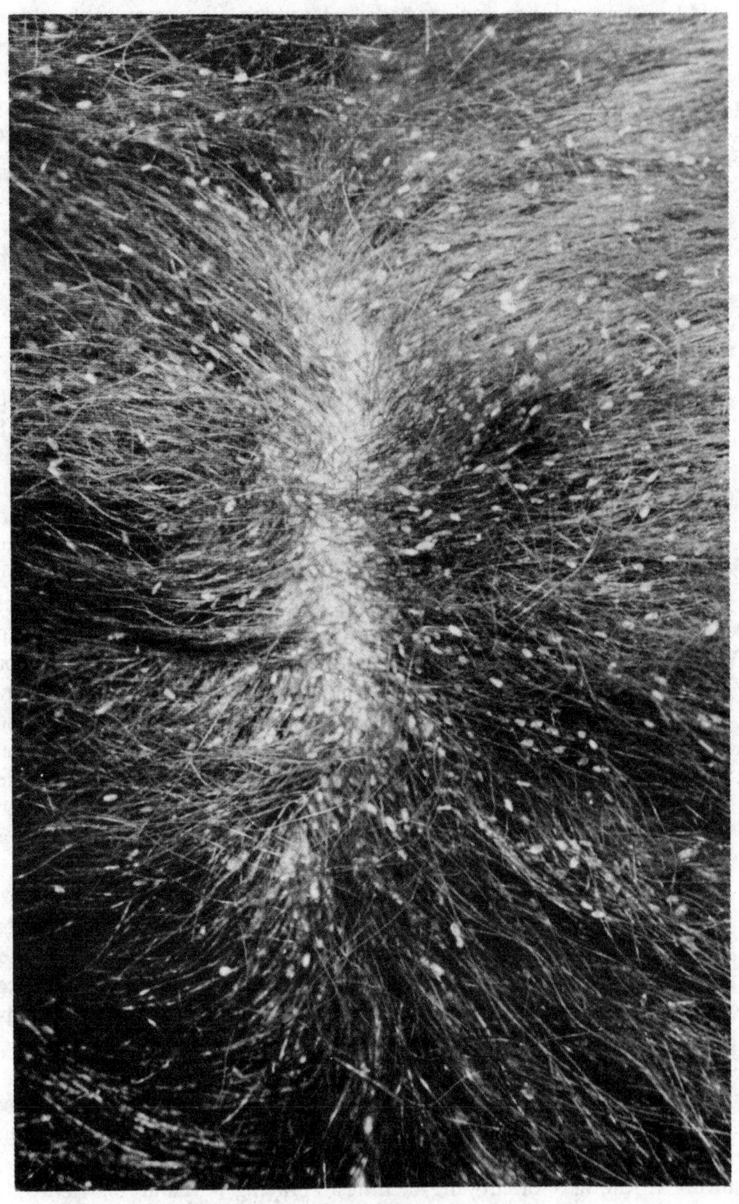

Fig. 61
Severe lice infestation showing lice eggs at the base of mane hairs.

the eggs, it is necessary to repeat the spraying in 14 days. Various insecticides are used in dips or sprays but the organic phosphorus compounds such as *Diazinon, Asuntol, Nankor* and *Ethion* now recommended for the control of cattle lice, are to be preferred. The manufacturer's instructions should be carefully followed. Various insecticide dusts are used where it is undesirable to wet the horse during cold weather, but, as better results are obtained with thorough spraying, it is desirable to spray in the autumn so that the horse enters the winter free from infestation.

The stable or shed in which the horse is accommodated should be thoroughly cleaned down and bedding and sweepings burned. The woodwork and floor should then be well sprayed with an effective insecticide, paying particular attention to spaces between boards. Care should be taken that excess of spray is not left in depressions, and that the premises have thoroughly dried before being re-occupied. Treatment of harness, rugs, brushes and other contaminated articles should not be overlooked.

LIGAMENTS — DAMAGE TO

Ligaments are the strong fibrous bands that unite bones across joints. There are a great number of ligaments in the body and when injuries occur then ligaments may be damaged.

Causes Trauma to a particular area may result in damage to ligaments. The ligaments in the lower leg are most commonly damaged as they are most subject to stresses associated with racing, jumping etcetera.

Symptoms In the early stages there are the usual signs of inflammation — heat, pain and swelling associated with a joint. In more long standing cases of ligament damage there may only be swelling in an area due to scar tissue formation. In some cases, for example, rupture of the peroneus tertius, there may be a change in the action of the leg. When this ligament ruptures, the stifle and hock move independently. In very severe damage to ligaments around joints, there may be dislocation of the joint. The most commonly damaged ligament in the horse is the suspensory ligament, which is situated between the cannon bone and the flexor tendons. When this is damaged there may be lameness of the affected leg.

Treatment In most cases of ligament damage rest periods up to 12 months are necessary for healing to occur. In some cases a plaster cast may be necessary to provide support for an injured leg.

MANGE

Other than leg mange caused by the mange mite *Chorioptes equi*, the only other type of mange which affects horses in Australia is that known as otacariasis or ear mange, caused by the mange mite *Psoroptes hippotis.* It has been recorded in Queensland and New South Wales but is not yet of economic importance. Treatment with BHC is said to be effective.

Sarcoptic mange or scabies in horses, which is prevalent in overseas countries, does not occur in Australia.

See *Leg Mange*

MASTITIS (Inflammation of the Udder)

Mastitis means inflammation of the mammary gland, regardless of the cause. This condition is comparatively rare in the mare, although sometimes the udder becomes painfully distended prior to or after foaling and a doughy swelling, pitting on pressure, extends forward along the abdomen. This may recede or a more serious condition develops, when one or both glands become enlarged, hot, tense and painful and the milk dries up or is replaced by a watery or reddish fluid. The mare walks lamely, goes off her feed, has a temperature and shows all symptoms of a general constitutional disturbance.

Cause The latter condition is of bacterial origin and its severity depends on the type of infection. Sometimes the infection leads to gangrene of the udder or results in death from septicaemia.

Treatment In the early stages, hot fomentations and active massage with a little olive oil in the palm of the hand, and frequent drawing off of milk by hand may bring about rapid improvement. If this fails, professional attention should be obtained immediately, as infection is likely. When the disease persists, milk samples should be submitted to a veterinary laboratory, preferably by a veterinarian, for a determination of the type of infection. Subsequent treatment with antibiotics will depend largely on the laboratory report. If an antibiotic cream is to be injected into the udder, it should be noted that the mare has 3 separate ducts opening on the summit of each teat and each has to be carefully injected.

MELANOMA

A melanoma is a malignant neoplasm or tumour which contains melanin, a black or dark brown pigment. These occur more frequently in old grey

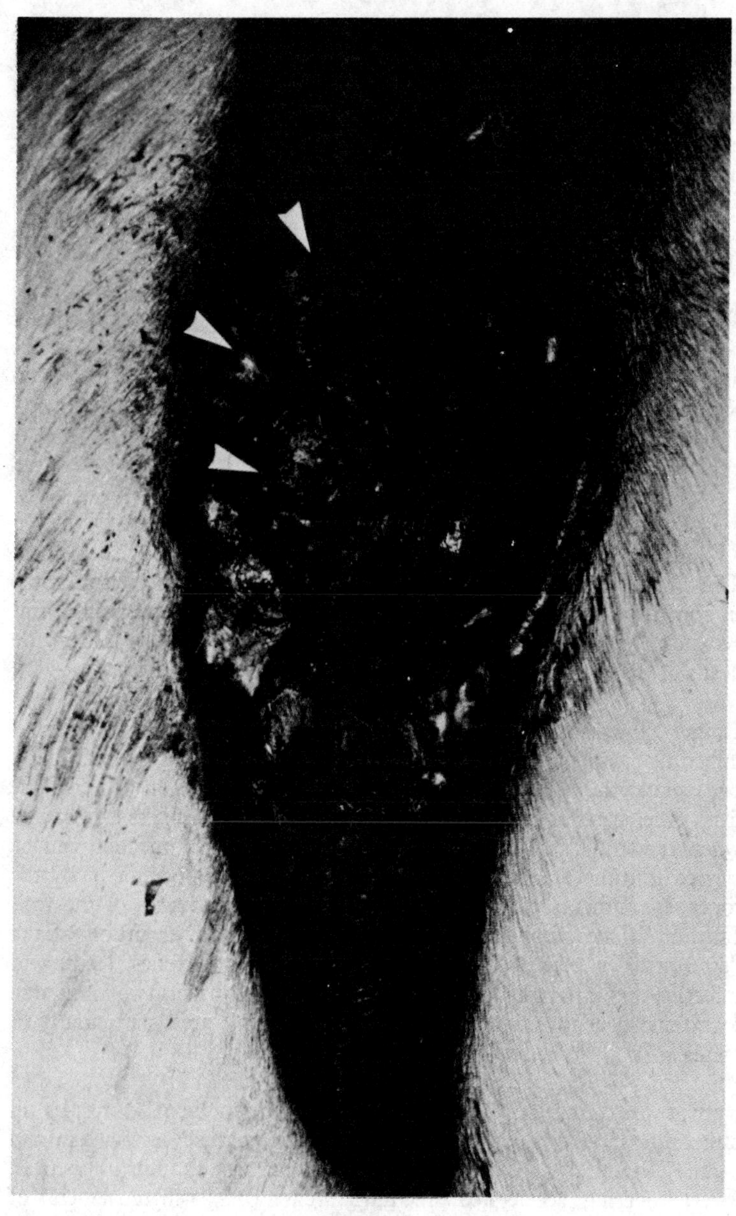

Fig. 62
Melanomas (arrows) under the tail of a 12-year-old grey mare.

horses, although they do occur in horses of other colours, especially in horses after 10 years of age when the coat begins to turn white. The condition is associated with abnormal pigmentary deposits. The tumours commonly occur under the root of the tail and sometimes on the upper surface, and about the anus, sheath and crest. From these situations, they spread to neighbouring lymphatic glands and then, by metastasis, to the spleen, lungs and other internal organs. Melanomas in the horse are much less malignant than those in man and horses may survive for up to 10 or 15 years after developing a melanoma.

Treatment In the early stages surgical removal is possible. It should be realised, however, that many horses survive a number of years following the appearance of a melanoma. Unfortunately there is no accurate way of predicting the survival time of the horse following development of a melanoma.

METRITIS (Inflammation of the Uterus)

The term used to describe inflammation of the uterus (womb) is metritis. In the mare, acute metritis most commonly occurs after foaling, but occasionally it occurs in late pregnancy when it usually results in the death of the foetus and sometimes also of the mare.

Cause Inflammation of the uterus is generally the result of bacterial infections, which usually occur at normal or assisted foaling, more particularly the latter, but can also occur by the extension of infections from other parts of the genital tract. Unless great cleanliness is observed when rendering assistance to a mare at foaling time, infection can be carried into the uterus by the hands or arms of the operator or by the ropes, instruments or other apparatus used to assist birth of the foal. Further, if the mare fails to "clean" properly and a portion of the "afterbirth" is retained in the uterus, this soon putrefies, leading to infection and inflammation of the uterus. Metritis can also be found due to extension of infection from the external genital area, particularly in mares with a "sunken vulva" conformation.

Symptoms Acute inflammation of the uterus usually results in systemic as well as local symptoms and may cause septicaemia and death. Within 24 to 72 hours after foaling, the mare exhibits uneasiness; fever; shivering; accelerated breathing; arched back; stiff movements of body and looks back at the flanks. A discharge occurs from the vulva, which may at first be watery, reddish or yellow, but later becomes thicker and more abundant and may be foetid. The mare goes off her feed, loses

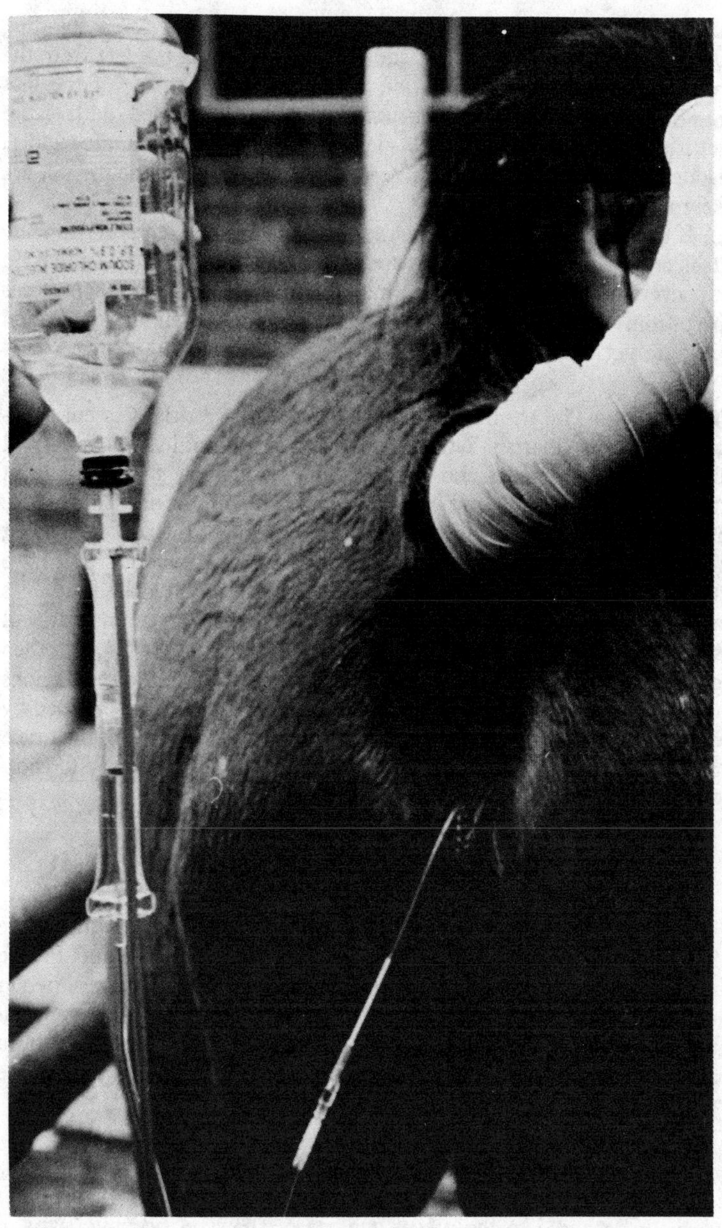

Fig. 63
Metritis in a mare being treated with antibiotic and saline infusion.

interest in the foal and may lose her milk. She maintains a standing position. Stiffness of movement and difficulty of lifting the feet from the ground indicate that inflammation of the sensitive laminae of the foot (founder) has occurred, this being commonly associated with acute metritis. Other complications, such as inflammation of the udder, bladder, vagina and, still more serious, peritonitis and pneumonia are likely to occur.

If the mare survives, chronic metritis may supervene upon the acute attack and be the reason why a mare does not subsequently get in foal. In less severe forms of metritis the mare may exhibit no other symptoms apart from a purulent discharge from the vulva when in season and failure to get in foal.

Treatment The treatment of an acute case of metritis is essentially a matter for a veterinarian. Satisfactory treatment cannot usually be carried out by the horse owner and usually more harm than good is done in attempting to douche out the uterus, frequently with inadequate instruments and lack of knowledge of the anatomy of the parts. Flushing out the vagina is a simple matter and will remove discharges that have passed through the cervical canal (neck of the uterus), but the fluid does not get into the uterus, the seat of the infection. A veterinarian will usually take a swab to determine the type of bacteria involved, and then undertake local and systemic antibiotic treatment. In chronic infections the uterus may be irretrievably damaged, and this can be ascertained by performing a uterine biopsy. This entails taking a small piece of the tissue lining the uterus with a special instrument called uterine biopsy forceps.

METRITIS — CONTAGIOUS EQUINE (CEM)

Contagious equine metritis or CEM appeared in Newmarket during the 1977 stud season in England. It was also found in Ireland and France during the same season. Importation of stallions from England resulted in the introduction of this disease into Australia. The infection is a venereal disease spread by the stallion from mare to mare and is caused by a particular type of bacteria which sets up a severe inflammation within the uterus.

Symptoms A profuse purulent and greyish coloured discharge appears 1 to 2 days following the mare being served by the stallion. The infection is usually localised to the uterus and mares show no systemic signs of illness. CEM may be suspected when a number of mares show these signs of discharge from the vulva several days after service by a stallion.

Treatment The most important phase of the treatment lies in identification of the specific bacteria causing this condition. This involves having the veterinarian take swabs, which have to be processed using specialised techniques, as the bacteria will not grow in the presence of air. Once the bacteria has been positively identified then local treatment, using drugs such as penicillin, is very effective. However, the infection is very difficult to clear completely and many mares and some stallions can become carriers of the infection without exhibiting any clinical signs themselves. Therefore, any stud that has had contagious equine metritis must undertake scrupulous preventative measures, which involve collection of sets of swabs from all mares from at least 3 oestrus periods to ensure that the bacteria is not present. Stallions should also be swabbed to determine if they are carrying the infection. Using these rigid preventative measures the disease has been generally overcome in the United Kingdom and was not found to be a major problem in the 1980 stud season in Australia.

MYOSITIS — ACUTE ("Tying-up" or "Cording-up")

The terms "tying-up" and "cording-up" are commonly used in racing stables to describe a muscular disorder, the cause of which is not thoroughly understood. The condition is similar to paralytic myoglobinuria, commonly known as "Monday morning sickness" which was once frequently seen in working draught horses, (see *Azoturia.*). It is sometimes called *atypical myoglobinuria.* The disease is seen more particularly in race horses and light horses under heavy exercise or training. It can also occur in the heavier breeds of horses. Whereas paralytic myoglobinuria (azoturia) commonly occurs when the horse is put to work following a short period of idleness whilst being maintained on full working rations, "tying-up" or "cording-up" occurs following strenuous exercise, or after a hard day's work, in horses that are in training and being fed rations consistent with the work performed.

Symptoms The term myositis means inflammation of a muscle and this is essentially what happens. A group of muscles over the loins and croup are affected, accompanied by pain, lameness and disinclination to move. The muscles are rigid and the affected horse, when forced to move, does so with great difficulty. Other symptoms are rapid respiration, dilated nostrils, profuse sweating and sometimes the passing of coffee-coloured urine. The latter is not as consistent as in azoturia. When forced to walk, affected horses improve and often recover quickly, in contrast to the collapse and paralysis which occurs when cases of azoturia are exercised. The mortality rate is negligible and most affected animals make an uneventful recovery. It is possible to determine the extent of the muscle damage and follow its resolution with the aid of certain blood tests.

Treatment Lack of basic knowledge as to the cause of the condition makes treatment difficult, but some research indicates the possible value of selenium and vitamin E in the treatment and prevention of the disease. Various drugs are used by veterinarians in symptomatic treatment and include preparations which produce relaxation.

Pending the arrival of the veterinary surgeon, the horse should be well rubbed down, rugged if necessary, and quietly walked about with periodic rests. After an attack of "tying-up", the horse's training programme must be reduced and it is essential that the amount of grain in the diet be reduced. The horse should be given a gentle exercise programme which is gradually built-up over the next month, and during this time the amount of grain is slowly increased in the diet. Blood tests to determine the level of muscle enzymes are useful in monitoring the horse's progress.

NAVEL-ILL

See *Joint-ill*

NAVICULAR DISEASE

Navicular disease is a condition causing fore leg lameness and is due to damage of the blood supply to the navicular bone. The navicular bone rests against the back of the central part of the third phalanx (pedal bone) at the back of the foot. The bone above the second phalanx, sometimes referred to as the short-pastern bone, articulates with the coffin bone and the navicular bone. The navicular bone is covered with cartilage and the deep flexor tendon of the foot runs over it to join on to the pedal bone. The disease, which causes a chronic progressive fore limb lameness, is most common in light horses, being seldom seen in heavy breeds and is almost invariably confined to the front feet. It appears to be more commonly seen in horses that are infrequently exercised and is seldom found in young horses.

Cause Although a number of causes have been postulated no definitive cause has been found. Some of the suggested causes include poor conformation, particularly horses with short upright pasterns, contracted

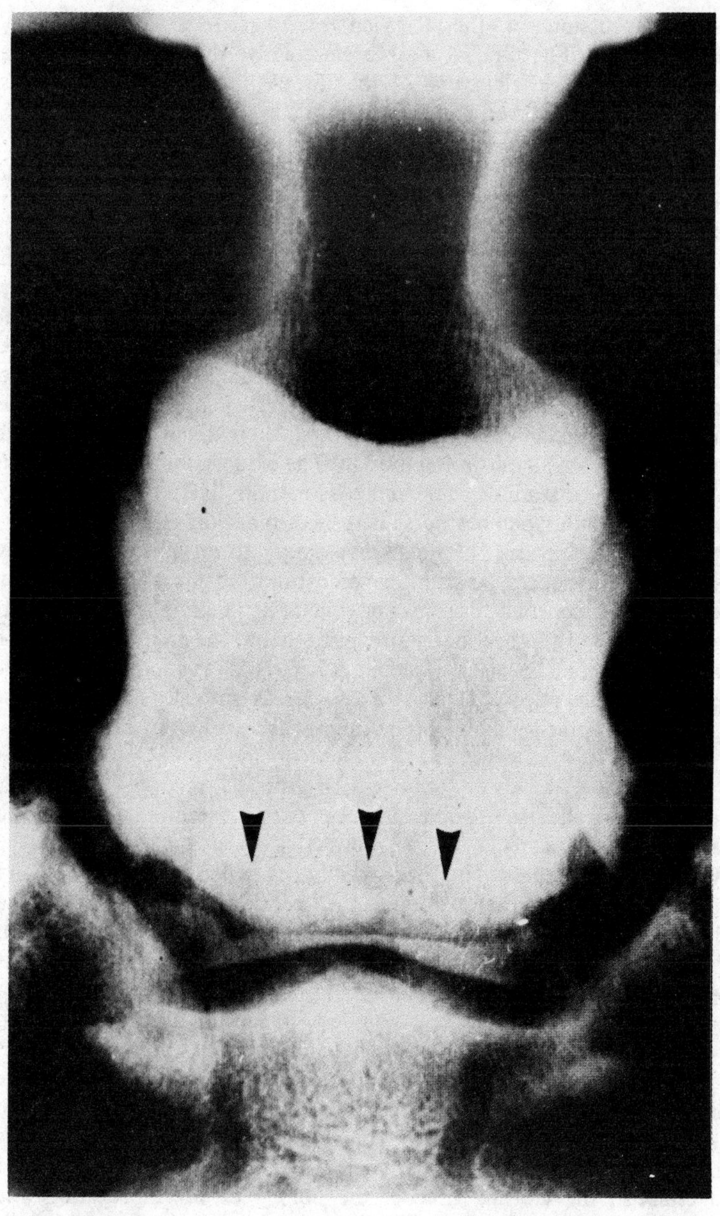

Fig. 64
X-ray of the foot and pastern of a horse showing changes in the navicular bone (arrows) indicating navicular disease.

heels, concussion of the feet on hard ground, and hereditary predisposition. The type of work performed by the horse may have a bearing on the development of the disease, as navicular disease is frequently found in working quarter horses in the United States.

Symptoms The symptoms of navicular disease usually develop slowly. An early symptom is "pointing" of the fore foot when the horse is standing at rest. The foot is placed in a position slightly in advance of the other fore foot, with the heel only just touching the ground. When both fore feet are affected, each is alternately pointed. Whilst "pointing" is a common symptom, it is not absolutely characteristic of navicular disease, because "pointing" may be shown in other painful conditions below the fetlock. Slight lameness is shown early in the course of the disease. The horse may take a few lame steps or appear stiff when first worked in the morning, but the lameness then disappears. Alternatively, it may start off sound and become lame during the day. The stride is shortened and there is a tendency to stumble. The lameness is more likely to be shown on hard ground and when the horse is turned in a short circle.

The following day the horse may appear to be quite sound. This intermittent lameness persists for some time but eventually lameness becomes more constant. Pain may be evident by pressing with the thumb in the hollow of the heel or by firm pressure on the frog with a pair of farrier's pincers. The gait is altered; changes in the form of the foot become evident, due to the fact that the horse continually saves the heels, and in due course the horse becomes unfit for work.

Treatment Few cases of navicular disease recover. Treatment generally only alleviates the condition but does not result in a cure. In the early stages of navicular disease corrective shoeing can alleviate the symptoms of lameness. The shoes used have a rolled toe, raised heel and are chamfered from the quarters to the heel on the solar surface of the shoe in such a fashion that the heels are spread when weight is taken on the foot. This shoe is most successful in show and pleasure horses as it is generally too heavy for use in galloping or trotting horses. The use of pain relieving drugs prescribed by a veterinarian can also be effective in prolonging the life of the horse. These medications cannot be used in racehorses and trotting horses and so tend to be of most use in pleasure horses. A new treatment involves the use of an anticoagulant drug to attempt to overcome the decrease in blood supply to the bone. This treatment is rather expensive as frequent blood tests must be performed to establish the clotting time of the horse's blood. In addition, the medication results in relief of lameness, only as long as the horse is receiving it. There is also some hazard to the horse as the increase in clotting time in the blood makes the horse susceptible to possible haemorrhage following cuts and bruises. However, this treatment has been used with success in England in treating hunting, jumping and show horses.

If none of these treatments is successful, or appropriate, for the particular horse, then cutting of the nerves to the navicular bone will result in relief of symptoms of pain and lameness. This operation is only to be used as a last resort as there are several complications associated with it. Whereas it may be used in trotting horses, the rules of racing prohibit this operation being performed on galloping horses.

NURSING A SICK HORSE

Although the sulphonamide and antibiotic drugs have greatly contributed to the treatment of disease, good nursing still plays an important part in restoring a horse to health and should not be neglected, as it is a valuable adjunct to the use of modern drugs. Without detracting from the importance of skilled veterinary attention, it can be said that many a horse has been saved by the good nursing of an attentive groom or owner.

The comfort of the patient is very important. Horses affected with certain respiratory diseases, such as pneumonia, will not lie down because they can breathe better standing up. Under these circumstances, bandaging the legs below the knees and hocks with Newmarket bandages gives leg support and warmth, which adds to the comfort of the animal. The bandages should be removed twice a day and the legs well rubbed before re-adjusting.

An unstabled horse should be placed in a fresh clean grass paddock, well protected from prevailing winds and, if the weather is cold, it should be lightly rugged by day and more heavily rugged at night. Water should be readily available. If the horse is accustomed to being stabled, it should for preference be placed in a loose box or shed away from other horses, well bedded down with straw, and disturbed as little as possible. Good ventilation without draughts is essential, fresh water should be provided, and rock-salt be available in the manger.

With few exceptions, illnesses are accompanied by a rise in temperature and a tendency to constipation. The horse is consequently disinclined to eat, and invalid foods of a laxative nature, such as a well-prepared bran mash, are called for. Instructions for the preparation of this mash are given under *Bran Mash.* It is necessary that the bran mash be freshly prepared and if it is found that the horse has not eaten it all, the remainder should be discarded, the manger or box thoroughly cleaned and a fresh mash prepared. The object is to tempt the horse to eat to keep up its strength and, if possible, to overcome constipation without drenching.

Freshly-cut green food is usually attractive to a stabled horse. Other light, nourishing feeds which are easily prepared and which should be fed fresh, and in small quantities and often, are:

Oatmeal gruel, prepared by mixing 500 g of oatmeal with a little water to form a paste and then adding this, with a little salt, to 4.5 litres of water and heating, stirring continuously until it boils, after which it should be allowed to simmer until it is of uniform thickness. Many horses will eat this in preference to a more sloppy mixture.

Linseed tea, prepared by boiling slowly 250 g of linseed in 4.5 litres of water, and stirring repeatedly, until the grains are quite soft and it becomes the consistency of jelly. This is a very valuable article of diet for a sick horse, 250 to 500 g being added daily to other feed.

Scalded oats, prepared by pouring boiling water over 1 to 2 kg of crushed oats in a clean bucket, adding a little salt and allowing to stand for 15 minutes. This may be fed in small quantities or added to bran mashes.

A sick horse should not be worried by the routine of grooming. Nevertheless wisping, hand-rubbing, and sponging the eyes, nostrils and dock contribute to the animal's comfort.

OSSELETS

Osselets is a term used to describe a traumatic arthritis of the fetlock joint.

Causes This condition is most commonly found in young horses in their first or second season of racing. It appears to be a wear and tear disease and is found more commonly in horses with an upright pastern conformation.

Symptoms Heat, pain and swelling associated with the fetlock joint is seen, usually in one or both fore legs. There is also lameness of the affected leg(s). X-rays are necessary to determine if any chip fractures have occurred within the joint.

Treatment Anti-inflammatory drugs such as *phenylbutazone,* together with rest, are important in resolving this disorder. A 3-month rest period is usually necessary.

OSTEOCHONDROSIS DESSICANS (OCD)

Osteochondrosis dessicans or OCD is a disease affecting various joints and has become recognised only in more recent years. The disease is one

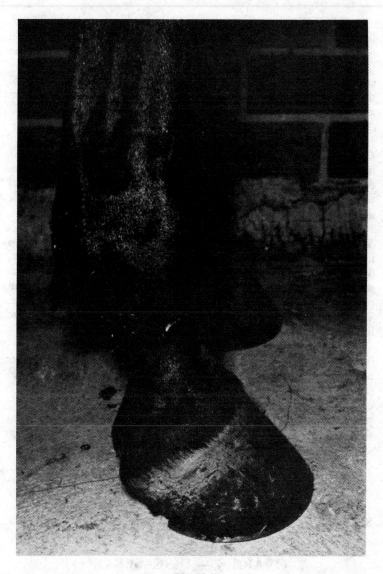

Fig. 65
Swelling over the front of the left fetlock joint associated with osselet formation.

affecting all animal species, including man, and is most common in very fast growing individuals. It affects a number of joints, the most common ones being the shoulder and the fetlock in the fore leg and the stifle and the hock in the hind limb. OCD results in a defect within the normally smooth cartilage lining of the various joints and so results in lameness of the affected limb. Yearling and 2 year old horses are the only age groups affected.

Causes The condition is associated with rapid growth rate in young horses. Therefore, there may be a certain genetic predisposition to it in certain lines of horses. There is also the impression that the widespread use of anabolic steroid injections in young growing horses may be associated with an increase in the frequency of the condition.

Symptoms The main symptom is lameness of the affected leg which is usually quite severe. There may be swelling of the affected joint, depending on which joint is involved. For instance, involvement of the stifle or hock usually results in swelling of that part, whereas involvement of the shoulder usually results in no visible external signs of joint damage. The condition may be suspected when there is a sudden onset of severe limb lameness unassociated with any trauma.

Treatment It is essential to make a definitive diagnosis of this disorder and to do this x-rays are necessary. From the x-rays the degree of joint involvement can be ascertained and the prognosis given. Where there is only minor joint involvement a rest period of 9 to 12 months usually results in healing of the affected area. In more extensive joint involvement there is little chance that the horse will ever be sound. Surgery is also possible in some specific cases and can produce good results.

OSTEOMYELITIS

See *Bone, Infection of*

OVARIES — DISEASES OF

The ovaries are situated at the end of the uterus in mares and can vary in size from the size of a walnut to the size of a tennis ball. They produce the ova or eggs which, when fertilised by sperm, result in conceiving. The ovaries also produce various hormones which are responsible for the cyclical nature of the mare's "heat periods". Disorders of the ovaries are

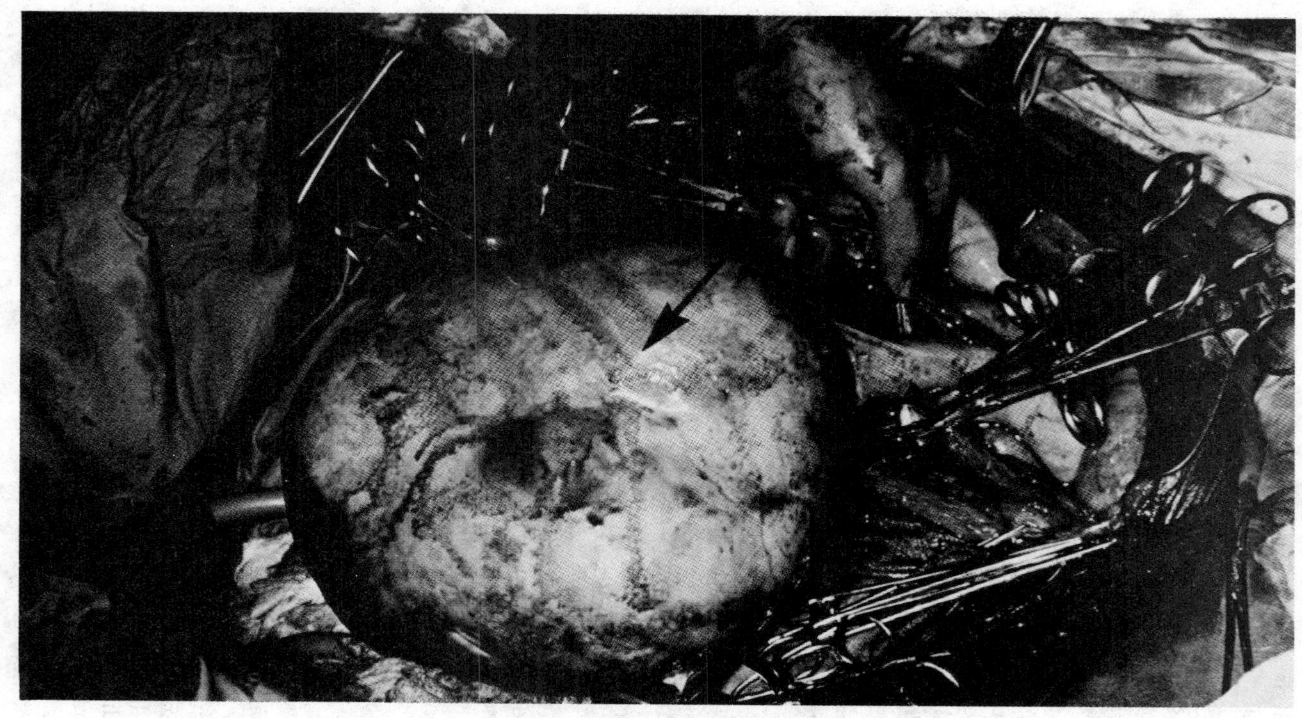

Fig. 66
Granulosa cell tumour of the ovary. These tumours cause a change in behaviour of the mare with more aggression being shown. This tumour weighed 4 kg after removal.

reasonably common and can produce infertility problems or abnormal cyclical reproductive activity.

Causes The causes of most dysfunction of ovaries are unknown. Two major hormones influence the mare's reproductive behaviour: *Follicle stimulating hormone (FSH)* is produced in the brain and stimulates the ovary to produce the follicles, one of which will eventually become the ova. If inadequate amounts of this hormone are produced the mare will not cycle. *Luteinising hormone (LH)* overrides the activity of FSH and results in rupture of the follicles and release of the ovum. If inadequate amounts of LH are produced in the brain the follicles will not rupture and the mare will continue to cycle in the so called "nymphomaniac" mare.

Treatment A veterinary surgeon can perform a rectal examination and together with the history can determine the type of hormone that may be required. It should be remembered that many mares will not cycle during the early part of the breeding season. This is due to the breeding season being artificially set, and the true breeding season is several months later. Therefore, most mares will reach the peak of their fertility during November, December and January.

PARALYSIS

Broadly, paralysis means loss of nerve control over any of the bodily functions, but the term is usually used to describe loss of muscle function or of sensation, caused by injury to nerves or other interference with the nervous system.

Paralytic affections are of two kinds, the complete and the incomplete. The former includes those in which both motion and sensibility are affected; the latter, those in which only one or other is lost or diminished. Paralysis may be general or partial. When only a small portion of the body is affected, such as the face, a limb or the tail, it is referred to as local paralysis.

Causes Most commonly, an injury to the neck or back with resultant damage to the spinal cord causes paralysis. Some nerves are very superficial and, therefore, local injuries and kicks can result in local paralysis. The radial nerve is easily damaged in its course over the shoulder and when paralysed results in loss of use of the affected fore limb. More recently, it has been shown that a particular virus (herpes virus) infection can cause a hind limb paralysis.

Treatment In view of the fact that there are so many causes and different types of paralysis, professional aid should be obtained as soon as possible. Until such assistance is available, the horse should be kept quiet and, if necessary, secured in such a way that it cannot suffer serious injury from accidents. In most cases there is little treatment that can be undertaken and time is necessary to see if nerve regeneration takes place.

PARASITES — INTERNAL

The horse harbours a variety of internal parasites, some more harmful than others. Probably no individual animal is ever entirely free of some of them but, unless heavy infection occurs, the less important species do no real damage to the horse, especially if it is well fed and kept under good conditions. On the other hand, certain parasites can be extremely harmful and be responsible for death of the animal. The majority of worm parasites of the horse develop in the digestive tract, although some of them, such as the so called redworms or bloodworms, spend part of their life history in other parts of the body.

Infection with internal parasites can be responsible for such common troubles as poor condition, rapid tiring when working and digestive disturbances. There are few horse owners who have not had some first-hand experience with worms in horses, but considerable misunderstanding exists as to the damage done by the various types of parasites. The commonest misunderstanding is to attribute the poor condition of the horse to the larger parasites which can be readily seen in the droppings or at a post-mortem examination, whereas the trouble is more likely to be due to other very small parasites which are less readily recognised.

A complete classification of horse parasites is not justified here, nor would it be very helpful to the horse owner. The commonest parasites of the horse in this country are the redworms or bloodworms, large roundworm, stomach worms, pinworms, tapeworms and the larval stage of the bot fly. The latter parasite has been dealt with under *Bots*. Of the parasites listed, those that are responsible for the greatest amount of ill health in horses and which not infrequently cause death are the redworms, especially in foals. Next in importance is the large roundworm.

Redworms or Bloodworms There are several varieties of the so called redworm or bloodworm which have the common generic name of *Strongylus*. Their life histories and the effect they have on the horse are similar. The mature worms are from 12 mm to 5 cm in length and about the thickness of the lead in an ordinary pencil. The colour is whitish-brown if free in the bowel, but red if they have sucked blood, hence the common names. Infective larvae are picked up and swallowed by the horse when

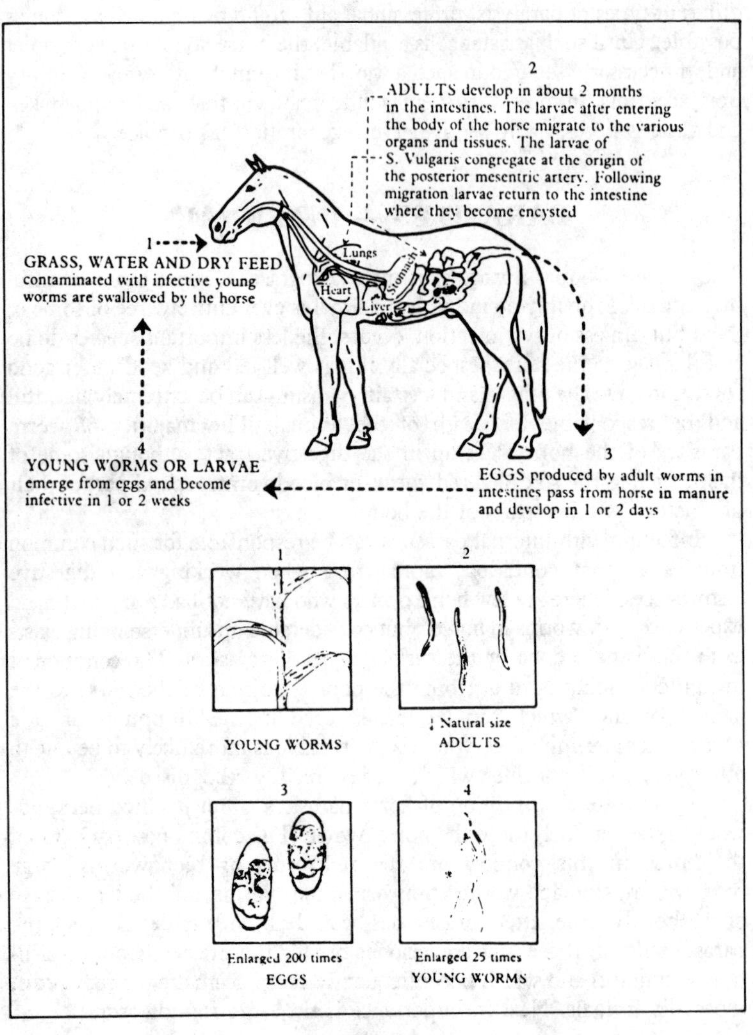

Fig. 67

Life history of redworm, *Strongylus vulgaris.*

(F. Thorp and R. Graham, University of Illinois, College of Agriculture)

grazing. After casting off their protective skins, the larvae burrow into the wall of the bowel, enter the bloodstream and are then carried to the liver, lungs and elsewhere. The larvae may enter the walls of the arteries, causing much damage and large blood clots. After some months, the worms migrate back to the bowel wall and wander through and into the bowel, eventually becoming adults, male and female, 7 to 8 months after the larvae were swallowed. Large numbers of eggs are laid in the bowel and passed out in the droppings.

The wandering immature redworms, particularly those of *Strongylus vulgaris,* damage liver, lungs and bowel wall. While in the blood vessels, the worms cause thrombus formation (clots within the blood vessels) which may interfere with the supply of blood to the intestines, resulting in digestive upsets and attacks of colic. Sometimes the wall of the blood vessel becomes so weakened by the activities of the worms that it ruptures and the horse dies of internal haemorrhage. When the arteries supplying blood to the hind legs are affected, a horse may sway and even fall when doing hard work.

Adult worms feed on the lining of the bowel and large numbers cause loss of blood, irritation to the bowel, indigestion, intermittent diarrhoea, constipation and even rupture of the bowel.

Horses of all ages are subject to the ravages of redworms, foals becoming infected as soon as they commence to graze.

Treatment

A number of drugs have been found to be effective against *Strongylus,* including *Thibenzole, Telmin, Camben, Byfield, Equiban* and *Rintal,* many of which are available in paste form. However, it has been recently found that a number of worms have become resistant to *Thibenzole*-type drugs. Therefore, *Telmin, Camben, Rintal* and *Thibenzole* preparations may not be effective if resistant worms are present.

Prevention

Avoid overstocking of paddocks with horses and adopt rotational grazing if possible. Other stock may be run in the paddock being spelled, as the redworms only infect horses.

Yards and stables should be kept free of droppings and particular attention should be directed to the protection of foals by treating the mares before the foals are born, to reduce the risk of their becoming infected from the pasture soon after birth. If a number of horses are run on a property, or horse breeding is carried out, an organised plan of campaign should be adopted to minimise the harmful effects of these serious parasites. Such a campaign is best carried out under the supervision of a veterinarian.

The Large Roundworm The common large roundworm, *Ascaris (Parascaris) equorum,* which infects the horse is quite a large worm, measuring from 15 to 35 cm in length and 12 mm in diameter. It resembles an earthworm in shape, is yellowish-white in colour and is commonly seen in the droppings of infected horses. It does not do as much harm as redworms, which are not so commonly seen, but can be very troublesome in foals.

The adult worms live mainly in the small bowel, where the females lay large numbers of eggs which are passed out in the droppings. These do not hatch on the ground and become infective larvae, as in the case of the redworms. In 10 to 14 days the larvae develop inside the eggs which are subsequently picked up by the horse when grazing or licked up by the foal in the stable or yard. In the intestine, the egg covering dissolves and the larvae emerge and burrow into the wall of the intestine, enter the bloodstream and are carried to the liver. Here they feed and grow and subsequently re-enter the bloodstream and are carried to the lungs. The larvae later enter the air passages of the lungs and are coughed up into the throat and swallowed back into the stomach. They pass on to the small intestine, where they grow rapidly. At the end of 10 weeks, they are mature and the females start laying eggs, thus starting the life cycle again. The whole life cycle inside the horse takes 2 to 3 months to complete. The eggs may survive many months on pasture and in stables.

Harmful Effects

Young horses up to 2 years of age and especially foals, suffer most from roundworm infection. Older horses seem to develop a resistance to the parasite. Bronchitis and even pneumonia occur in foals as a result of the migration of the immature roundworms to the lungs. This would depend largely on the extent of the infection. Later, as the adult worms develop in the small intestine, unthriftiness, stunted growth, harsh coat, scouring, rapid tiring and digestive trouble result. These parasites are sometimes so numerous that they block up the small intestine and give rise to colic which may kill the animal. They occasionally cause perforation of the bowel, resulting in fatal peritonitis.

Treatment

For many years, carbon bisulphide has been widely used for the removal of large roundworms from horses and has the additional advantage that it is also effective against the larvae of the bot fly ("bots") in the stomach of the horse. The drug must be administered expertly in a gelatine capsule or by stomach tube, and therefore its use usually requires the services of a veterinarian. The dose rate is 5 ml. per 50 kg body weight. Dose for foals (8 weeks) 10 ml, yearlings 10 to 15 ml, adults 20 ml. The horse should be starved, but given access to water, for 18 to 24 hours before giving the drug, and for 4 hours afterwards. The treatment

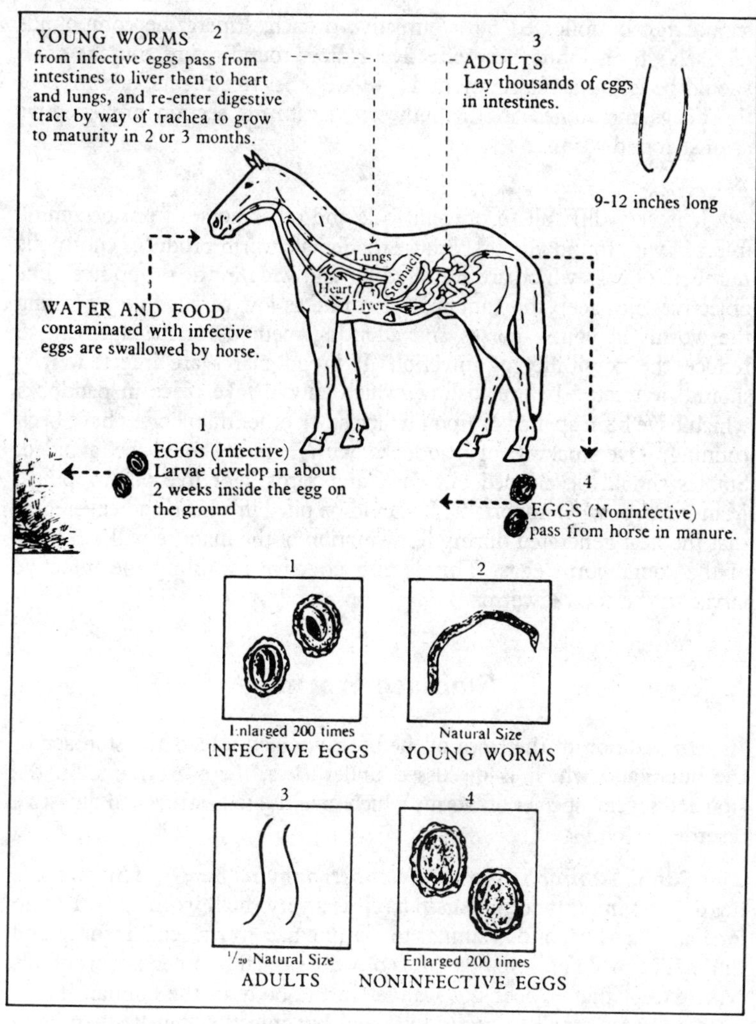

Fig. 68

The life history of large roundworm, *Parascaris equorum.*

(*F. Thorp and R. Graham, University of Illinois, College of Agriculture*) should not be followed by a purgative drench. Piperazine compounds have also been found very effective against roundworms but their use should be left to a veterinarian. There are other treatments, and most of the drugs mentioned in the redworm treatment section are effective against roundworms.

Prevention

It is very difficult to prevent foals and other horses from becoming infected with roundworms, because the female worm produces enormous numbers of eggs which are scattered far and wide in the droppings. The objective is to keep the contamination rate as low as possible by killing the worms in young horses and adopting methods of management to reduce the possibility of infection. If brood mares are infected, they should be treated before foaling, which should take place in paddocks which have been spelled or upon which stock other than horses have been running. Overstocking of paddocks with horses should be avoided. Stables should be cleaned out daily and yards kept free of droppings. Manure disposal is important. It should be piled in a heap and covered so that the heat generated during fermentation of the manure will kill most of the roundworm eggs. This is also effective in killing the infective larvae of the the redworms.

Stomach Worms

In addition to the larva of the bot fly which infects the stomach of the horse and which is discussed under *Bots*, there are found in the stomach several species of worms which give rise to gastritis and digestive disorder.

The Small Stomach Worm (Trichostrongylus axei) This worm is not of great importance in Australia. It is a very small worm, 6 to 12 mm long and hair-like, and is similar to the fine hair worm seen in sheep and cattle. The mode of development is broadly similar to other worms of this type, except that it does not wander in the body of the animal. These worms are too small to be readily seen, but infection can frequently be diagnosed at post-mortem examination by the appearance of a number of isolated, raised, button-like areas on the lining membrane of the stomach. Heavy infections with these parasites can cause rapid loss of condition in the horse.

Large Stomach Worm (Habronema spp.) The most troublesome worms infecting the stomach of the horse are the so called large stomach worms of the *Habronema* species. Actually, there are 3 species of this type of worm which infect horses in Australia. They are all slender white

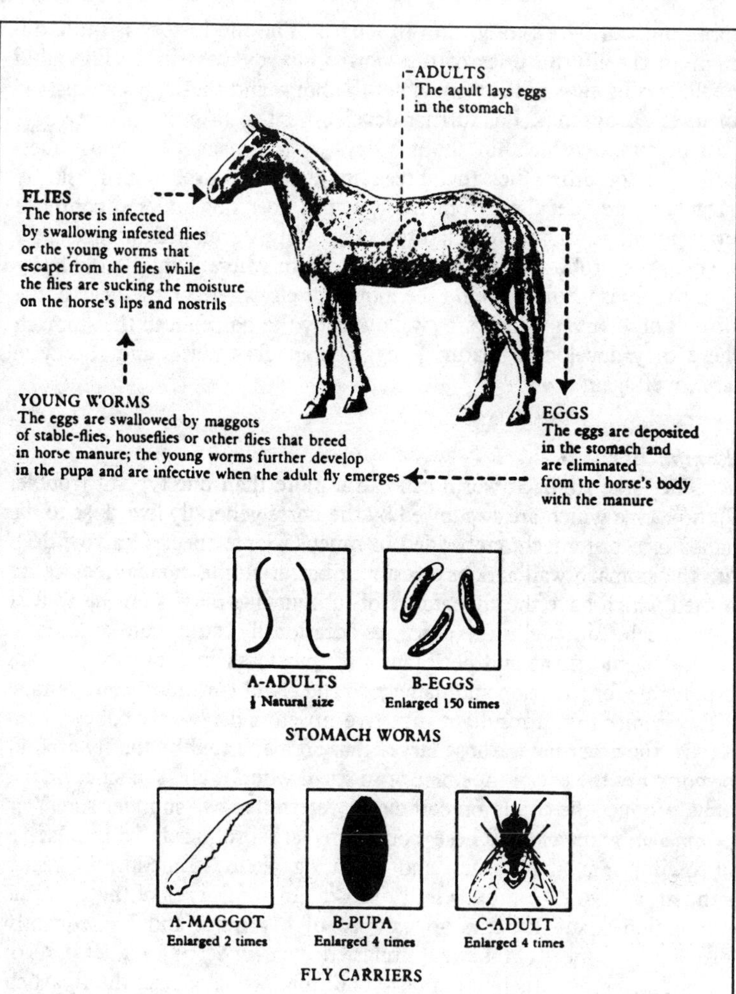

Fig. 69
Life history of large stomach worm, *Habronema spp.*
(F. Thorp and R. Graham, University of Illinois, College of Agriculture)

worms measuring 12 to 30 mm in length. The life history is quite different to the life histories of the worms already described. The adult female lays its eggs in the stomach of the horse and these eggs are passed out in the droppings. For further development to take place, these eggs must be swallowed within about 8 days by the maggots of house flies, stable flies or other flies that breed in horse manure. Within the fly maggot, a larva develops from the egg, but does not undergo complete development until the fly matures. The fully developed larva is now found in the proboscis (snout) of the fly, from where it infects the horse when the fly is feeding around the mouth or elsewhere on the head of the horse. Those larvae which are swallowed by the horse reach the stomach where they develop to maturity, egg-laying takes place, and the cycle starts over again.

Harmful Effects

The large stomach worm can cause more than one type of trouble. Those larvae which are swallowed by the horse generally live close to the glands of the stomach, embedded in mucus. Some species burrow deep into the stomach wall and, as a result of bacterial infection, abscesses are formed which have the appearance of tumour-like masses on the wall of the stomach. Although these abscesses occasionally cause acute conditions, such as haemorrhage and perforation of the stomach, generally they are responsible for irritation and damage to the glandular mucous membrane of the stomach with resultant digestive upset, and possibly colic.

On the other hand, those larvae that are deposited by the fly around the corner of the eye of the horse or in small wounds and scratches on the body, produce the condition commonly referred to as "summer sores" or *habronema granuloma.* These conditions are produced by the larvae burrowing into the tissues and irritating them, sometimes causing granulation tissue or proud flesh to form. In the corner of the eye, this granulation tissue has the appearance of a growth and is frequently mistaken for cancer of the eye. Similar effects may occur on other parts of the body wherever there are moist conditions which attract the fly, such as the sheath of a horse, wound surfaces and even the pasterns and fetlocks.

Treatment

The treatment of large stomach worms (*Habronema spp.*) involves the administration of carbon bisulphide or *Neguvon* by stomach tube. This treatment should only be carried out by a veterinary surgeon. A complex compound known as *Safersan,* which releases carbon bisulphide in the stomach, has been found very effective against *Habronema spp.* It should also be administered by a veterinarian.

Prevention

The control of the small stomach worm is along the lines of good stable and yard hygiene, involving constant disposal of manure in the manner already described, the avoidance of overstocking of horse paddocks, and routine treatment where necessary.

In the case of the large stomach worm (*Habronema spp.*), the same general considerations apply regarding hygiene but it is also important to break the life cycle by preventing flies from breeding and by destroying them. This can be done by the effective disposal of manure by piling it in heaps and covering it so that the heat generated will destroy the parasitic eggs or fly larvae, or by placing the manure in fly-proof pits. In and around the stables and yards, flies may be destroyed by regular spraying with an effective residual insecticide during the summer months.

Pinworms The pinworm (*Oxyuris equi*) is a slender, whitish, thread-like worm, commonly seen around the anus of the horse. The female pin-worm measures up to 15 cm in length and has a fine pointed tail. The male is very small, about 2.5 cm long. Actually pinworms do not do a great deal of harm and only rarely do heavy infections lead to loss of condition.

The immature forms of these worms inhabit the caecum and large colon of the horse, where they develop without migration elsewhere in the body. The mature female wanders down or is carried with the dung to the rectum and does not normally leave the body completely, but at intervals wriggles partly out of the anus and deposits eggs, together with a sticky material. This enables the eggs to adhere in clusters to the skin around and below the anus. When egg laying is complete, the female dies. Development within the egg is rapid. In 24 to 36 hours a motile larva is present, and the eggs are infective in 3 days. The eggs are rubbed off or drop to the ground, where they are later picked up by horses when grazing.

Harmful Effects

Due to the irritation caused by the sticky material surrounding the eggs, the horse rubs its hindquarters against posts and fences, thus removing the hair from the tail. Close examination will reveal the egg masses around the anus.

Treatment

The anthelmintic medications mentioned in the section on redworms are effective against pinworms.

Prevention

Thorough daily grooming will remove eggs from the anal region before they become infective.

Tapeworms Tapeworms do occur in the horse but they are not common, nor are they of much importance. These worms are flat, segmented and vary according to the species from 2.5 to 30 cm in length and up to 12 mm in width. They are found in the small intestine. As the worms mature, segments containing eggs are shed and passed in the droppings where they are sometimes seen. The intermediate host is a small mite found on pastures, which is ingested by the horse when feeding. The damage caused by tapeworms in horses is so slight that treatment is not warranted. Regular treatment against other internal parasites will offset any damage likely to be done by tapeworms.

PARTURITION — FOALING

Mares in this country are usually allowed to foal in a clean, well-grassed paddock in which there is adequate shelter and a plentiful water supply. It is best that the mare be left alone and disturbed as little as possible, whilst at the same time keeping her under close observation.

The signs of approaching parturition include a gradual enlargement of the udder about 3 to 6 weeks before foaling. A sticky secretion oozes away from the teats as long as 8 to 10 days before the birth, but sometimes not until close to foaling. This forms a wax-like coating around the teat openings (waxing-up). The belly drops, the flanks fall in and the loins may become depressed. Swelling of the vulva is noted, which increases as foaling approaches. Finally, the mare becomes uneasy, has an anxious look, stops feeding, switches and elevates the tail, strains and may lie down and get up again several times. As the time of parturition approaches, the lips of the swollen vulva swell out and a copious slimy discharge is shown. There may be considerable variation in the periods at which some of the above signs are shown. It has been recently found that the calcium level in the mare's milk is closely related to the time of foaling. The calcium level in the milk gradually increases over the last week or 2 and can be measured by a veterinarian to determine if foaling is imminent.

The Act of Foaling The mare frequently foals when she is down. In other cases, the act is accomplished standing. Violent contractions of the womb and abdominal muscles take place and the "water bags" appear and burst, followed normally by the fore feet of the foal, with the nose between them, and then, after a few more expulsive efforts of the mare, the foal is expelled. The whole act may be over in 5 to 10 minutes. The navel cord, which connects the foal to the membranes, is ruptured when the foal falls to the ground, or when the mare rises if she has been down.

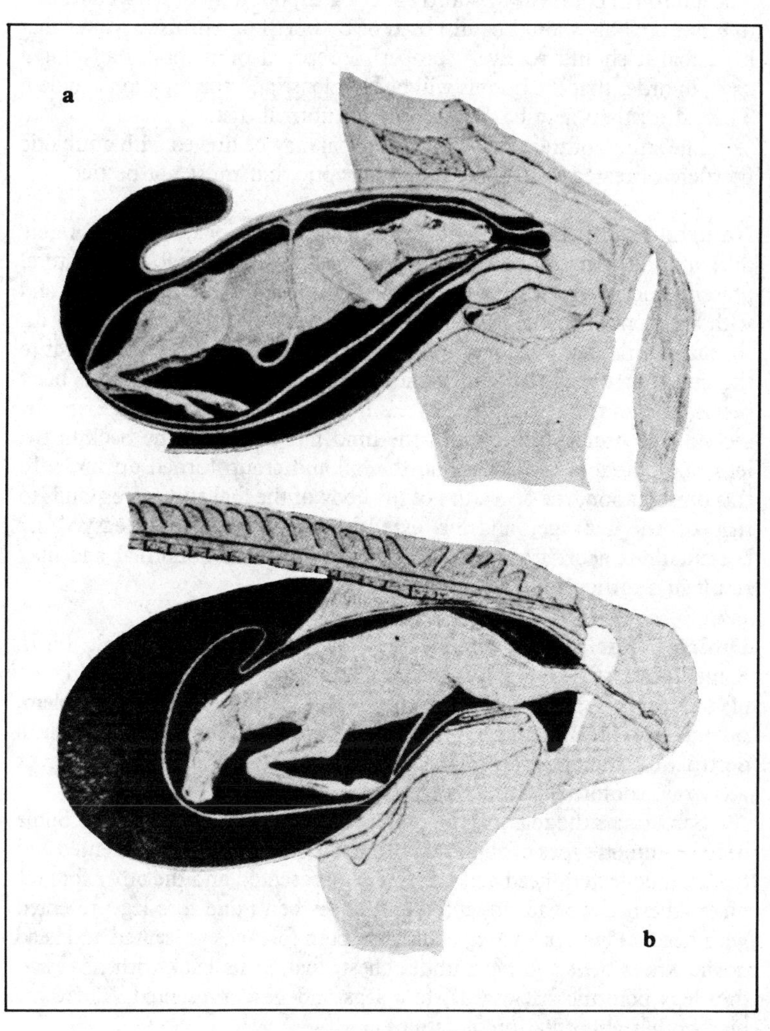

Fig. 70
Normal Presentations of the Foetus **a.** Vertebro-sacral presentation **b.** Lumbo-sacral presentation
(from "Diseases of the Horse." United States Department of Agriculture)

The afterbirth comes away shortly afterwards, but may be delayed from 3 to 6 hours. This should be disposed of by burial or burning. Mares that have foaled should receive a properly prepared bran mash daily for 3 days, in order that the bowels will be kept loose and constipation avoided. Thereafter, they may be placed on their normal diet.

The stump of the navel cord of the foal may be dusted with antibiotic powder or treated with some mild antiseptic, but must not be tied.

Natural Presentation With natural presentations, there is rarely difficulty at parturition. When there is a single foal, the natural presentation is with the fore feet first, the nose between the knees, and with the front of the hoofs and knees and the forehead directed upwards. In this way the natural curvature of the body of the foetus corresponds to the curve of the womb and genital passages, particularly of the bony pelvis, and so the foal passes out easily. When there is a twin birth, the second foal usually comes with the hind feet first, and the back of the legs, the points of the hocks and the tail and croup turned upwards. In this presentation, the curvature of the body of the foal still corresponds to that of the passage, and its expulsion may be just as easy. Any presentations apart from these 2 may be said to be abnormal and may result in a difficult birth.

Difficult Parturition There are many causes of difficult birth. Sometimes birth commences before relaxation of the pelvis and dilation of the cervix. Narrowness of the pelvic outlet can be a problem, particularly in underdeveloped mares, or there may be mechanical obstruction due to overweight, pressure of tumours, constipation or abnormal conformation.

Sometimes the foal may be presented in an abnormal position. Some of the common types of abnormal presentation are fore legs presented and the head deflected; head and one fore leg presented and the other fore leg under the body; head presented and knees bent; one fore leg presented with head and other fore leg bent back; both fore legs presented and head down; knees bent and head under chest; foal on its back with head and fore legs pointing backwards; four legs and head presented. There are many other abnormal presentations.

Although most mares foal normally and rapidly, difficult and delayed presentations are serious and require skill and care in handling. Whereas a layman can often overcome some cases of difficult parturition in a cow, similar assistance given to a mare is likely to be disastrous. Difficult parturition in a mare is a matter for a qualified veterinary surgeon. In an emergency, and should professional assistance not be available, an attempt might be made to rectify a minor abnormal presentation. The greatest cleanliness must be observed. The whole arm and hand of the

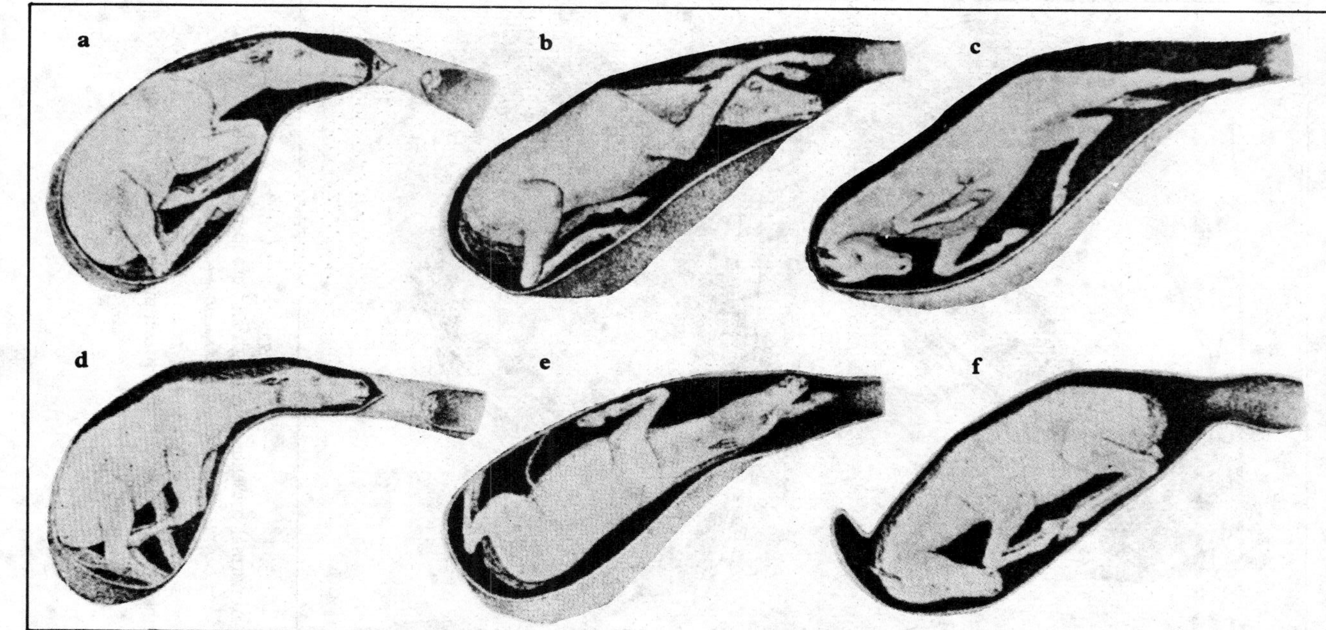

Fig. 71

Abnormal Presentations **a.** Anterior presentation: limbs bent on breast. **b.** Anterior presentation: limbs on the neck. **c.** Posterior presentation: right leg bent on itself. **d.** Anterior presentation: limbs bent on abdomen. **e.** Anterior and dorsal presentation: left leg bent on itself. **f.** Posterior presentation: croup and hock deviation.

(from "Diseases of the Horse." United States Department of Agriculture)

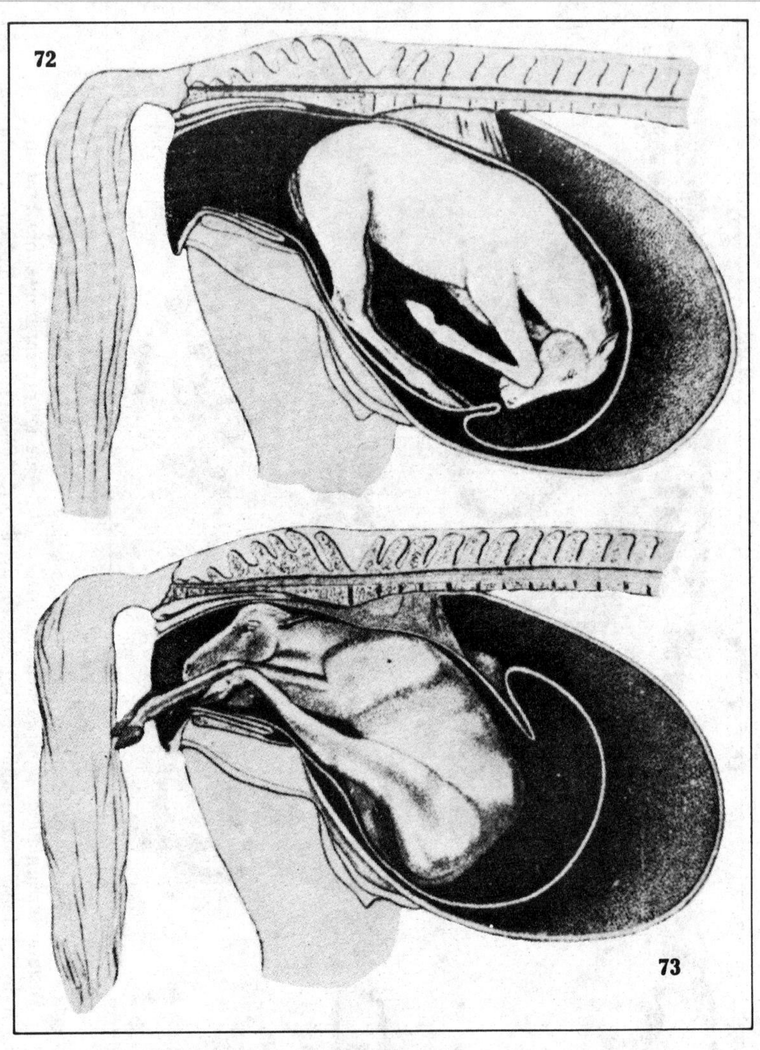

Fig. 72
Abnormal presentation. Thigh and croup presentation.
(from "Diseases of the Horse." United States Department of Agriculture)

Fig. 73
Abnormal presentation. Anterior presentation. Hind limb deviation.
(from "Diseases of the Horse." United States Department of Agriculture)

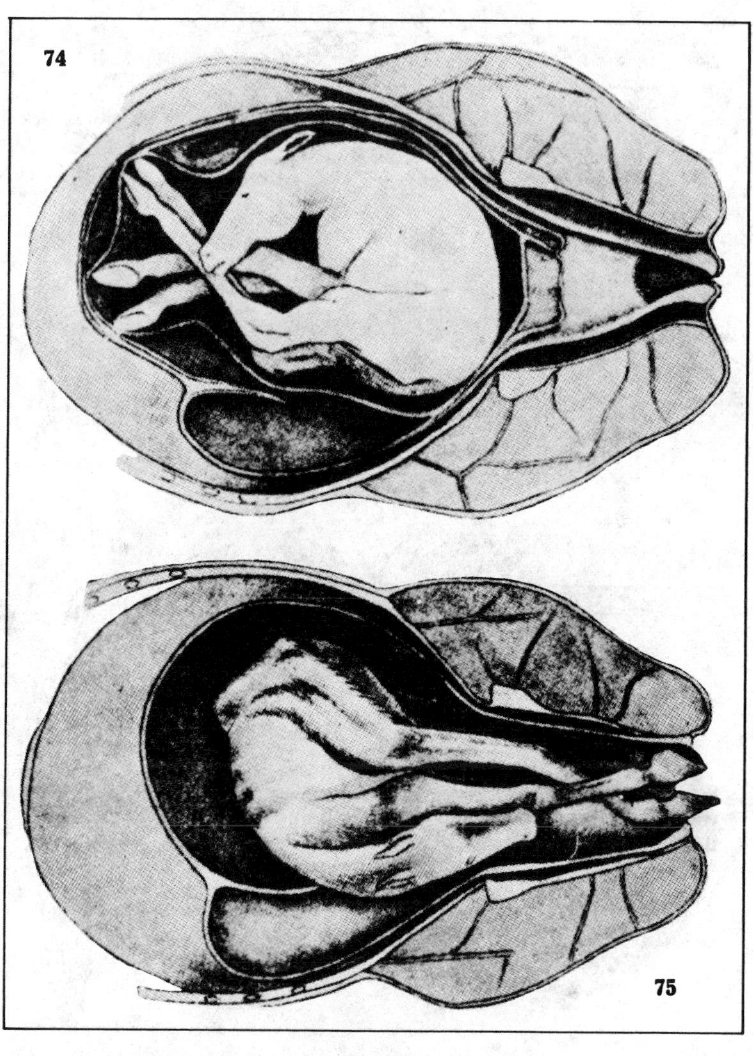

Fig. 74
Abnormal presentation. Transverse presentation—upper view.
(from "Diseases of the Horse." United States Department of Agriculture)

Fig. 75
Abnormal presentation. Sterno-abdominal presentation—head and feet engaged.
(from "Diseases of the Horse." United States Department of Agriculture)

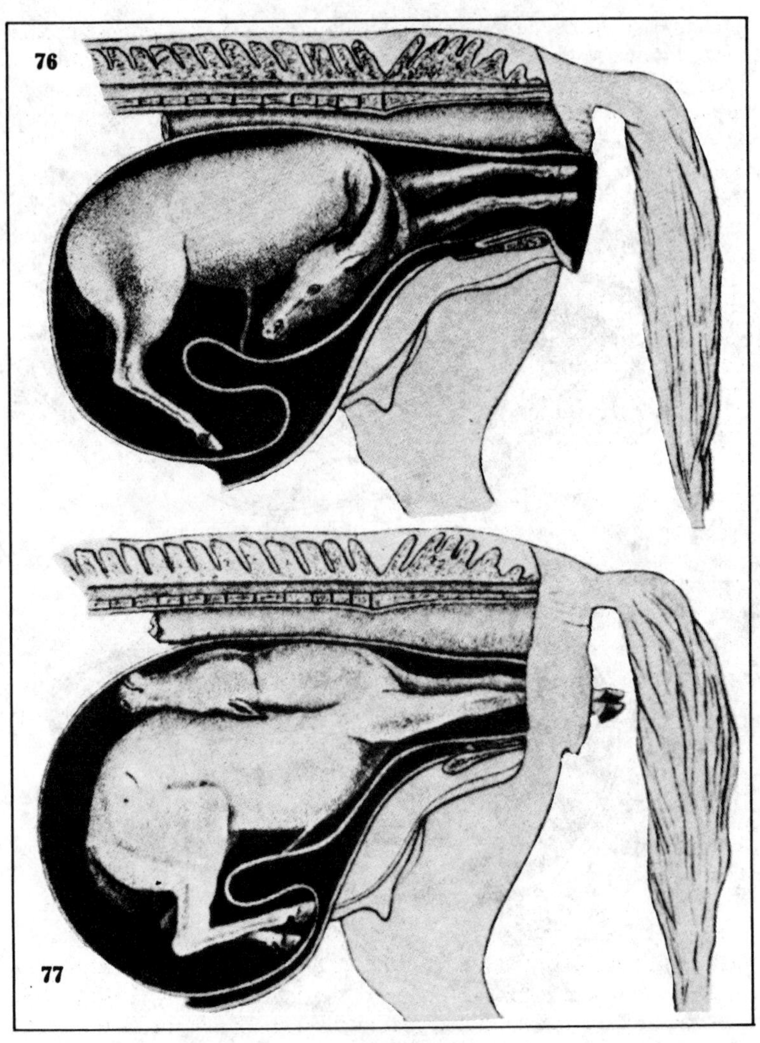

Fig. 76
Abnormal presentation. Head turned on side.
(from "Diseases of the Horse." United States Department of Agriculture)

Fig. 77
Abnormal presentation. Head turned on back.
(from "Diseases of the Horse." United States Department of Agriculture)

operator should be thoroughly washed with soap and warm water and then smeared with petroleum jelly. The nails must be cut short. The hand should be inserted with the thumb and fingers drawn together in the form of a cone. Whether lying or standing, the head of the mare should be downhill, and the hindparts raised as much as possible. This facilitates the exploratory examination and manipulations. Any traction should always be downwards towards the mare's hocks, pulling when she strains and resting when she rests.

PEDAL BONE — FRACTURE OF

The pedal bone is the bone contained within the foot of the horse. Due to the concussion that the foot sustains when it strikes the ground, the pedal bone is subject to injury. The most severe injury to the pedal bone occurs when it is fractured.

Symptoms Most horses will become acutely and severely lame after the injury. In many cases fracture of the pedal bone occurs during a race and the horse will appear lame immediately after the race. The lameness will become very severe as the horse cools down, until, within half an hour or an hour, the horse will not take any weight on the affected leg. Pain is evidenced when the hoof is squeezed with a pair of pincers or tapped around the wall with a farrier's hammer. However, many horses, within 24 to 48 hours, will improve to a stage that they hardly appear lame on the affected leg at all.

Treatment For healing of fractures of the pedal bone a rest period of at least 12 months is necessary. After the fracture is sustained a bar-shoe with quarter clips should be applied to stop expansion of the foot and to keep the pedal bone as rigidly immobilised as possible. This shoe should be changed every 6 to 8 weeks to allow foot trimming and to prevent contraction of the heels, and at least 6 months of immobilisation of the foot in this type of shoe is required. At the end of 6 months further x-rays can be taken to check on the progress of healing of the bone, but in most cases the fracture line will not have healed before 12 months have passed. With horses under 3 years of age the prognosis for healing of pedal bone fractures is quite good, with most fractures healing within a 12-month period. In horses older than 3 years of age the prognosis is very poor and where the fracture extends right to the coffin joint, complete healing seldom occurs. In such cases surgery can be performed to insert a stainless steel screw through the hoof wall into the pedal bone to stabilise the fracture line. The operation is usually very successful, but there is an increased risk of infection due to difficulty in sterilising the hoof wall.

(See Fig. 78 on p. 154)

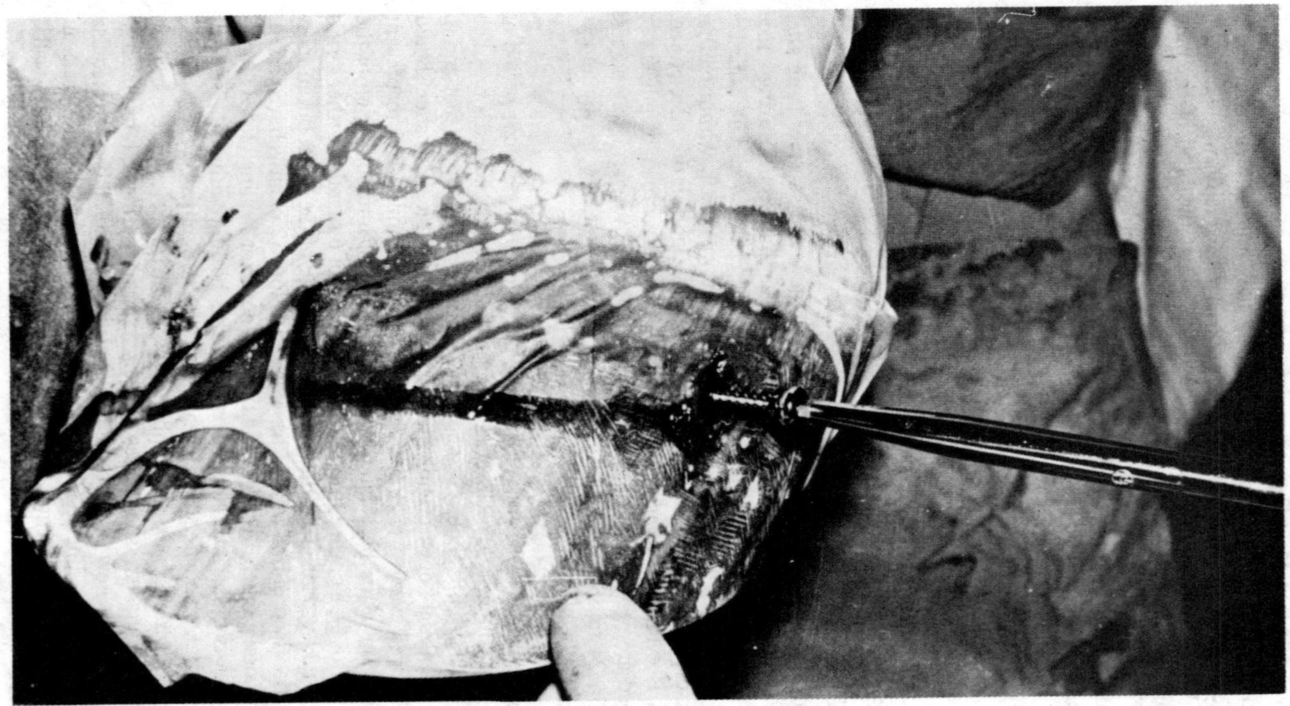

Fig. 78
Insertion of a screw into the foot of a horse with a fracture of the pedal bone.

PEDAL OSTEITIS

This condition is a common cause of lameness in shallow-footed horses or horses working on very hard ground. It is essentially an inflammation of the sole surface of the pedal bone.

Symptoms Horses are frequently lame in both fore legs and have a gait which appears as though they are stepping on hot bricks. If the sole of the foot is tapped with a hoof hammer or squeezed with a pair of pincers, a painful reaction will be found. This reaction may be localised to the heels or be apparent over the whole sole.

Treatment Corrective shoeing is necessary to ensure that the shoe is not bearing weight on the sole, inside the white line. In addition a leather or rubber pad should be inserted under the shoe to reduce concussion to the foot. If the condition is very acute anti-inflammatory drugs, such as *phenylbutazone*, may be useful.

PERIOSTITIS

Periostitis means inflammation of the surface of the bone and its covering membrane, the periosteum. Probably the most common type of periostitis is that found in racing stables and is known as "sore shins". It may be followed by inflammation of the bone itself (*osteitis*), which shows as a roughened bony surface generally to the front of the cannon bone. Sore shins are usually seen in the fore legs, particularly in young racehorses in training, and are due to concussion. Any local injury to bone will result in periostitis and the condition of "splints" is initially a periostitis.

Symptoms The horse walks in a sore and tender manner, especially after a gallop on hard ground. Signs of inflammation, as shown by soreness, may be obscure at first, but later there is a soft fluctuating swelling which eventually becomes hard. During the early stages, the swelling is painful to the touch; the horse keeps shifting its feet if both legs are affected, or points the toe and bends the fetlock joint if the trouble is only in one leg.

Treatment Cold applications either by hosing or the application of ice poultices, followed by warm application and hand rubbing, are usually sufficient to cut short mild attacks. *Antiphlogistine* applied under a light bandage is useful. The horse should be rested from work, but may be given light exercise on soft ground. Although blistering and firing are carried out to treat periostitis, the treatments usually do more harm than good. Radiation therapy, using radioactive cobalt or radon packs, has been useful in preventing new bone growth often associated with periostitis. Anti-inflammatory drugs, such as *phenylbutazone* and cortisone, are also used by veterinary surgeons to relieve the inflammation associated with this disorder. Horses with periostitis should be given a rest period of 8 to 12 weeks and should be brought back into work gradually, exercising at first on soft ground.

PERITONITIS

Peritonitis means inflammation of the serous membrane lining the cavity of the abdomen and covering the organs. It is most frequently caused by damage to the bowel with resultant leakage of bacteria into the abdomen setting up inflammation and infection. Peritonitis can also occur during the course of certain infectious diseases.

Symptoms These include fever, distress, disinclination to move, stiffness of the abdominal walls, which are painful when touched; frequent passage of small quantities of urine with pain; attempts to lie down with bending of knees and hocks but failure to carry out the intention. Constipation is usually present and gut sounds cannot be heard in the abdomen. There is rapid pulse and the visible mucous membranes, such as those of the eyes and the nose, are congested. Death usually occurs within 1 to 2 days and there is extensive effusion of fluid into the abdominal cavity.

Treatment The services of a veterinarian are required to administer effective antibiotics systemically, following identification of the type of bacteria. Drainage tubes should be inserted into the abdomen to allow infected fluid to be removed and antibiotics to be instilled. Intravenous fluids must be used to replace lost fluids. From this it can be seen that treatment of peritonitis is both difficult and expensive, and despite intensive treatment most horses usually die.

PERVIOUS URACHUS (Leaking Navel)

Pervious urachus occurs in the newborn and is a fairly common condition in foals. Up to the time of birth, the urine is discharged through the urachus (a small ureter-like structure within the umbilical cord), into a membranous bag called the allantoic sac, one of the "water bags" surrounding the foetus. In this way, it is prevented from entering the inner "water bag", the amniotic sac, where it would mingle with the liquids directly surrounding the foetus and cause irritation. This structure usually closes when the umbilical cord is ruptured at birth, and the urine takes the normal course and is voided through the bladder and urethra. It sometimes happens that the closure of the urachus is imperfect and a continuous dribbling of urine from the region of the umbilicus of the young foal keeps the area wet, although, in addition, urine may still be passed in the natural way.

This is not a very serious condition and is readily treated by a veterinarian, but if the leaking persists for any great length of time, the moist condition around the umbilicus favours bacterial infection of the navel stump, leading to joint-ill and other troubles.

Treatment Most cases will correct themselves within a few days, but it is undesirable to delay treatment longer than this, when a veterinarian should be called in to cauterise the urachus. The navel cord must not be tied to correct this condition. More serious cases, especially when the entire contents of the bladder are being passed through the urachus, will require surgical intervention.

PHOTOSENSITISATION (Trefoil Dermatitis)

Photosensitisation develops when the animal is sensitive to the rays of the sun due to the presence in the bloodstream of certain photodynamic or sensitising substances of plant or chemical origin. These predispose the unpigmented skin to the harmful effects of ultra-violet rays. On rare occasions even pigmented skin is affected. Plants capable of producing light sensitisation are referred to as photodynamic plants.

Horses are affected only with simple or primary photosensitisation and apparently do not suffer from the type asociated with damage to the liver as occurs in sheep. A dermatitis of the unpigmented areas of the skin of horses, without obvious liver damage, has been known for a long time following the eating of certain medicagos and trefoils such as *Trifolium pratense, T. hybridum, Medicago sativa* and *M. polymorpha.*

In the days when draught horses were used for farming, trefoil dermatitis was a fairly common condition on the white portions of the skin, but particularly on the white fetlocks and legs of Clydesdale horses, in seasons of luxuriant herbage growth and much bright sunlight. Because aphids were frequently present on the trefoil and these were also seen on the white legs of the horses, the disease was commonly referred to as "aphis disease". Whilst the work of many investigators has not shown any association between aphis infestation and the toxicity of the trefoil plants, scientists working on the pigments of aphids have found a photodynamic substance in the aphids, and it is now suggested that this agent may be absorbed from the aphids eaten with the plants, which may contribute in some way to the development of the disease.

Symptoms The lesions of photosensitisation in horses occur mainly on the white or unpigmented parts of the skin such as the legs, the nose and face and in piebald horses on the white portions of the neck and body. The skin on the unpigmented areas is at first red, becomes thickened owing to the presence of fluid in the deeper layers and fluid may ooze from the surface. Itching occurs and the parts often become covered with crusts or scabs of dried exudate and blood. Quite commonly, as a result of the animal biting or rubbing the affected parts against logs and fences, large, raw areas are produced. These may become dry and cracked, or, following secondary infection, exude pus. Dead, leathery skin may be shed in large flakes. In white-muzzled horses, lesions occurring about the mouth may interfere with feeding.

Treatment On the first signs of photosensitisation, horses should be removed to another pasture, free of trefoils and clovers and containing plenty of shade, the last being very important. If practicable, the horses should be stabled or shedded and hand-fed. Treatment will vary according to the severity and extent of the lesions. Zinc cream or calamine lotion may be used to relieve itching. Hard crusts may be softened and their removal facilitated by raw linseed oil and lime water (50-50). If the lesions have become infected, they should be treated as infected wounds—see *Wounds*.

When horses have to be left in the open, an attempt should be made to darken the unpigmented areas of the skin to give some protection from the sun. This may be done by mixing lamp black or soot with equal parts by weight of petroleum jelly and smearing this over the affected portions of the skin, and other unpigmented areas if practicable. A fairly strong solution of potassium permanganate (*Condy's crystals*) will also darken the skin. Unfortunately, most pigments do not last long. Internal treatment is of little value, but if the horse is stabled, a laxative drench may be given to advantage. Antihistamine and cortisone injections may be of some use in early cases. Severe cases may need veterinary attention.

PLEURISY

Pleurisy or pleuritis is an inflammation of the serous membrane lining the chest cavity and enveloping the lungs. It is not a common disease in horses except for its association with pneumonia, and as a complication of respiratory tract infections. It may also be caused by a penetrating injury through the chest wall or a rib fracture. The condition may be acute or chronic.

Symptoms The symptoms of acute pleurisy usually commence suddenly and often the first indication of the disease is that the horse is disinclined to move or turn around due to pain in the chest. There may be shivering, temperature, dullness, fast and shallow respiration and loss of appetite. The animal often sweats, is uneasy and may show mild signs of colic. Pressure or tapping over the chest between the ribs induces pain. The horse is usually stiff and walks as though foundered. The breathing is abdominal, the chest hardly moving at all and inspiration is short and jerky, the expiration longer. These latter symptoms indicate pain in the chest due to friction between the dry, inflamed, pleural surfaces of the chest and the lung. Application of the ear to the chest wall over the sensitive area may detect a dry-friction murmur. The horse prefers to stand rather than lie down. There may be a short, suppressed cough. After a few days, when effusion occurs, the patient appears to improve. The temperature drops somewhat, the pain decreases and the horse eats a little. The friction sound disappears as the exudation in the chest cavity builds up, moistening the pleural surfaces. Percussion or tapping with the fingers on the chest reveals a horizontal line of dullness which gradually rises higher in the chest as the fluid accumulates. The course of the disease varies. In mild cases, the fluid undergoes absorption and the case may terminate favourably in a week to 10 days, although some adhesions of the pleurae may remain. In the more severe cases, when the quantity of effusion is large, the process of absorption is retarded. Respirations now become more frequent and rapid and the horse has an anxious and haggard expression and gradually weakens. Swelling may appear under the chest, extending to the abdomen and even the legs. In unfavourable cases, particularly when the pleural fluid contains pus, death usually occurs in 2 to 3 weeks.

Recovered animals sometimes have permanent disability due to adhesions in the chest cavity, the bands of fibrous tissue causing embarrassment to the free movement of the lungs. Such cases become "short in their wind" and "grunters".

Treatment Pleurisy does not respond well to home treatment, although good nursing and general care of the patient contribute greatly to recovery. Veterinary assistance should be obtained in order that appropriate treatment can be carried out early. This involves insertion of a needle into the chest to determine the type of fluid and whether bacteria are present. It may be necessary to insert a drainage tube into the chest to allow antibiotics to be infused and excess fluid to be removed. If intensive treatment is given many horses will survive.

PNEUMONIA

Pneumonia is an inflammation of the lung substance caused by various agents such as viruses, bacteria, parasites, fungi, or the aspiration of dust and other foreign substances into the lungs. It is commonly complicated by inflammation of the bronchioles and/or pleurisy, and occurs as a complication of a number of specific diseases. Predisposing causes include inclement weather, fatigue, poorly-ventilated stables and sheds, bad sanitation and transportation with associated fatigue and lowered resistance.

Aspiration pneumonia is caused most frequently by careless or incompetent drenching, such as raising the head too high, giving the drench too fast, or interfering with the throat region to make the horse swallow. Drenching a horse when it is suffering from laryngitis or other respiratory conditions, attempting to drench an animal when it is down, and passing a stomach tube into the windpipe instead of the gullet are other causes. The disease produced is a necrotic or gangrenous pneumonia and is usually fatal.

The various forms of pneumonia are not discussed, but the general symptoms of all types of the disease are given below.

Pneumonia in the horse, apart from aspiration pneumonia, occurs mainly in foals or young horses and in old and debilitated animals.

General Symptoms These are rises in temperature, not uncommonly reaching 41 °C; increased pulse rate; rapid shallow respirations which are abdominal in character; cough; nasal discharge; loss of appetite and great depression. When the temperature is very high, the horse sweats profusely. The nostrils are inflamed and dilated, the mucous membranes of the eyes are red, and the horse stands with head stretched forward, appearing to be afraid to lie down, and usually remains standing. In the early stages of pneumonia, if the ear is held close to the chest, or a stethoscope is used, a gurgling sound may be heard, due to the air being forced through inflammatory liquid in the air sacs. After 12 to 24 hours, listening over the same area may reveal no sound owing to consolidation of that portion of the lung.

The course of primary, acute pneumonia varies, but in the horse it is usually less than a week after which, if the animal is going to recover, the general symptoms described above subside, the cough becomes loose and the appetite returns. If improvement does not occur within the first week, the prognosis is poor and death is likely. Some cases continue as a chronic pneumonia and make a partial recovery. With early diagnosis, prompt and correct treatment and good nursing, the prognosis is more favourable.

Treatment It is important to determine the specific type of bacteria causing pneumonia. Once this is done an appropriate antibiotic can be administered under the supervision of a veterinarian. Treatment with antibiotics is necessary until the temperature has been normal for 24 hours, which usually entails a 5 to 10 day course of treatment.

Supportive treatment combined with good nursing should not be neglected. Warmth and protection from adverse weather conditions are necessary for the patient, but in favourable weather an unhoused animal is best kept in the open, rather than confined to a badly ventilated stable or draughty shed. A blanket may be placed under the rug to provide extra warmth, and the legs can be bandaged with Newmarket bandages. Soft and nutritious food should be offered in small quantities and varied. Freshly prepared bran mashes, carrots and chopped greenstuff may all be tried in turn. The object is to tempt the horse to eat and so maintain its strength. An adequate and fresh water supply should be readily available.

POISONING

Plant Poisoning Other than Kimberley horse disease and Birdsville disease, which occur in Northern Australia, cases of poisoning of plant origin are far less common in horses than they are in sheep and cattle. Generally, horses are rather selective grazers and are not so prone to eat poisonous plants as are other grazing animals.

The effects produced by eating poisonous plants vary according to the poison they contain. Some plants cause rapid death owing to the toxic action of the poison. Others are highly irritant to the digestive system causing gastro-enteritis followed by death, whilst others again affect the nervous system or cause locomotory disturbance (staggers and incoordination of movement). Other plants cause photosensitisation, which has been discussed under *Photosensitisation.*

It is frequently difficult, from the symptoms shown by the animal, to differentiate plant poisoning from other common diseases, and the fact that there are poisonous plants in the paddock does not mean that the horse has eaten them. Diarrhoea or scouring, for example, is an indication of gastro-intestinal disorder and, although it may be produced by plants containing irritant poisons, it is also a symptom of bacterial infections and may even be caused by eating indigestible feedstuffs. Plants containing prussic acid or nitrate can cause sudden death, but there are a number of other causes of collapse.

It is necessary, in connection with a suspected case of plant poisoning, to enquire closely into the history of the horse or horses, how hungry they were when turned into a paddock, and to find evidence that they had eaten poisonous plants in sufficient quantity to cause toxicity. If mortality has occurred, a post-mortem examination may help in arriving at a diagnosis.

Stomach contents can be collected and forwarded in a suitable container, preferably a screw-top jar, to a botanist, who may be able to identify the plants which have been eaten. A space should be left at the top to allow for gas formation and a little pure formalin added to reduce fermentation. Specimens of suspected poisonous plants, pressed between newspaper, should also be sent with the stomach contents.

Treatment

The poisonous properties of many plants are not known, which renders treatment difficult. Antidotes are available for only a few kinds of plant poisoning and, to be effective, the diagnosis must be correct and the antidote administered quickly. Professional assistance should be obtained without delay if poisoning is suspected. A drench of 250 g of Epsom salts and 125 to 250 g of sodium bicarbonate (baking soda) may be of assistance in some plant poisonings. Tannin, in the form of tannic acid (15 g), or strong tea, counteracts many poisons.

See also *Kimberley or Walkabout Disease* and *Photosensitisation*

Mineral Poisoning

Arsenic Poisoning

Cases of mineral poisoning occur from time to time in horses. Of the mineral poisons, arsenic is the one most commonly responsible for mortality in cattle and sheep in Australia, and has caused deaths of horses. The usual sources of arsenic are sheep and cattle dips from which horses may drink, weed killers, vermin killers, mixtures for painting skins, empty arsenic containers and mining or industrial residues. Pastures that have been poisoned by arsenic from recently dipped sheep and cattle, or vegetation that has been sprayed with arsenical weed killers are sources of poisoning. Horses have suffered from arsenical poisoning from over-dosing with tonic medicines containing arsenic, and also from application of arsenical preparations to the skin.

Symptoms

There are at least four distinct forms of arsenical poisoning, namely *acute, sub-acute, nervous* and *chronic.* In the first category may be included those cases in which death occurs within 36 hours after eating or drinking the arsenic. The symptoms shown are slobbering at the mouth, thirst, loss of appetite, colicky pains, diarrhoea, coldness of the extremities, paralysis of the hindquarters and collapse. Some of these symptoms may not be exhibited and, when a large dose of soluble arsenic has been consumed, the horse may die before the signs of enteritis are shown. In the sub-acute form, the symptoms are somewhat similar but more prolonged;

the more prominent are diarrhoea, loss of appetite and disinclination to move. The course of the disease in these cases may extend over 2 to 3 days to a week. In the less frequent nervous form of arsenical poisoning, the foregoing symptoms are almost entirely absent. There may be muscular tremor and inco-ordination, but frequently the animal collapses suddenly without any premonitory symptoms. In such cases, the arsenic appears to paralyse the action of the heart by some direct effect upon the nervous system. The chronic form, sometimes seen in man, is rather rare in stock under Australian conditions. It occurs in other countries where animals are grazed in the vicinity of smelting works and where the water and pasture have become contaminated with arsenic. It can occur, however, where pastures have been contaminated by the drippings from sheep and cattle which have been dipped in an arsenical solution, or on pastures which have been sprayed with an arsenical weed killer. The symptoms shown in this form are poor appetite, intermittent diarrhoea and constipation, wasting, swelling of the joints and loss of hair. There may be reddening of the eyes and swelling of the eyelids and also inflammation and ulceration of the mouth extending sometimes to the muzzle.

Treatment

In the case of acute poisoning, treatment will be of little value unless promptly carried out. Veterinary surgeons have at their disposal a preparation known as *B.A.L.* (British Anti-Lewisite) which, if injected promptly in correct dose rates, has been found a useful antidote for arsenic and some other metallic poisonings. Sodium thiosulphate (photographic hypo), as used for the treatment of arsenical poisoning in sheep and cattle, can also be used for horses. One litre of milk or limewater can be given as a drench and repeated in 2 hours. The whites of 12 eggs may also be given. Good nursing is very important and, provided treatment is commenced early and is carried out by, or under the supervision of a veterinarian, good results can be anticipated, at least in the less acute cases of arsenical poisoning.

Lead Poisoning

This form of poisoning does not occur as frequently in horses as in cattle and, since the advent of new formulations for paints, is not as common in the latter animals as it was. Acute lead poisoning is very rare, but, as lead is a cumulative poison, horses may suffer from the chronic form if they have, over a period, been drinking water that has been standing in new lead pipes, in old lead paint barrels or similar containers. It has occurred when horses have grazed on pastures which have been contaminated by lead residues from smelting works. Horses, unlike cattle, are less liable to lick lead-based painted surfaces, discarded storage batteries, lead foil, pipes and fittings, unless they are suffering from some mineral deficiency. There are cases on record where the source of lead has been from lead arsenate used as a spray in gardens or orchards.

Symptoms

In acute lead poisoning, there are symptoms of abdominal pain, staggering, grinding of the teeth, depression, twitching, especially of the eyelids, champing of the jaws, convulsions and collapse. Chronic lead poisoning leads to loss of appetite, emaciation, constipation and, in some cases, to paralysis of the lower lip and paralysis of part of the larynx, resulting in "roaring".

Treatment

The modern treatment for lead poisoning is the use of a complex therapeutic agent sold under the proprietary name of *Calcium Versenate,* which removes absorbed lead from the tissues. The drug is administered in solution by slow intravenous injection over several days and would require the services of a veterinarian.

POLL EVIL

See *Fistulous Withers and Poll Evil*

POLYPS

These are tumours or growths with narrow bases which sometimes occur in cavities like the nose or throat. The name refers to the shape of the growth and has nothing to do with its structure. Most polyps are non-malignant. In the nose, the stem or base of the tumour is generally attached to the membrane high up in the nasal chambers, and when small it cannot be seen. Occasionally it increases in size until it can be observed within the nostril. Sometimes, instead of hanging down towards the nasal opening, it falls back into the pharynx. A polyp may also be attached to the fauces (opening of the back part of the mouth) and the body of the tumour then falls into the pharynx. In this situation, it may seriously interfere with breathing.

Symptoms When in the nose, these growths cause a peculiar snoring noise, a discharge from the nostril, which may be blood-stained if the tumour is injured, or foetid if the turbinate bones are involved. If the growths are in the throat, the symptoms depend on their location. Interference with breathing is a general symptom, especially if the tumour falls into the pharynx.

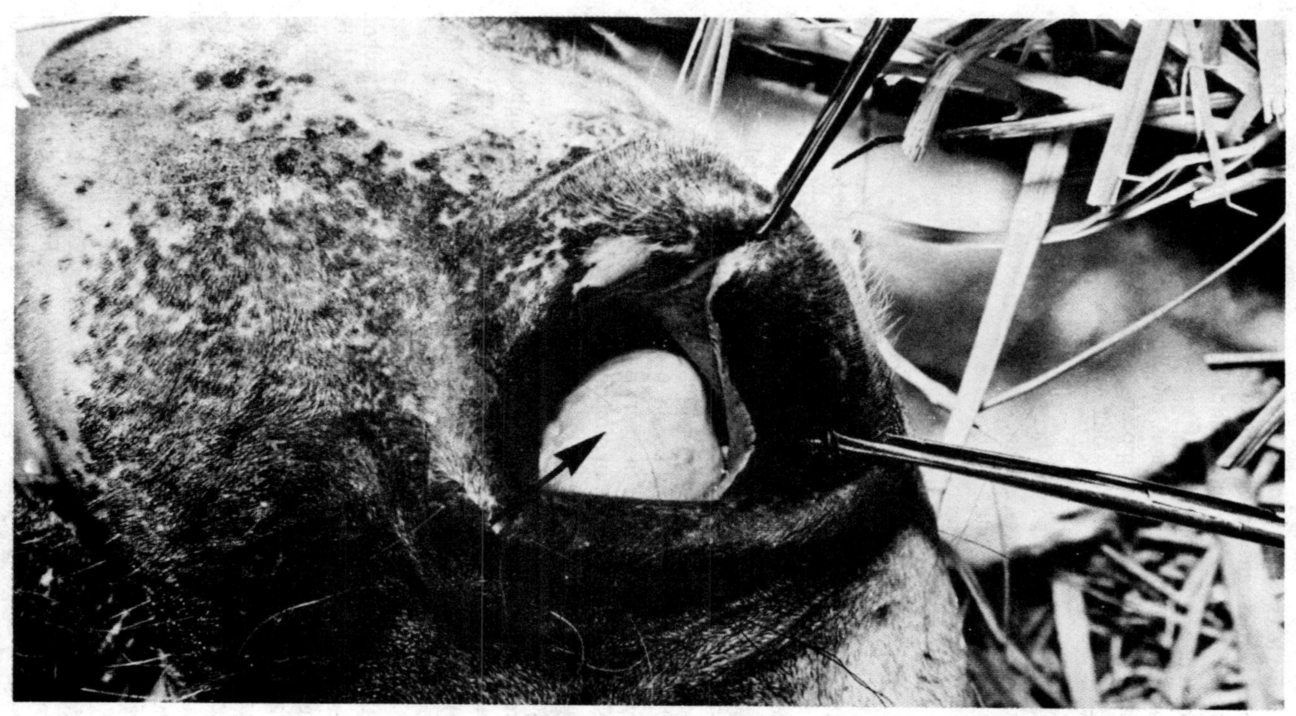

Fig. 79
Nasal polyp (arrow) obstructing normal respiration.

Sometimes it falls into the larynx, causing most alarming symptoms. The animal coughs or tries to cough, saliva flows from the mouth, breathing is performed with great difficulty, and accompanied by a loud noise. The animal appears as if strangled and often falls to the ground exhausted. When the tumour is coughed out of the larynx, the animal quickly recovers and soon appears to be quite normal. These sudden attacks and quick recoveries point to the nature of the trouble.

Treatment These polyps, because of their shape, are comparatively easily removed by a veterinarian, except when located high up in the nose where access is difficult.

PREGNANCY

Pregnancy or gestation is the period during which the female carries its young and when the foetus is undergoing development. The breeding season for horses in Australia starts in September and extends to December or early January. This is because mares normally come into *oestrus* (heat) in the spring and early summer months. At other times the appearance of *oestrus* in mares is irregular, but it can occur at any time of the year. Mares come in season 6 to 9 days after foaling and are commonly mated again at this period. The heat period lasts from 3 to 7 days, but is most variable. In some mares it may be shorter and in others it may last 2 or 3 weeks. From the time a mare goes off *oestrus*, a period of 16 to 17 days elapses before the next *oestrus* period starts, and, unless the mare is served and gets in foal, this cycle continues throughout the breeding season. The gestation period for mares is about 340 days (325 to 355) or approximately 11 months. This may vary even more, when it is usually associated with some disease of the genital organs.

Indications of Pregnancy As the mere fact of service by the stallion does not ensure pregnancy, it is important that the result should be determined as soon as possible. A veterinarian can make an accurate diagnosis of pregnancy in a mare by rectal examination, or by laboratory tests on samples of blood or urine. When this is not done, it is usual to accept the cessation of *oestrus* as evidence of pregnancy, but this is not an infallible sign. Sometimes the mare shows signs of *oestrus* after she has conceived. These symptoms usually only last about a day. Other mares may cease to show signs of *oestrus* and yet have failed to get in foal. An early sign of pregnancy is the altered behaviour of the mare. She usually becomes more docile and tractable after conception and may exhibit other signs, such as change in attitude to other horses. From 20 days onwards a veterinary surgeon is able to palpate the foetus through the wall of the rectum, but this is not easy at this early stage. Pregnancy diagnosis is usually performed at 42 days. Somewhere between 10 and 20 per cent of mares will not carry the foal to term despite having been in foal when tested at 42 days. Enlargement of the abdomen may be noted at about the fifth month and is more pronounced at 6 months. Slight falling-in beneath the loins and hollowness of the back are suggestive signs, although they are not always present. Swelling and firmness of the udder, with smoothing out of wrinkles, occur at intervals during gestation. A steady increase in weight, of 500 g to 1 kg daily, from about the fifth month is an indication of pregnancy. After the seventh or eighth month, movement of the unborn foal may be detected by pressing firmly with the palm or knuckles of the hand against the abdominal wall in front of the left stifle, especially after the mare has had a drink of water or while she is feeding. The indications of approaching parturition have been described under *Parturition.*

PURPURA HAEMORRHAGICA

This is a non-contagious disease which is also known as petechial fever. It may occur following an attack of strangles, influenza or other acute infectious disease. It may also follow upon a deep-seated infected injury, or when a horse is affected with fistulous withers or poll evil. Occasionally it occurs as a primary disease.

The disease damages the walls of the small blood vessels leading to escape of plasma and blood into the tissues. The formation of haemorrhages and the accumulation of dropsical fluid in various parts of the body are characteristic of the condition. It is a serious disease and has a high mortality rate.

Cause Although the disease has been recognised for a long time, its exact cause is not yet known. Several theories have been advanced. One is that it occurs as the result of a hypersensitive reaction to the protein of streptococcal organisms.

Symptoms The disease usually appears quite suddenly with, at first, the appearance of small haemorrhages or petechiae on the visible mucous membranes of the nostrils, eyes, mouth and lips of the vulva in mares. This is followed by the development of a dropsical swelling of the nostrils extending over the nose, and sometimes of the eyelids which may later involve the whole head, which then becomes greatly enlarged. The legs swell, and swellings may occur along the belly and on other parts of the body. These swellings tend to disappear quite suddenly and then to reappear later. They are cold and painless and, if pressed with the finger, an indentation remains for a while. On their surface the skin may be tightly stretched and sometimes oozes a pale straw-coloured fluid. Blood may ooze from the haemorrhagic areas and a nasal discharge is quite common. There is variable fever and the horse loses its appetite and becomes weak. The oedematous swellings and haemorrhages may extend internally, leading to pulmonary oedema, or when the intestines are involved, cause a severe attack of colic. Both of these conditions are usually fatal.

The course of an uncomplicated case of the disease is 8 to 10 days when some cases terminate favourably. In other cases recovery may occur after 1 or 2 relapses extending over several weeks. Many horses die well within this period from asphyxia (when oedema of the head is severe), oedema of the viscera, broncho-pneumonia, blood loss, or secondary bacterial infections. The mortality rate is variable, depending on the severity of the cases, but is estimated at approximately 50 per cent.

Treatment There is evidence to show that the high mortality rate from purpura haemorrhagica is greatly reduced by good treatment and nursing. The treatment therefore requires the co-operation of the veterinary surgeon and the horse owner. Blood transfusions and antibiotic treatment, together with cortisone injections, usually give the best results. Intravenous injections of calcium gluconate (100 to 200 ml of 7.5 per cent solution) daily, have been found useful. No medicine should be given by the mouth owing to the risk of mechanical pneumonia. Good nursing is essential. The horse should be made as comfortable as possible and kept warm, either in the open or in a well-ventilated stable, but the legs should not be bandaged and care is necessary to avoid chafing the swellings with rugs. Clean drinking water should be readily available and kept fresh by frequent changes. To maintain the horse's strength, tempting laxative foods should be fed, such as freshly prepared bran mashes to which scalded oats and sliced carrots may be added. A little green lucerne is useful. If feeding is difficult, owing to swelling of the lips and nose, sloppy foods such as gruels of oatmeal and linseed can be offered. Gentle massage of the swollen limbs, careful grooming with a soft body brush and light exercise are helpful in reducing the oedematous swellings. Care is necessary during the convalescent period to prevent a relapse and a long period of rest is desirable.

QUEENSLAND ITCH

A skin disease of horses known as Queenland itch has been recognised in Australia for a long time, but the cause was not understood and the empirical treatment carried out was not very successful. It was known,

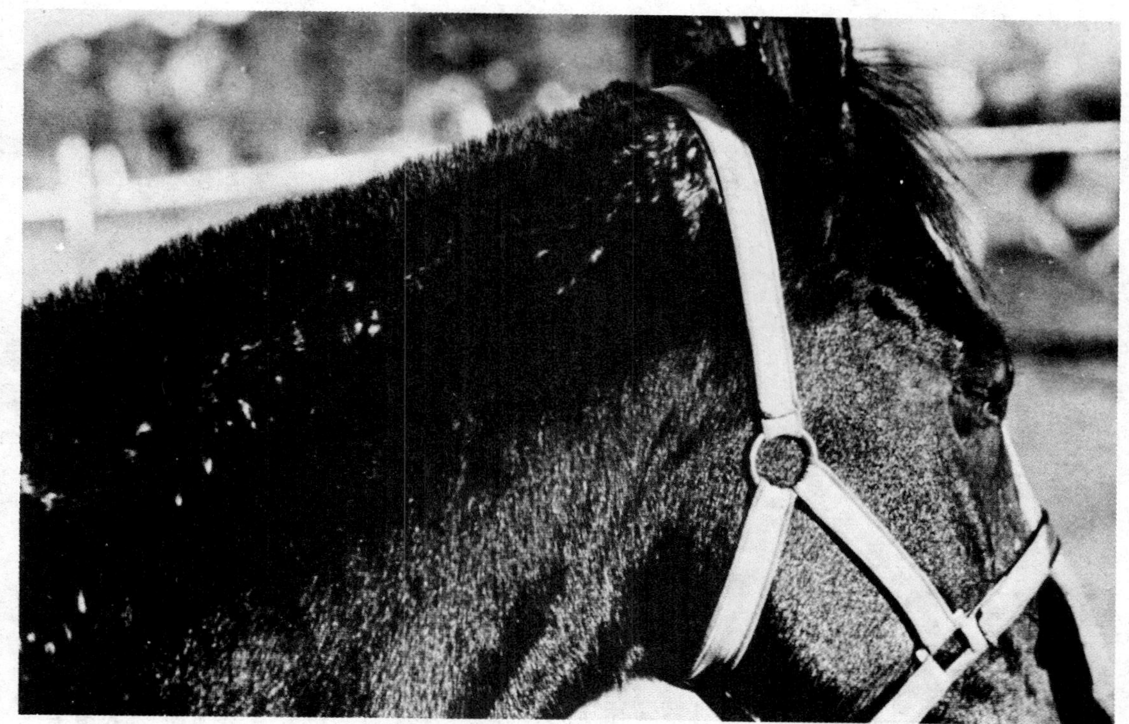

Fig. 80
Queensland itch. Hair loss and skin irritation around mane and neck.

however, that when affected horses from the coastal districts of Queensland and New South Wales were sent inland, the disease cleared up. Research work having shown the cause of the disease gives the answer as to why this occurs.

The disease occurs mainly in the summer rainfall areas of the continent, particularly in the coastal and subcoastal regions of Queensland and northern New South Wales, but also elsewhere in coastal or near-coastal regions. It seldom occurs inland.

Cause The disease is caused by the hypersensitivity of some horses to the bites of the sandfly, *Culicoides robertsi.* All horses are not affected by the sensitising substance injected by the sandflies. Susceptible horses, however, show signs of the disease from early summer until the cooler weather approaches. All types, colours and ages of horses are affected by this allergic dermatitis, which is often mistaken for a form of mange.

Symptoms The lesions are mainly confined to the upper parts of the body including the butt of the tail, rump, along the back, withers, crest, poll and ears. Rarely are lesions found on the sides of the body, the neck, face or legs. Usually the first symptoms shown are the formation of small papules or pimples on which the hair stands erect. The hair on these pimples is brittle and gradually falls out. The itching caused is variable and occurs particularly at night. When severe, the animal rubs the part on any suitable object such as fences and trees and bites at the part if it can reach it, thus aggravating the condition and causing large hairless patches on the body. In chronic cases, the skin becomes thickened and may form into ridges. There is no constitutional disturbance and the appetite is unimpaired, except when secondary bacterial infection of the lesions occurs. Loss of condition may occur as a result of the prolonged irritation and interference with feeding.

Treatment Frequent intramuscular injections of antihistamines have been shown to relieve the irritation caused by Queensland itch, but would be too costly for general use. The application of antihistamine ointments or creams to the affected areas will relieve the itching and assist cure and subsequent growth of hair.

Prevention of the disease lies in spraying susceptible horses once a week with a weak solution of a product such as *Gammawash* (I.C.I.), 1 in 1,000 concentration. Rugging horses with light rugs in the late afternoon also helps in preventing the sandfly bites.

QUIDDING

When a horse chews its food partially and then drops it from the mouth, it is said to be *quidding*. This generally results from irregular or diseased teeth, or when permanent teeth are pushing the temporary teeth out from the gums. It may also result from abrasions of the membranes of the mouth and tongue or more severe injury to the latter. It can arise from paralysis of the throat or some other condition such as a sore throat, which causes difficulty in swallowing.

Treatment Quidding is, of course, only a symptom and not a disease. The mouth and throat should be inspected, preferably with a mouth-gag. Dental irregularity must be corrected either by rasping or, if necessary, the extraction of a diseased or projecting tooth (see *Teeth*). Injuries to the mouth and tongue will need attention as will a sore throat. Under certain circumstances, as in the cases of injuries to the mouth, it may be necessary to feed only soft or liquid foods for a few days.

QUITTOR

Quittor is the name given to a discharging wound of the foot, usually at the heels or quarters, opening above the coronet and discharging pus from one or more sinuses.

Causes The condition results from an infected injury such as a tread on the coronet, a suppurating corn, a punctured wound of the foot and so on. The suppuration usually results initially from a necrotic lateral cartilage.

Symptoms A quittor causes intense pain and lameness. A greyish-coloured pus, often streaked with blood, is discharged almost constantly at the swollen coronet. It is not uncommon, however, for one discharging site at the coronet to heal up, to be followed by pus breaking out at another place. If not checked by efficient treatment, the pus continues to burrow downwards involving other structures.

Treatment Drainage of pus from the area is the problem in the treatment of quittor. In some early cases, opening up the wound to afford simple drainage, antiseptic treatment and the intramuscular injection of antibiotics may bring about favourable results. Repeated hot fomentations and poulticing may be applied to advantage in certain cases.

Most cases of quittor need expert surgery under an anaesthetic to remove all diseased tissue, including sometimes the whole of the lateral cartilage. Frequent dressing of the surgical wound is then necessary and the convalescent period may be quite prolonged. Cartilage is poorly nourished by blood and once it is injured and infected, necrosis or death of the part commonly occurs, hence the difficulty of bringing about a cure without surgery. Healing cannot take place until the area or areas either slough away or are surgically removed.

RECTOVAGINAL FISTULA

A rectovaginal fistula is an abnormal communication between the rectum and the vagina occasioned by an injury during foaling. It is usually due to one of the foal's feet sticking through the roof of the vagina and rectum, causing a tear and a communication between these two cavities.

Symptoms The injury is usually noticed at, or soon after, foaling, although it does not appear to cause the mare undue distress. It is usually noticed that the mare is passing faeces through her vagina and that a tear is present.

Treatment In the case of minor lacerations, these can be relatively easily repaired. Surgery is necessary to repair the damaged tissues and this is usually performed 3 to 4 weeks after the injury to allow swelling and infection to subside. In extensive lacerations, surgery is extremely difficult and often 3 to 4 operations are necessary.

RETENTION OF AFTERBIRTH

The afterbirth or "cleansing" refers to the foetal membranes (placenta) in which the foetus develops in the uterus (womb), which serve as a connection between it and the mother. It is composed of three parts, the *chorion*, the *amnion* and the *allantois*, which are expelled when, or soon after, the young animal is born. The term placenta refers to the special area of the membranes through which the blood circulation of the mother nourishes the foetus.

Retention of the afterbirth in the mare is much less frequent, but much more serious than in the cow. In the mare the afterbirth is normally expelled regularly a few hours after the foal is born, but if the mare has not "cleaned" properly within 6 to 8 hours, action must be taken to remove the membranes manually, otherwise infection is likely to occur. Owing to the speed with which the membranes decompose, and the risk of death of the mare or the development of metritis and acute laminitis, a veterinarian should be called immediately. If a veterinarian is not available and the horse owner is obliged to attempt to remove the

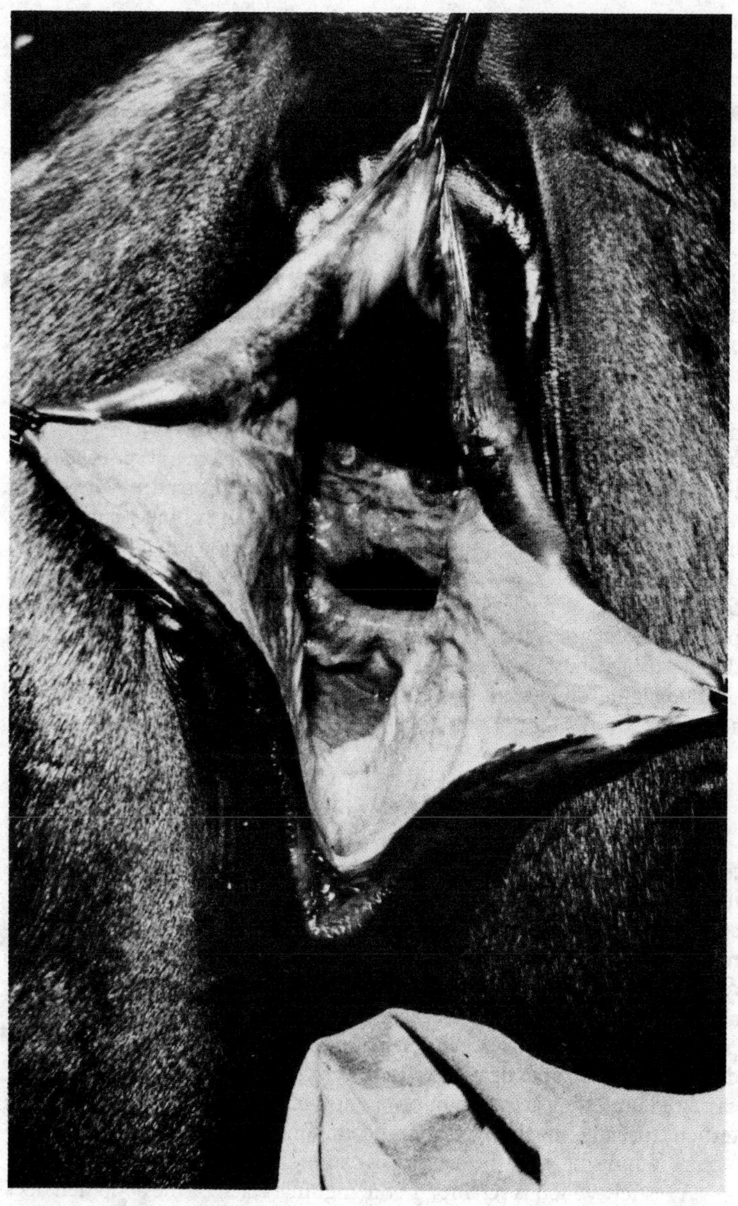

Fig. 81
Rectovaginal fistula from trauma during foaling resulting in communication between the vagina and rectum.

membranes, the greatest cleanliness and antiseptic precautions must be taken.

If portions of the membranes are protruding, it may be possible to remove them without introducing the hand into the uterus, thus avoiding introduction of infection. Examine the part hanging out and separate the more bulky, comparatively thin, and whitish-grey portion from the lesser, thicker and reddish-coloured portion. Collect within the hand as much of the reddish and thicker portion as possible. Wrap this around the thinner greyish membranes so that the free portion of the reddish membrane, now outermost, represents the layer previously adherent to the wall of the uterus. Now commence to twist the afterbirth, keeping the reddish portion outermost, and at the same time exerting gentle traction to keep the membranes moving steadily through the vulva. This torsion is continued slowly until all the afterbirth has been removed. If this is done hurriedly, haemorrhage is likely to occur. In order to be sure that the whole of the afterbirth has been removed, spread the membranes out and find the opening of the sac at the end which first protruded. Now pour 4.5 litres of water into this opening and lift up the membranes sufficiently high to let the water run into the uterine horns. These should be intact so that the afterbirth holds water and appears something like a pair of trousers tied at the ends of the legs. If any portion is missing it will be necessary to pass the thoroughly-cleaned hand (with short-cut fingernails) and arm into the uterus and horns in order to gently remove the retained portions.

Douching out the uterus with weak antiseptic solution is not now advocated.

RIG

A rig is a horse in which one or both testicles have failed to come down into the scrotum. In the foal, the descent of the testicles is often complete at birth, but it frequently happens that one testicle or both may be retained for months in the inguinal canal or in the abdomen. In other cases the testicle may descend normally but return into the canal or abdomen. This may occur because the ring through which the testicle passes is large, and the testicle small and soft and not yet closely anchored down by the scrotal ligament. It is for this reason that colts are not castrated until they are 12 months old or more. Indefinite retention of one testicle (usually the left) is not uncommon. This condition is termed "cryptorchidism" and the animal is commonly referred to as a "rig".

A testicle which is retained in the inguinal canal or the abdomen does not produce fertile spermatozoa because of the body temperature to which it is exposed.

If only one testicle is retained, the stallion may still be fertile, but if

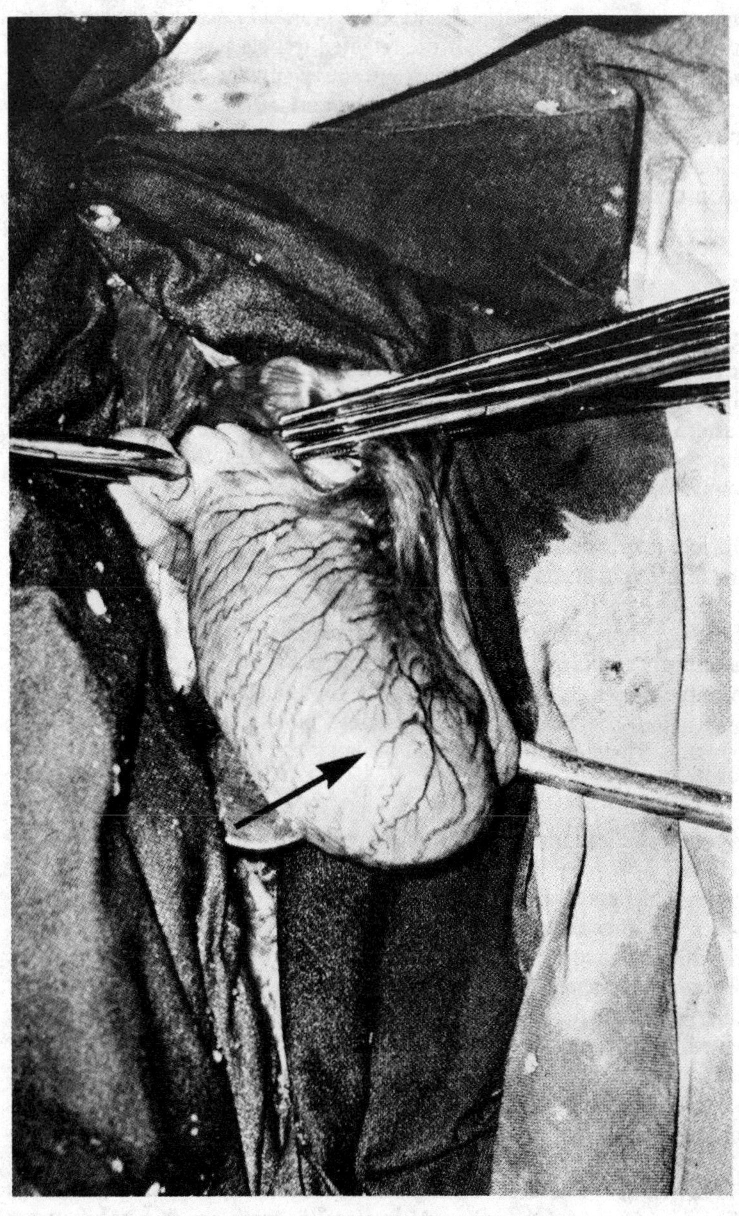

Fig. 82
Surgery to remove a testicle from the abdomen of a rig.

both are retained, he will be sterile. A cryptorchid horse is a nuisance and is often difficult to handle. If the retained testicle has not descended by the time the colt is 2 years old, a veterinary surgeon will be required to remove the undescended testicle. It is important that if the horse is a rig the testicle that is descended is not removed before the undescended one, as this frequently leads to confusion about which testicle was retained when cryptorchid surgery is being performed.

RINGBONE

Ringbone is an exostosis (bony outgrowth) occurring along the pastern. It is referred to as high ringbone when occurring between the long and short pastern bones, and low ringbone when occurring between the short pastern bone and the pedal bone. Usually an enlargement of the pastern is noted externally. If the bone growth encroaches on the coffin or pastern joints this is called articular ringbone. Low ringbone must not be confused with sidebone, which is a hardening of the lateral cartilages of the foot and is dealt with under *Sidebones*. Ringbone is more common on the fore feet than on the hind feet.

Cause Heredity plays an important part in the cause of ringbone, and an upright conformation of the legs induces liability to the disease. Other possible causes are heavy working of a young horse before the process of ossification has fully occurred; bruises; blows; sprains or injuries of tendons, ligaments and joints. All the latter are secondary to heredity and conformation.

Symptoms Lameness may or may not be present, depending on whether or not the joint is involved. In non-articular ringbone there may be no lameness at all. The lameness of ringbone is especially manifested when the affected animal is required to step from side to side. Marked flinching then occurs when weight is borne on the affected leg, even though no lameness may be revealed when the animal goes in a straight line. The lameness is frequently irregular at first, but finally becomes more or less constant and is accompanied by a plainly-visible, bony enlargement of the pastern. In the early stages of low ringbone, there may be heat and pain at the hoof-head, and bending of the joint causes increase of pain.

Treatment The treatment of ringbone is generally unsatisfactory. Firing and blistering were used to treat the problem, but results were unsatisfactory. In the early stages radiation therapy has been extremely successful in arresting growth of the bony tissue. A long rest on soft

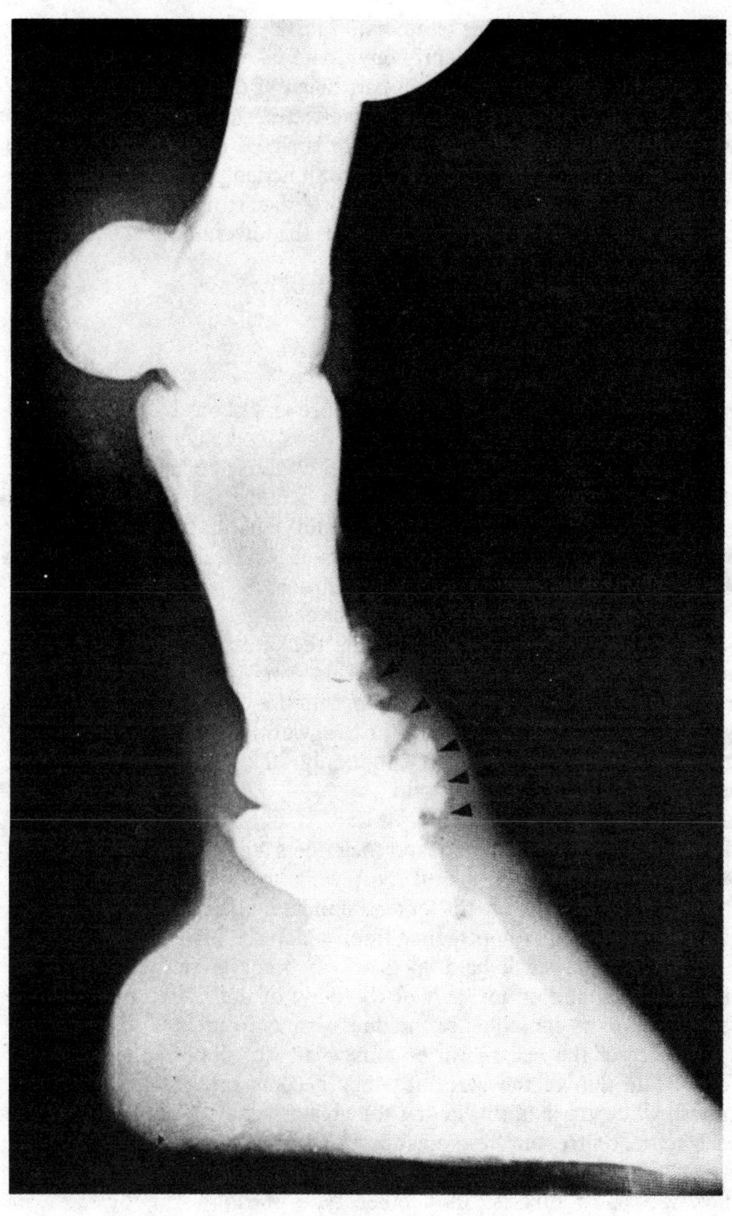

Fig. 83
X-ray of a horse with high ringbone showing damage to the pastern joint and extensive new bone production (arrows).

ground is essential after this treatment. The usual outcome of the disease is the formation of sufficient bony material to cause ankylosis, or complete fusion of the bones of a part or all of the involved joint, thus destroying the free action of the affected joint. In such cases, serviceability rather than complete cure is aimed at. Specially-designed shoes can be fitted for such cases, in conjunction with changing of the proportions or angles of the hoof by appropriate trimming. Neurectomy (cutting out a piece of nerve) to desensitise the lower limb may be carried out to prolong the usefulness of the horse.

RINGWORM

Ringworm is a contagious skin disease brought about by the growth of fungi on the skin and at the roots of hairs, and may be caused by a number of species. The disease is spread by direct contact with infected animals or contaminated objects such as bedding, harness and saddles, grooming kits, horse blankets, rails and fences. It can be a very troublesome disease when large numbers of horses are brought together as occurred during the 2 world wars. Fungal spores are very resistant and may survive in stalls and sheds for a year or longer. Spores can also exist on the skin of animals without causing the disease, so that apparently-healthy animals can act as carriers. Minor abrasions of the skin surface may favour infection. The incubation period after a natural infection is generally from a week to a month. Ringworm is readily transmissible from animals to man. It most commonly affects young horses of the yearling and 2 year old age group.

Symptoms When the hairs and their roots are invaded by the fungus of ringworm, the hairs break off short. Small bare areas are then formed which later spread from the outer boundary, thus giving the area its characteristic circular appearance from which the name is derived. Not infrequently, the small bald spots which occur in the early stages of ringworm, on almost any part of the body of the horse, are apt to be regarded as of no consequence and due to minor injuries. The subsequent appearance of the lesions varies somewhat according to the species of fungi. The skin of the bare area may become raised and scurfy, and greyish-white crusts form, giving the area a scaly appearance. The area heals in the centre, but fresh areas occur around the outside edge. Itching is not great, although the horse may show some signs of irritation by rubbing against objects. In another type of ringworm, pustules are formed below the crusts and the itchiness is much greater. It is not uncommon for ringworm lesions to join up and form large irregular-shaped bare areas over the head and body.

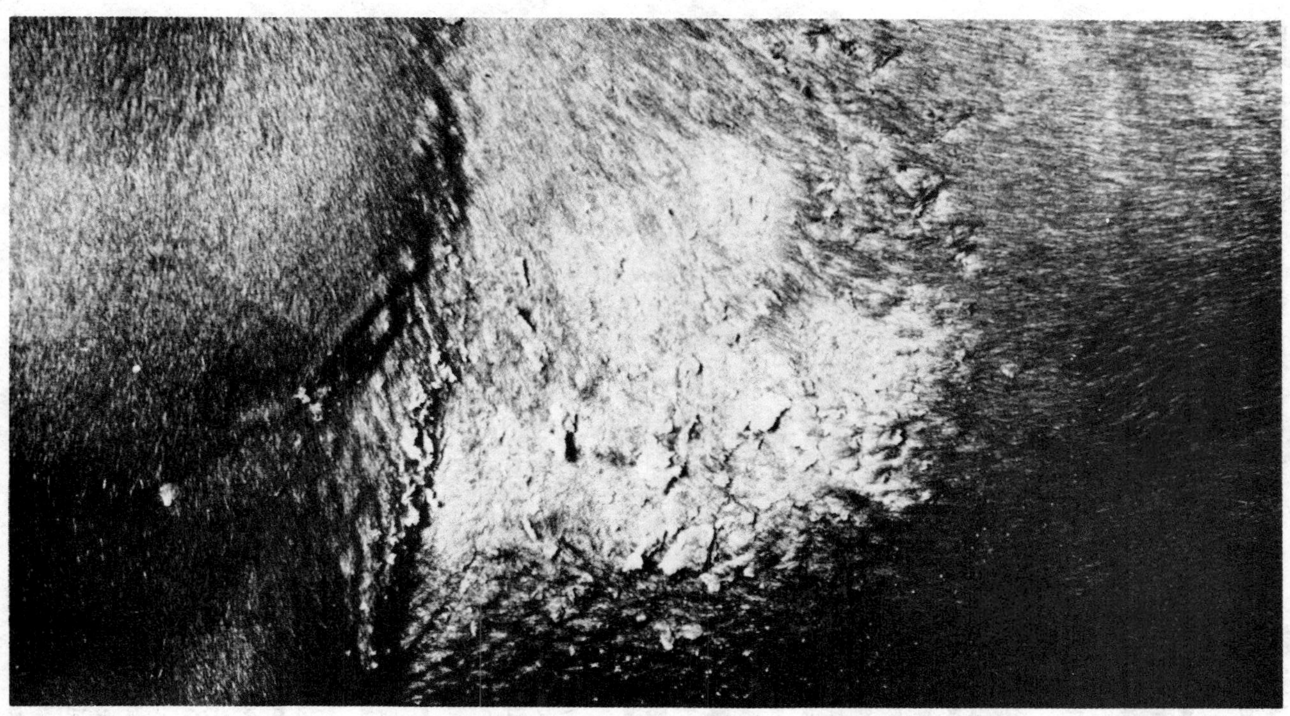

Fig. 84
Scurfy appearance of the skin in the girth region of a horse with ringworm.

A definite diagnosis of ringworm can be readily made from examination of skin scrapings under a microscope.

Treatment Because ringworm is a self-limiting disease and spontaneous recovery is likely to occur over a period, doubt has been expressed as to the value of any treatment for ringworm. Nevertheless, treatment, if well carried out, will arrest the spread of the disease and this can be important.

There are many iodine-based preparations on the market for the topical treatment of ringworm and most have to be well dabbed or sprayed on the affected areas. Where the disease is detected early and there are only a few lesions, the hair round the region should have tincture of iodine applied to it. Whitfields Ointment, or 10 per cent ammoniated mercury ointment, and many other dressings are used, but none has been shown to be outstanding. There are a number of new anti-fungal agents on the market which are said to be effective in the treatment of ringworm, but which should be used under veterinary supervision. *Captan*, a new fungicide used for the treatment of plant fungi, has been found to be very useful for the treatment of ringworm. A newer fungicidal preparation called *Natamycin* has been shown to be effective where other treatments are not successful. In many cases the disease will clear spontaneously within 6 to 12 weeks, and when only a few lesions are present no treatment may be necessary.

Control In addition to the measures outlined under "treatment", affected horses should be treated as soon as they are found and segregated until the lesions have healed. The premises of stabled horses and all grooming equipment, harness, saddles and rugs should be cleaned and disinfected.

ROARING AND WHISTLING — LARYNGEAL HEMIPLEGIA (Broken-wind)

These are chronic conditions which are characterised by an unnatural noise that can be heard when the horse is breathing deeply from exertion. The only difference is the pitch of the note, which is higher in whistling than in roaring. The noise is made during inspiration of air into the lungs and in severe cases may be accompanied by difficult or laboured breathing. The condition is seen most commonly in thoroughbred and other light horses, particularly those over 16 hands in height. It is rare in ponies and mules. The incidence is greatest in animals 3 to 6 years old.

Cause There is still debate concerning the cause of roaring, but most authorities agree that the condition is hereditary. Roaring results from degeneration of the left recurrent laryngeal nerve, giving rise to partial or complete paralysis of the muscles on the left side of the larynx.

Symptoms In chronic roaring there is no sign of any disease of the larynx, although an experienced veterinarian may, by palpation, be able to detect evidence of the wasted condition of the muscles in question. Unless the muscles on both sides of the larynx are affected, the horse shows no symptoms when at rest, but if a light horse is galloped some distance, or a draught horse made to pull a heavy load uphill, the roaring or whistling sound on inspiration is soon evident. As the condition becomes worse the horse will make the roaring noise at slower paces and will lack stamina due to insufficient air entering the lungs. Veterinarians have a special instrument called a rhinolaryngoscope with which it is possible to see the paralysed cartilage and vocal cord of the larynx.

Treatment There is no medicinal treatment for chronic roaring or whistling as it is impossible to restore the degenerated nerve or the wasted muscle. Various operations are carried out to overcome the roaring, the most recent of which involves insertion of a prosthetic material into the larynx to simulate the action of the paralysed muscles. Success rates with this operation are in the region of 60 to 70 per cent. This surgery is usually combined with the older operation of stripping the lining membrane from the little pouch which lies between the vocal cord and the laryngeal wall.

RUPTURE

See *Hernia*

SALIVARY CALCULI (Cheek Stones)

A calculus ("stone") is sometimes formed in the duct of the parotid salivary gland (*Stenson's duct*), along the side of the face of the horse. It appears as a hard, sharply defined, slightly movable swelling and may attain considerable size. The salivary duct is usually distended behind the swelling and, when the flow of saliva is entirely shut off, the gland beneath the ear becomes enlarged. Inflammation is seldom present, but infection may occur and lead to abscess formation.

Treatment A minor operation is necessary to remove the calculus, but this should be carried out by a veterinarian.

SANDCRACK

A sandcrack is a fissure in the horn of the wall of the foot which commences immediately below the coronary band and extends part of the way or right down the wall. These fissures are narrow, and, as a general rule, they follow the direction of the horn fibres. They may occur on any part of the wall, but the common situations are directly in front of the hoof, when they are termed toe cracks, or to the side of the hoof, when they are known as quarter cracks. True toe cracks are most common in the hind feet, whereas quarter cracks nearly always affect the fore feet, where they are seen more commonly on the inside quarter of the foot. The term "*complete sandcrack*" means that the crack extends from the coronary band to the ground surface. This occurs more commonly in a toe crack than in a quarter crack, which is generally incomplete. The seriousness of sandcracks depends on whether they are superficial, involving only the outer parts of the wall, or whether they are deep, involving the whole thickness of the wall and penetrating to the soft tissues beneath.

Cause Faulty conformation predisposes a horse to sandcrack, but any horse having dry, brittle hooves is liable to develop the trouble. Furthermore, anything that interferes with the proper secretion of horn at the coronet, such as an injury sustained from a tread, from over-reaching or other accidental wounding of the coronary band, can lead to the condition. Overgrown toes of the hind feet may lead to continual pressure on the coronary substance by the small pastern bone, thus interfering with its function and causing sandcrack. Excessive rasping of the outer surface of the hoof, which renders the horn brittle; alternate changes from damp to dry conditions of standing; excessive dryness and unskilful shoeing, are some of the other predisposing causes. Concussion from fast work on hard roads and jumping, especially in association with other factors, plays a part in the causation of sandcracks and more particularly quarter cracks.

Symptoms The presence of the crack in the horn is the most obvious symptom. When the crack is superficial, lameness is not shown, but when it is deep, pinching of the soft structures may occur, or infection supervene, causing lameness. Extensive injury to the coronet immediately above the sandcrack causes swelling, which may ultimately give rise to the condition known as false quarter. Various complications can occur following infection of a deep sandcrack.

Treatment Sandcracks are treated according to their location and extent. In a simple case, where the crack is superficial and close under the

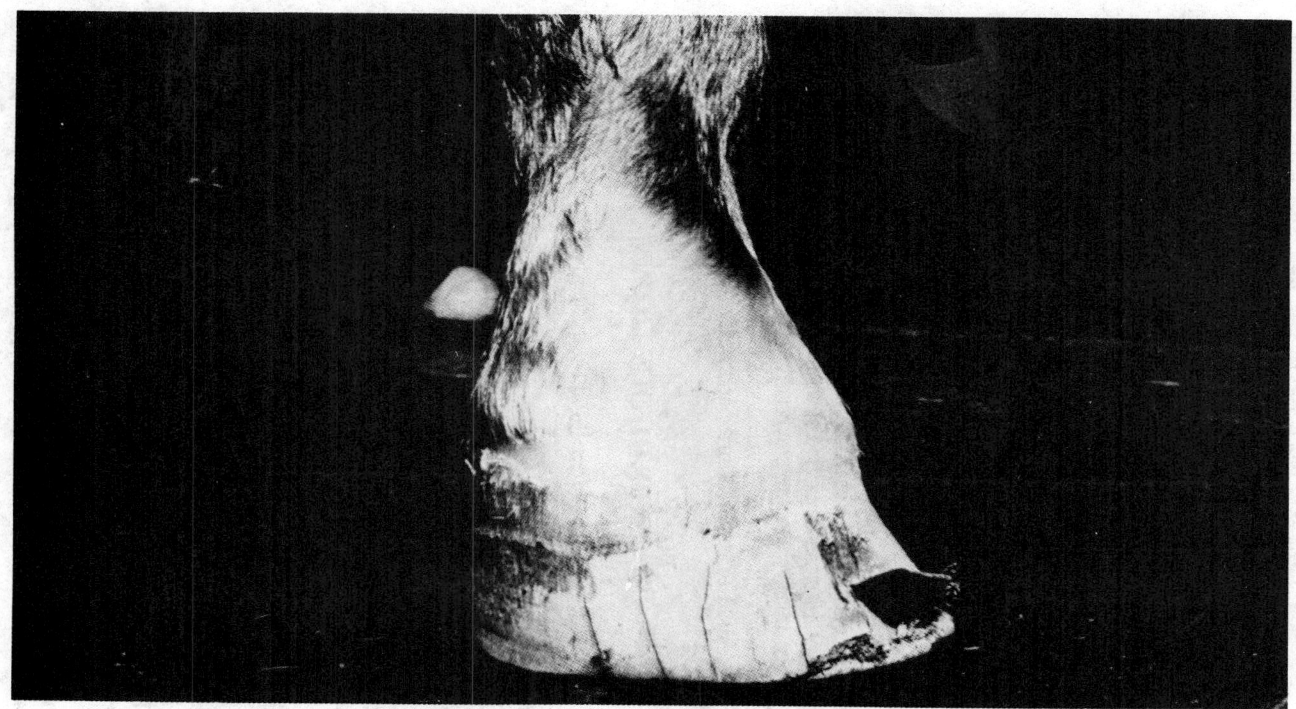

Fig. 85
Sandcracks in the front of the hoof.

coronary margin, blistering of the coronet will stimulate horn growth sufficiently to overcome the crack. Alternatively, the coronet may be clipped immediately above the crack and a horizontal line made 2.5 cm long and about 6 mm deep with a hot iron just below the coronary band through the upper end of the crack. Afterwards the blister should be applied to the coronary band above the sandcrack. This blister might be repeated to advantage in a fortnight. Before shoeing, the ground surface of the foot where the crack would normally end should be cut away to relieve pressure.

In complicated cases, where infection has occurred and there is acute lameness, hot antiseptic foot-baths, or the application of poultices are indicated to reduce the inflammation and help to control the infection. Antibiotics are used to greater advantage in infected cases, and for this reason these cases should receive veterinary attention. If the crack is very complicated and has refused to yield to other forms of treatment, a surgical operation can be carried out under an anaesthetic, when a portion of the horn involved in the crack is removed. A long spell is necessary until new horn fills the uncovered space. Acrylics, a form of plastic, are now being used to repair injuries and defects in horses' hooves.

SCIRRHOUS CORD

This is a hard fibrous enlargement of the cut end of the spermatic cord in castrated horses.

Causes The condition is caused by infection of the stump of the spermatic cord by *Staphylococcal* or *Streptococcal* organisms at the time of, or shortly after, castration. Chronic abscesses with thick fibrous walls are produced, interspersed with a mass of granulomatous tissue, the whole of which may weigh 3 to 4 kg. This type of infection usually occurs when horses are not properly exercised after castration.

Symptoms The first symptom is usually incomplete healing of the castration wound, some swelling in the region, and the discharge of thick pus. This discharge may cease after a while, but the swelling continues to increase slowly in size. The swelling causes a stiff, straddling gait, and may be felt as a hard mass in the groin, connected above with the cord.

The infected mass can proliferate over several years and in some cases a horse castrated as a yearling may not show signs of a problem until he is 3 or 4 years old. In these cases the horses may present with hind leg lameness or a stiff gait, and the infected cord will have moved into the abdomen where it can be felt on rectal palpation.

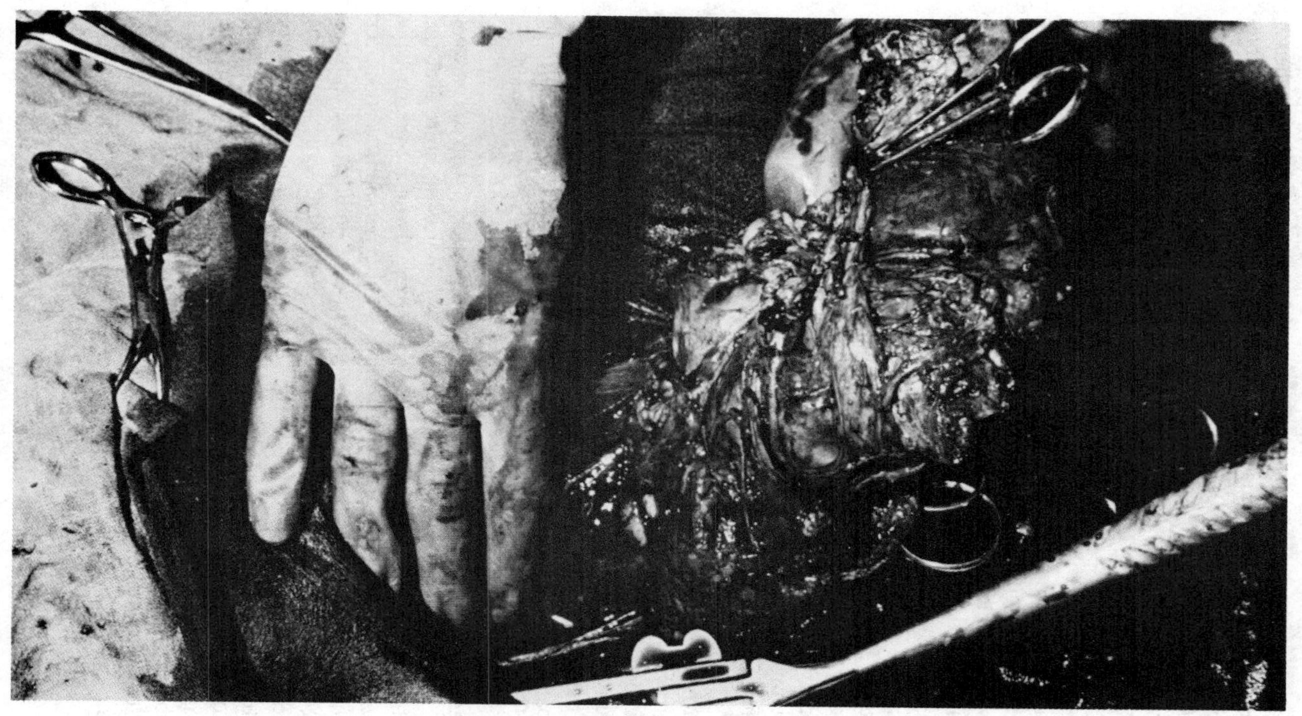

Fig. 86
Surgical removal of a scirrhous cord after infection of a castration wound. The infected tissue weighed 3 kg.

Treatment The treatment is surgery under an anaesthetic. Arrangements should be made for the operation to be carried out before the mass has become too large, otherwise it may be impracticable, or cause systemic complications.

SEEDY-TOE

Seedy-toe is a condition of the hoof in which there is a separation between the inner and outer parts of the wall, usually at the toe, but occurring elsewhere round the foot. It is a defect in the horn of the wall. The space is partly filled with degenerated crumbly horn, and the cavity may not be seen until the foot is pared after removal of the shoe.

Cause There has been much speculation as to the cause of seedy-toe, but basically it would appear to be associated with some abnormality of the coronary band following an injury, and interference with the horn-secreting substance. Bacteria and fungi, which have been reported as causing the condition, would appear to be secondary invaders.

Symptoms Seedy-toe does not usually cause lameness. This does occur, however, when the separation is large and dirt and small stones have become wedged into the space and thus cause pressure on the sensitive laminae. The cavity may be detected in the shod horse by tapping the foot on the outside with a light hammer. Once the cavity is exposed by paring the foot, the extent of the separation can be ascertained with the blade of a pocket knife or a thin nail.

Treatment A small cavity can be cleaned out, packed with cotton wool and tar and the foot shod in such a way as to relieve pressure over the area. The usual treatment for a more extensive seedy-toe is to remove the outer crust of apparently healthy wall over the separation, clean up the area thoroughly, swab with strong tincture of iodine, and apply a Stockholm tar bandage which will need protection in some way. The bandage should be renewed from time to time. A more convenient way of protecting the exposed area is to cover it with a fluid rubber preparation or other special waterproof preparations which are available. The coronary band should receive attention to stimulate horn growth by rubbing with a stimulating liniment twice a week or by application of blister. Special shoeing is desirable to relieve pressure over the affected area.

SESAMOID BONES

The sesamoid bones are 2 small, floating bones placed at the back of the fetlock joint in each limb. They are attached to the suspensory ligament and, with it, assist in keeping the lower end of the cannon bone in place on top of the sloping pastern bone, thus supporting the fetlock under stress.

Sesamoiditis Sesamoiditis is inflammation in the region of the sesamoid bones at the back of the fetlock joint, usually due to injury to the bones themselves, or to the various ligaments associated with them.

Cause

The condition may result from a blow, or from tearing of the attachments of the suspensory ligament to the sesamoid bones by strain or concussion, as may occur in jumping and, to a lesser degree, in flat racing.

Symptoms

Lameness of the affected leg and swelling at the back of the fetlock joint are the main symptoms. The swelling is hot and tender to the touch and the horse is inclined to walk on the toe. Diagnosis is not always easy and the condition is commonly mistaken for sprained fetlock or tendons. X-rays are necessary to differentiate sesamoiditis from fractures of the sesamoid bones.

Treatment

Sesamoiditis does not respond well to treatment, mainly because there is commonly tearing away of some of the fibres of the suspensory ligament from the sesamoid bones. The lameness may disappear with rest, only to return when the animal is worked. In the early stages, continuous cold water applications with a hose, or cold-water bandages, are helpful in relieving the pain and lameness. This may be followed by the application of an elastic adhesive bandage over a thick layer of cotton wool, the bandage extending from well below the fetlock joint to within about 7 cm of the knee or hock. Special shoes with high heels relieve pressure on the affected parts. Radiation therapy is sometimes useful to prevent the new bone growth associated with sesamoiditis. A rest period of at least 6 months is necessary before putting the horse back into work.

Fractures of Sesamoid Bones Fractures of the sesamoid bones occur under similar situations to those producing sesamoiditis. The symptoms tend to be very similar, however, horses with fractures of the sesamoid bones are usually more severely lame and have a greater degree of swelling at the back of the fetlock.

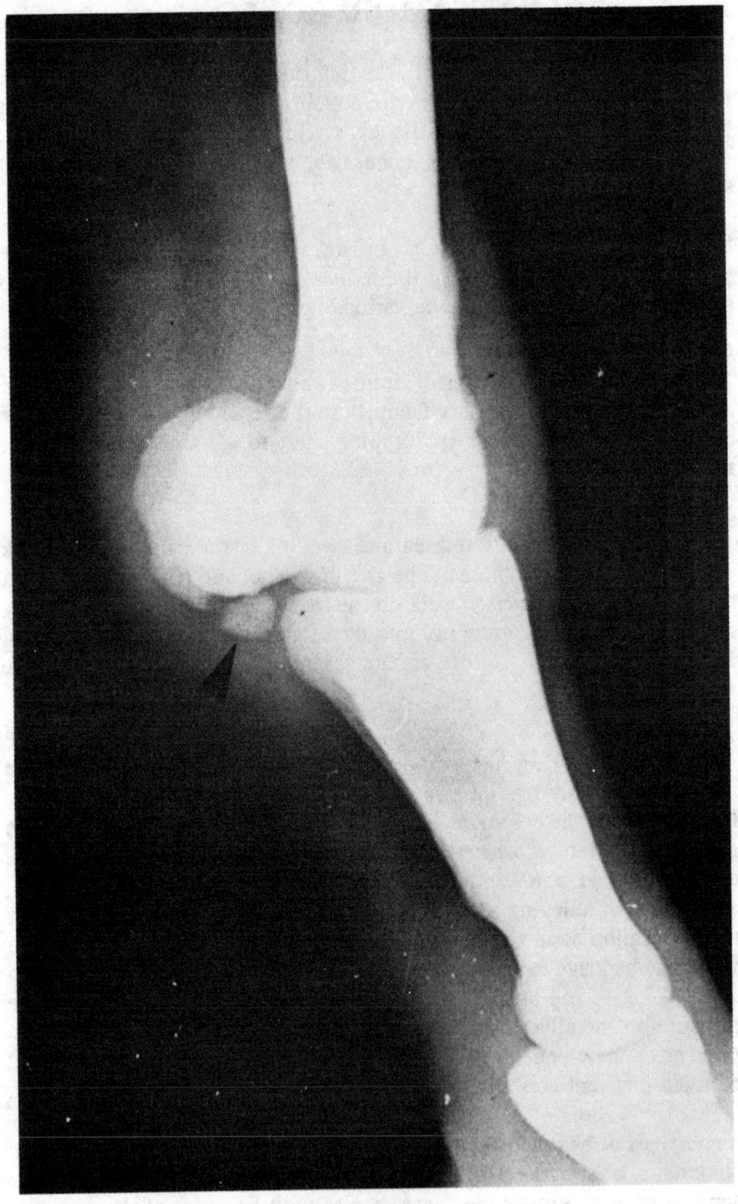

Fig. 87
X-ray of the fetlock joint showing fracture of the base of the sesamoid bone (arrow).

Treatment

X-rays are essential to diagnose the presence of a sesamoid bone fracture. If a small piece of bone is fractured from the top of the sesamoid then surgery can be performed to remove the fractured piece, and this is usually successful. However, if more than one-third of the bone is fractured then the prognosis is very poor due to substantial damage to the suspensory ligament. These types of fractures require up to 12 months to show signs of healing and even then tend to heal incompletely. Where both sesamoid bones in 1 leg are fractured this may lead to collapse of the fetlock joint, which will have no support. In such cases prolonged plaster casting, or even fusion of the fetlock joints surgically may be necessary.

SHOEING

The shoeing of horses which work on hard ground is a necessary evil. Many foot troubles will be avoided if the following rules are observed as nearly as possible when shoeing a horse:

1. Bring the wall of the foot down to what it would be if natural wear had occured
2. Fit the shoe to the outline of the foot, as rasping the outside of the wall makes it weak and brittle.
3. Never run the rasp over the outside of the wall, as it has a waterproof coat to keep in the necessary moisture and to keep out external moisture.
4. A sole cannot be too thick; it is there to protect the inner foot.
5. The bars should not be cut away; they are weight carriers, and the shoe should rest on them.
6. The frog should not be cut away; it is a cushion whose strength and function depend on it being level with the ground surface of the shoe.
7. The shoe should have a true and level bearing on the wall and bars.

SHOEING PRICKS

Lameness commonly occurs from a shoeing nail having been driven too close to or into the "quick" (*sensitive laminae*). An expert farrier knows at once when this has happened, but an amateur horse-shoer may continue to drive the nail right in.

Symptoms If the nail has pricked the sensitive laminae, lameness follows soon after shoeing. If, as is often the case, the nail has been driven too close, so that it causes pressure on, but does not prick the sensitive laminae, lameness may not be shown for up to a week afterwards. The latter condition is known as "nail-binding" and results in a bulging of the horn on to the soft structures, causing a bruise and inflammation due to the pressure. The offending nail can usually be detected by pressure with pincers or by gently tapping with a light hammer over each nail. If this is unsuccessful, the hoof should be washed and brushed with soap and water and dried. Then the shoe should be carefully removed, drawing each nail separately and examining them for evidence of blood-stain or dampness, and observing whether there is any discharge from the nail hole. The nails may not be moist and there may be no discharge observed if the horse has only been shod 2 or 3 days, but from 3 to 5 days after shoeing some pus is usually seen, and this will be more copious if the horse has been shod for a longer period.

The pain caused by these wounds is great. The horse rests the foot on the toe, raises and lowers the leg or holds it from the ground, flexes the leg and knuckles at the fetlock. Swelling of the fetlock and back tendons is frequently seen, and the foot is found to be hot.

Treatment If the nail prick is detected during shoeing, the offending nail should be withdrawn immediately, and the nail track treated with tincture of iodine or other suitable antiseptic. Another nail should not be driven in that place. If discovered later, the shoe should be removed in the manner described above, the offending nail detected, and the foot then soaked in a bucket of hot water to soften the horn and relieve pain. If the lameness is due to "nail-binding" and there is no evidence of infection, a few days of repeated soaking may overcome the condition. Paring down the sole in the vicinity of the nail hole can be carried out to relieve pressure. If, however, there is evidence of infection and pus formation, it will be necessary, after paring, to cut down over the nail hole, or at the site where pain is greatest on pressure, to permit free discharge. The wound should be syringed with a weak antiseptic solution.

The foot can now, with advantage, be immersed in a bucket of warm water to which some antiseptic, or 2 tablespoons of salt, has been added. The surgical opening must be kept free until all discharge has ceased, and the area protected with a pad of cotton wool or tow, soaked in antiseptic, and held in place by an improvised boot. A good plan is to protect the foot by using an Ezy-Boot. This also facilitates subsequent dressings. A warm kaolin poultice may also be applied in a similar manner. Any horse which has sustained a nail prick of the sensitive laminae should receive an injection of tetanus antitoxin. Neglected nail punctures, or those which have not been thoroughly treated, often lead to spread of infection within the foot and other complications. Veterinarians use antibiotics to control the infection.

SHOULDER LAMENESS

Shoulder lameness is not as common a condition as is sometimes thought, and many suspected cases of lameness in the shoulder are found to be due to injuries lower down the limb, such as navicular disease, and foot injuries. Nevertheless, there are genuine shoulder lamenesses. Sprain of tendons, muscles and ligaments, and inflammation of the shoulder joint occur. Injury of the suprascapular nerve results in a bulging of the shoulder and may be the cause of muscular atrophy or wasting, commonly called "sweeny". *Osteochondrosis dessicans* of the shoulder joint also occurs and is seen in yearling and 2 year old horses (see *Osteochondrosis dessicans*).

Causes Amongst the causes of shoulder lameness are a fall, accompanied by violent concussion; a mis-step following a quick muscular effort; a jump with faulty landing; a slip on a wet, smooth road and collision with another horse or other object.

Symptoms The diagnosis of shoulder lameness is sometimes difficult, and, although some of the symptoms of shoulder lameness are fairly definite, care is necessary not to confuse the suspected lameness in this region with trouble elsewhere in the limb. Lameness is more marked when the shoulder joint is involved than when the muscles alone are affected. Broadly, shoulder lameness is diagnosed by a restricted movement of the scapula (shoulder blade), marked lifting of the head as the limb is advanced, and a short step. The peculiar manner in which the leg is brought forward for another step in the act of walking or trotting is, in some instances, characteristic of injuries to the shoulder. The leg is brought forward with a bending round-swinging motion, and a shortening in the extension of the step. Lameness is often worse when travelling over soft ground, in contradistinction to foot lameness, when it is lessened. The foot is carried close to the ground due to the shoulder being insufficiently raised and stumbling is frequent, especially on uneven ground. Lameness is often worse when the horse is trotted uphill. When backed, the horse will often drag the foot of the affected limb.

Atrophy or wasting of the muscles of the shoulder should not be diagnosed immediately as injury to the suprascapular nerve, because it may be due to inactivity of the animal and disuse of the shoulder muscles because of a painful condition elsewhere in the leg.

Treatment Rest from work is the most important part of the treatment of shoulder lameness. Cold water applications from a hose, alternated with hot, wet blankets, are of value. Repeated massage over the affected area and the use of a mild liniment will be found beneficial.

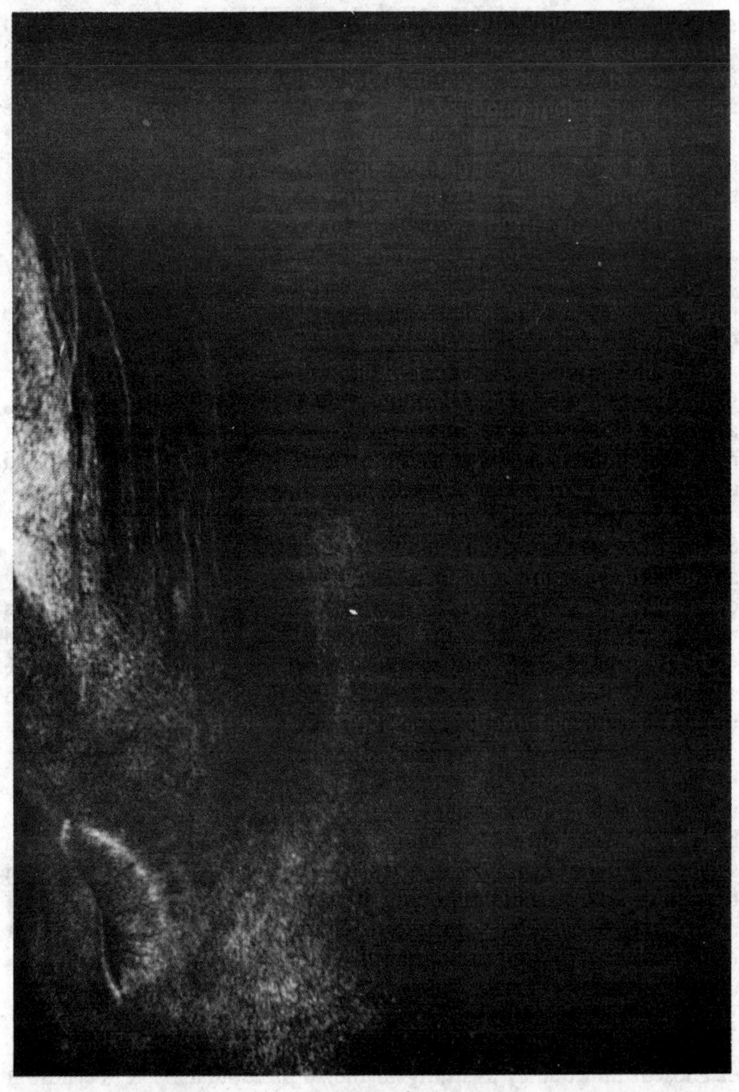

Fig. 88
Shoulder lameness. Wasting of the muscles over the left shoulder due to sweeney. Note the prominence of the shoulder blade.

Many shoulder conditions are the result of inflammation and so anti-inflammatory drugs can be used to relieve the pain and inflammation. Following this a spell of 3 to 12 months is necessary depending on the severity of the condition.

SIDEBONE

Attached to the wings of the pedal bone (coffin bone) within the hoof, and extending above the hoof at the coronet, are the lateral cartilages. These cartilages, one on each side of each foot, are normally very resilient, forming a shock-absorbing apparatus within the hoof. The formation of bone within these cartilages produces sidebones. Hardening of the cartilages has the effect of cramping the structures of the internal part of the foot and may eventually lead to lameness, although this is not common. Sidebones are especially frequent in draught types of horses and are not so prone to occur in light horses. They occur chiefly in the front feet and are usually bilateral.

Cause Although heredity plays a part in the development of sidebone, it is now considered that ossification of the lateral cartilages is a normal physiological process in the horse, especially in certain breeds. There are, however, a great many horses and ponies in which sidebone does not occur. Partial sidebone may occur in horses as they advance in age, and become complete in old age. Repeated concussion upon the pedal bone to which the cartilage is attached undoubtedly plays a part in the causation of sidebone, whilst contracted heels, ringbone, navicular disease, punctured wounds of the foot, quarter cracks, and even laminitis can be contributing causes.

Symptoms In many instances, sidebones are of slow growth and, being usually unaccompanied by acute inflammation, they cause no lameness until, because of their size, they interfere with the action of the joint. In the earlier stages of the condition there may be slight inflammation, when heat can be detected over the seat of the affected cartilage, and there will be slight lameness, which later disappears. Since the deposit of bony matter often begins in that part of the cartilage where it is attached to the pedal bone, the diseased process may exist for some time before it can be felt or seen. Later on, however, the cartilage can be felt to have lost its elastic character, and by standing in front of the animal a prominence of the coronary region at the quarters can be seen.

Treatment Should there be lameness in the early stages of the disease, this can be relieved by frequent soaking of the foot in cold water or by the

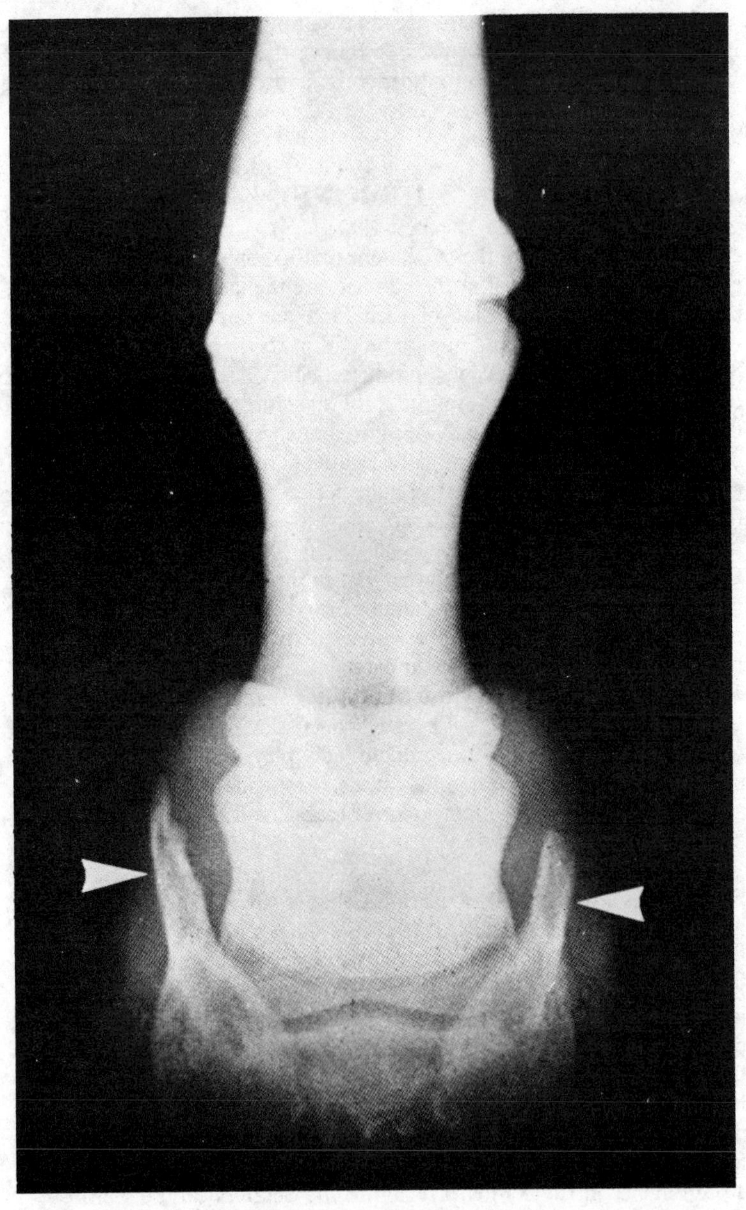

Fig. 89
X-ray of the foot showing sidebones (arrows).

use of cold water bandages. The treatment for later lameness, which may occur when the hoof is contracted, consists of lowering the heels (to allow good frog pressure), thinning the horn of the hoof below the sidebone with a rasp and applying a blister to the coronary region on the affected side. This allows expansion of the hoof, with relief of pressure within the hoof. Special shoeing can be carried out to expand the hoof. A veterinary surgeon can do more by an operation. Many horses have sidebones without causing them any inconvenience, particularly if they work on soft ground. If the sidebones fracture then the horse may show severe lameness.

SKIN DISEASES

See *Eczema, Leg Mange, Lice, Photosensitisation, Queensland Itch, Ringworm*

SLEEPY FOAL DISEASE (Actinobacillosis)

This is an acute, highly-fatal, septicaemic disease of newborn foals, caused by an organism now known as *Actinobacillus equuli*, but formerly as *Shigella equirulis*. This organism is common in the intestinal tract and tissues of normal mares, in which it does not cause disease.

Because foals may be observed sick at birth, or within a few hours and up to 3 days of birth, it would appear that infection of the foal occurs in the uterus of the mare, but could occur through the navel after birth. The disease is responsible for the deaths of many young foals in most countries, including Australia. The symptoms are sleepiness, lethargy, prostration, high fever, diarrhoea, rapid respiration, and the foal ceasing to suck its mother.

Many foals die within 12 to 24 hours. Those that survive the acute stage of the disease develop inflammation of the joints and abscesses of the muscles, and are lame. The latter animals usually die within a week, when post-mortem examination shows abscesses in kidneys and elsewhere.

Owing to the rapid onset of the symptoms and the development of septicaemia, treatment is difficult and calls for the early administration of specific antibiotics and supportive treatment by a veterinarian.

SORE BACKS

See *Back Disorders*

SORE SHINS

"Sore shins" is the term given to acute inflammation of the front of the large cannon bone of the fore leg. The same condition is sometimes seen on the front of the cannon bone of the hind leg. The trouble occurs more commonly in young horses when first put to work, especially in racehorses during the early weeks of training.

Causes In young horses, concussion appears to be the most important causative factor, because the symptoms are observed after exercise. The front of the cannon bone seems to be an area that receives a lot of the force of the galloping horse.

Symptoms In young animals, there is a hot, painful swelling in the front of one or both large cannon bones of the fore legs, and, much less frequently, of those of the hind legs. Lameness is present and the horse walks with a short stride. The swelling subsequently thickens, when the heat and pain are less. This is due to production of new bone which appears to strengthen the front of the cannon bone.

Treatment Rest is essential until all soreness and inflammation have disappeared. The acute inflammation may be relieved by cold packs or by hosing the affected legs. *Antiphlogistine,* or *Amoricaine* may be found useful to relieve the inflammation. Anti-inflammatory drugs, such as *phenylbutazone,* are also helpful. Although acute symptoms may have disappeared after 7 to 10 days, at least 3 months' rest is necessary to prevent recurrence of the condition. Blistering and firing are carried out on some horses, but appear to have no beneficial effects apart from enforcing a spell.

SPAVIN

Spavin means a disease of the hock of a horse, of which there are 2 common types, *bone spavin* and *bog spavin.*

Bone Spavin This occurs in two forms, true or "jack" spavin, and occult or hidden spavin. True bone spavin might be described simply as a chronic arthritis, which may eventually result in the union of the small bones at the inner and lower part of the hock, so that they become a solid mass. The enlargement caused by the exostosis (abnormal outgrowth of bone) is usually greatest on the inner side of the joint. It may be most easily observed by comparing the hocks one with another, standing outside each fore leg in turn to look at the inner sides of the hocks; or it

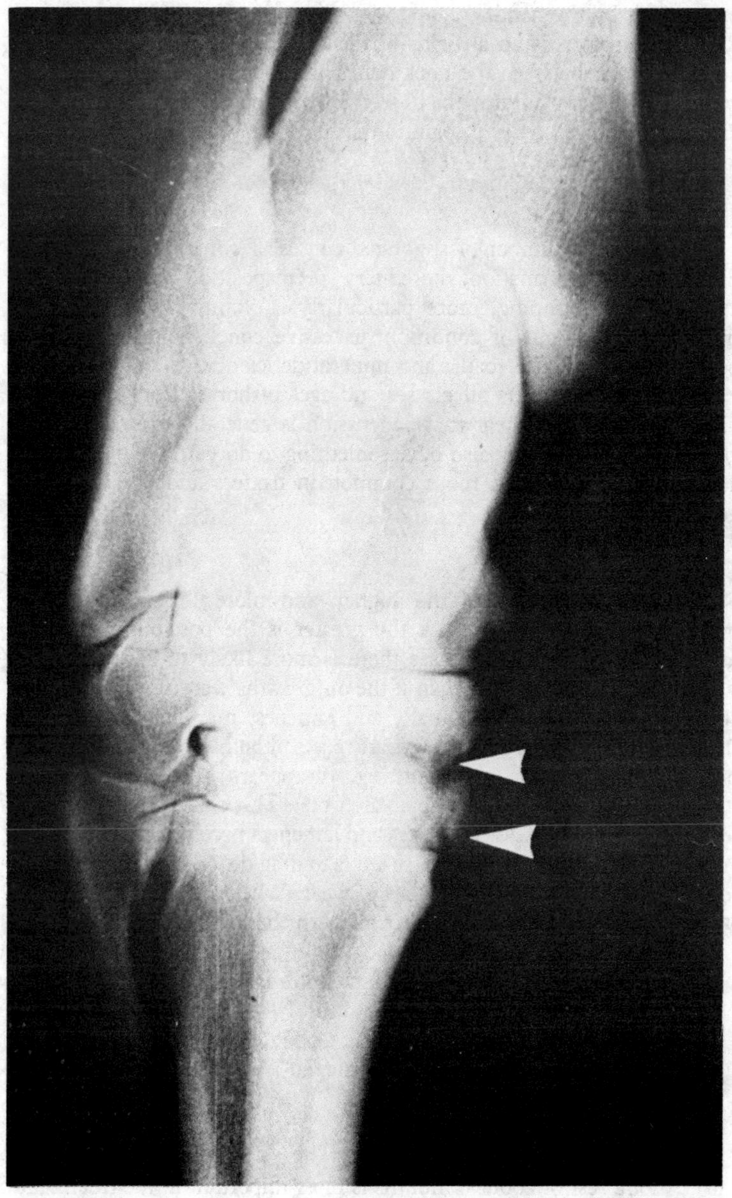

Fig. 90
X-ray of the hock of a horse with bone spavin showing destruction of the joint spaces (arrows).

may be felt by the hand.

Occult spavin is an arthritis of the articular surfaces (joints) of the hock bones, or between the hock bones and the cannon bone, but there are no visible bony outgrowths as seen in true bone spavin. It can only be diagnosed from evidence of pain in the hock joint and x-rays of the hock joint.

Causes

There are a number of suggested causes of bone spavin, including faulty hock conformation; hereditary predisposition; injury or over exertion as in jumping, more particularly in young horses when not trained or when out of condition; excessive concussion, as occurs in horses trotted on hard roads; and mineral deficiency.

Bone spavin affects all classes and ages of horses from 2 year olds onwards. It would appear that concussion is generally one of the main causes of spavin. It may also have something to do with the type of gait, as bone spavin is much more common in trotters and pacers than in gallopers.

Symptoms

In true bone spavin, the higher and more forward the bony outgrowths occur on the hock the greater is the possibility of severe lameness, because in such cases there is more likely to be interference with the action of the joint than if the outgrowths were at the side. Bone spavin usually develops gradually and lameness may be noticed before there is any bony enlargement. In early cases of both types the lameness is noticed first thing in the morning, disappears after the horse has "warmed up", only to return again after rest. This characteristic becomes less marked as the disease advances and lameness becomes more constant. As the disease progresses the horse tends to drag the toe, consequently the toe of the shoe or hoof shows signs of wear. When standing, the horse is inclined to rest the toe on the ground with the heel slightly raised.

A well-recognised test for bone spavin, although not infallible, is to lift the affected leg from the ground, holding the foot high so that the cannon bone is parallel to the ground for 1 to 2 minutes, and then have the horse trotted as soon as the leg is released. The lameness will then be greatly intensified and so assist in diagnosis. A comparison should be made with the other hock.

Treatment

A long rest of about 6 months is most important in the treatment of bone spavin. In the early stages, cold water applications by continued hosing may assist in arresting the progress of the inflammation.

The injection of *Healon* into the affected joints can result in relief of

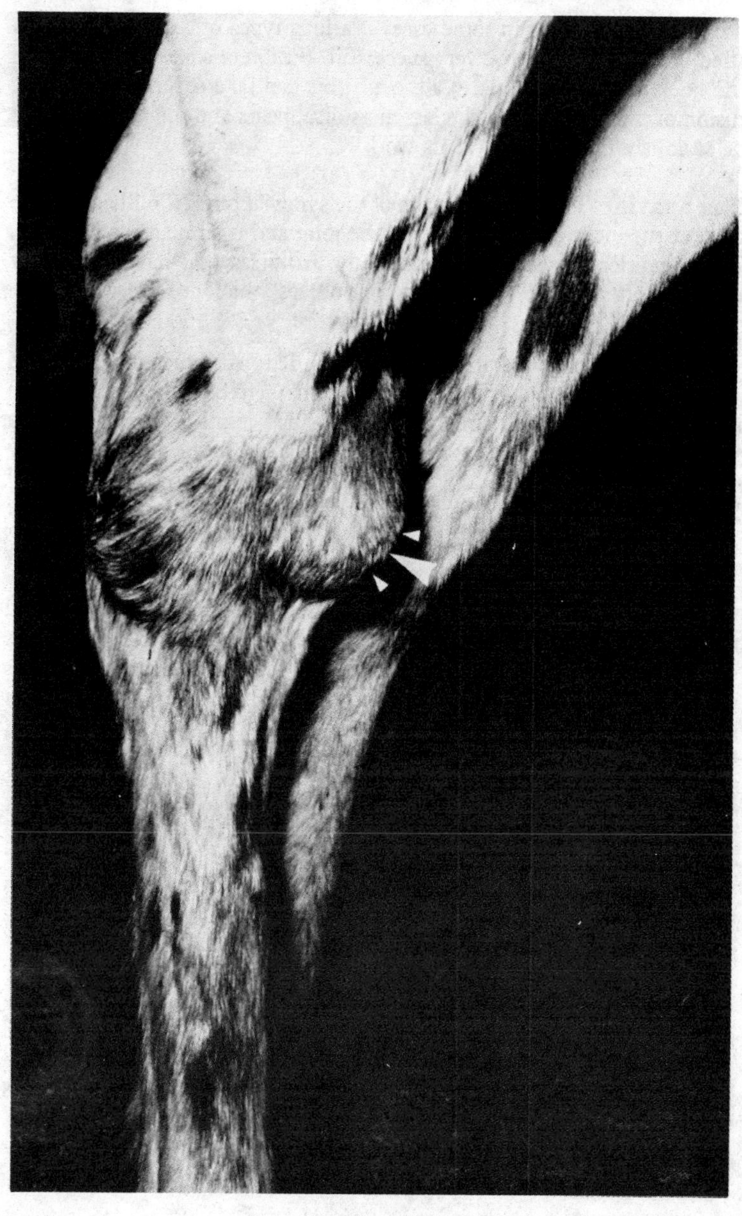

Fig. 91
Bog spavin (arrows) affecting the hock.

the signs of lameness in some cases. Various types of surgery have been tried, but none seem to be very successful. Fusion of some of the bones of the hock usually takes place, although this can take several years. Once fusion of the bones occurs the lameness disappears and the horse may not be seriously incapacitated in its work.

Bog Spavin This is a distension of the synovial bursa ("oil-bag") of the hock at the inner and upper part of the joint and is similar to a windgall. The condition is seen more commonly in horses that have straight or upright hocks. It also occurs in young horses which are overworked.

Causes

Although bog spavin is often regarded as indicating inherited weakness of the hock joint, the condition is frequently seen in aged stallions and breeding mares with well-shaped joints, when it is due to strain of the hocks. In young horses, it may be due to the greater elasticity of the joint structures and result from slipping backwards with the hind legs. Bog spavin is a chronic non-inflammatory effusion of fluid into the main hock joint.

Symptoms

The condition appears as a soft, fluctuating swelling about one-third the way down on the front and towards the inside of the hock. It is usually not hot to the touch and does not cause lameness. If there is lameness it indicates that the condition is complicated by inflammation and bone involvement. Therefore x-rays should be taken to determine if bone damage exists.

Treatment

Bog spavin is usually not a serious condition and sometimes disappears without any form of treatment. Rest is an essential part of the treatment. If there is no heat in the swelling and there is no lameness, it is unwise to attempt to reduce the size of the swelling, the best treatment being to turn the horse out into a well-grassed paddock.

In those cases that do not respond to rest and simple treatment the excess fluid in the joint capsule can be aspirated and steroid type preparations injected by a veterinarian. Following this a tight pressure bandage applied over cotton wool is necessary to keep pressure over the hock joint. With this treatment there is still only a 50 per cent success rate.

SPEEDY-CUT

Speedy-cut is the name given to an injury on the inner surface of the lower part of the knee, caused by the horse striking it with the inner portion of the shoe of the opposite foot, at fast pace.

Horses with faulty leg or foot conformation, or those which are very tired, especially if forced over rough ground, are most likely to sustain the injury. There may or may not be an actual cut in the skin, but in any case the bruise which results can be serious and the pain caused may bring the horse down. The leg swells and is very painful. When the blow is often repeated, as is common, a permanent enlargement remains.

Treatment and Prevention Hot fomentations, followed by the application of a cold water bandage, are recommended for a fresh speedy-cut. If the skin is cut, it should be treated as an open wound with mild antiseptics (see *Wound Treatment*).

To prevent speedy-cutting, shoe the opposite foot as close as possible at the inside toe and quarter, rasping off some of the wall if necessary, and rounding off the lower edge of the web of the shoe. Special speedy-cutting boots, or a pad of felt or rubber on the inner side of the shoe of the striking foot may be required.

When buying a riding horse, it is important to look and feel for old scars or enlargements from previous injuries.

A horse which continually "speedy-cuts" is dangerous to the rider.

SPLINTS

A splint is a bony outgrowth between the cannon bone and one or both of the small "splint bones". These are found on each side of the rear surface of the cannon bones of the fore and hind legs, and extend from the knee or hock to about the lower third of the main bone. The bony outgrowth results from inflammation of the fibrous membrane covering the bone, or of the ligamentous attachment between the cannon and the splint bone.

Young horses are most prone to splints, which occur more commonly on the fore legs and usually on the inside of the leg. Occasionally they appear on the outside of the leg. At times splints are found on the outside and inside of the hind legs.

During evolutionary processes, the horse developed from a 5-toed animal into one which moved on a greatly modified and developed structure corresponding to the original middle claw. Instead of walking with the claw flat on the ground, it eventually walked on the point, and this became enclosed in a hoof. In the process, most of the other bones disappeared.

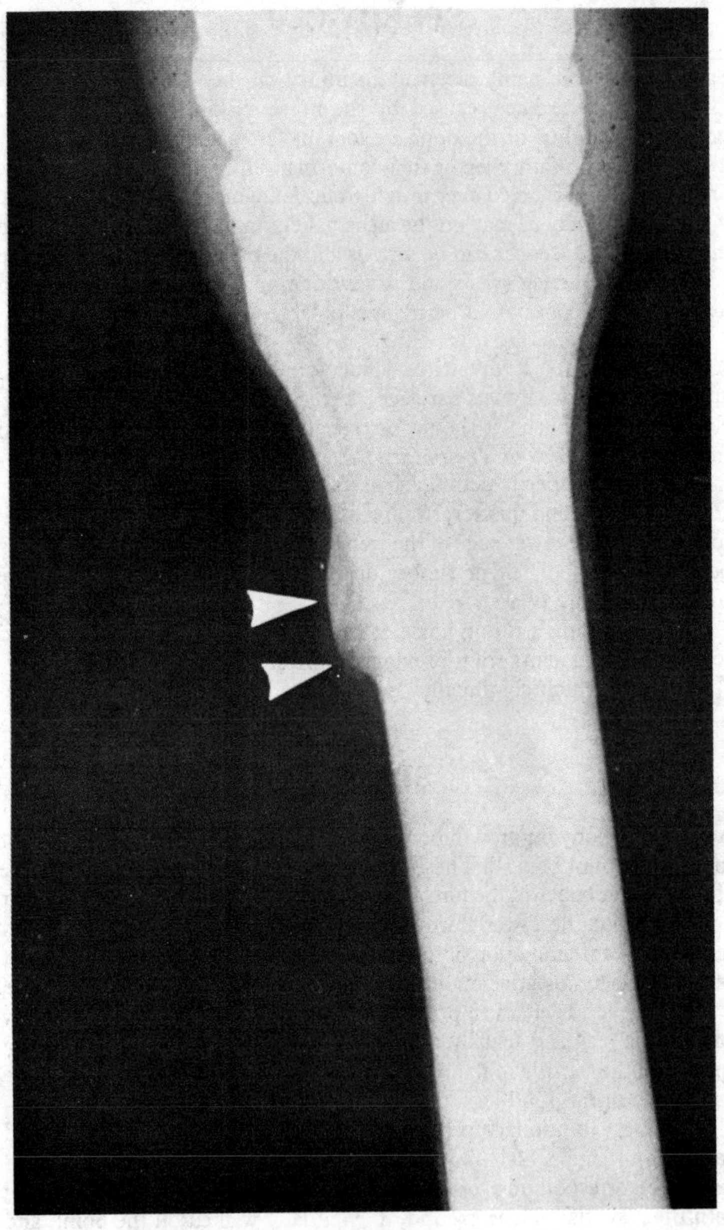

Fig. 92
X-rays of the cannon bone of a horse with a splint.

In the animal we know, the knee corresponds to the wrist, and the hock to the heel of the human, and the main bones below that have developed only from the central 1 of the original 5.

Just below the knee and the hock, on each side of the cannon bones, a remnant remains of the 2 adjoining bones. These are known as the splint bones. They form part of the joint with the knee or hock, but gradually diminish in size until they disappear about two-thirds of the way down the cannon bone.

In the young horse, the shafts of the splint bones are attached to the cannon bone by a ligament, which is gradually replaced by bone as the horse ages.

Strain on the joining ligament in young horses is the most common cause of trouble, but if this period is passed safely, the development of splints is not as likely.

Causes In the majority of cases, the bony deposit known as "splint" appears at the junction of the splint bone and the cannon bone — usually in young horses, before bony union has taken place between these bones. Sprain of the ligamentous attachment between the cannon bone and the splint bone, or injury to the membranous covering of the bone, is likely to give rise to an exostosis of bony material — a splint. Sometimes the exostosis is confined to the cannon bone, when it is usually due to a blow.

Fast movement on hard ground causes repeated concussion effects through the column of bones between the knee and the fetlock, and is a common cause of splints. The condition occurs quite commonly during the training of young horses or when they are first put to heavy work. Jumping is also a cause of splints, not so much because of striking the leg against a rail or fence, but from the concussion of landing on the other side of the hurdle. Horses with poor conformation and bad action are likely to strike themselves, producing mechanical damage leading to splints. The hind legs are much less exposed to the effects of concussion than the forelegs. Splints on the hind legs, when they do occur, seldom cause much trouble. The most common conformational fault associated with splints is where the cannon bone is set to the outside of the knee.

Symptoms Lameness may occur before any swelling appears on the bone. Careful examination should be made along the inside and the outside of the cannon bone for evidence of tenderness under pressure with the fingers. To examine a limb for splints, the knee or hock should be flexed with the cannon bone parallel to the ground and, with the thumb on one side and the fingers on the other side, pressed evenly from the knee downwards along the junction of the large and small bones. When splints are forming, a slight swelling may be felt. The inflamed part will be hot, and the animal will show pain by snatching the leg away when the part is pressed. A hind leg may be similarly examined.

Horses with splints may walk normally, but be lame at the trot. Lameness increases with exercise. The bony enlargements, which appear some time after lameness is shown, may develop to the size of a pea or a walnut and are sometimes of a longish and irregular form. The lameness occasioned by a recently-formed splint is in no way proportional to the size of the bony outgrowth. Small splints often cause severe lameness, while large ones sometimes occasion little or no inconvenience. There are a number of reasons for this, associated with the extent of the inflammatory processes, but the seriousness of splints depends mainly on their location. A splint which does not interfere with a joint, tendon, ligament or nerve, causes lameness only during the period of formation. When splints are near the knee or hock joints, or touching the back tendons, they are very troublesome.

Treatment In foals and yearlings, splints often disappear spontaneously, and treatment of these young animals should not be hurried. The mineral intake of the young horses should be checked and deficiencies or imbalance corrected. Rest is an essential part of treatment for splints and the lameness resulting therefrom, but a little regular walking exercise is desirable. This is best obtained if the animal can be turned out into a well-grassed paddock where it will obtain sufficient exercise while grazing. Reduction of recent splints can be assisted by a veterinarian injecting cortisone along the bone and application of a pressure bandage. To apply a pressure bandage, cotton wool padding is used over the area and then a crepe or cotton conforming bandage used to apply pressure over the region of the splint and cannon. If reduction of the splint has not occurred and lameness still persists after 4 to 6 weeks then x-rays of the area will be necessary to determine if a fracture of the splint bone exists. With simple splints a spell of 3 months is usually all that is required for natural resolution of the inflammation.

Prominent splints on the inside of the leg, which may be repeatedly knocked by the opposite leg, can be removed by operation. However, there is a very high rate of recurrence of these splints and a cosmetic result is not always achieved. Well formed splints seldom cause any lameness.

Finally, skilful shoeing is important to prevent striking and to effect a proper distribution of weight, thus preventing splints caused by mechanical injury.

SPRAIN OF TENDONS

See *Tendons — Sprained*

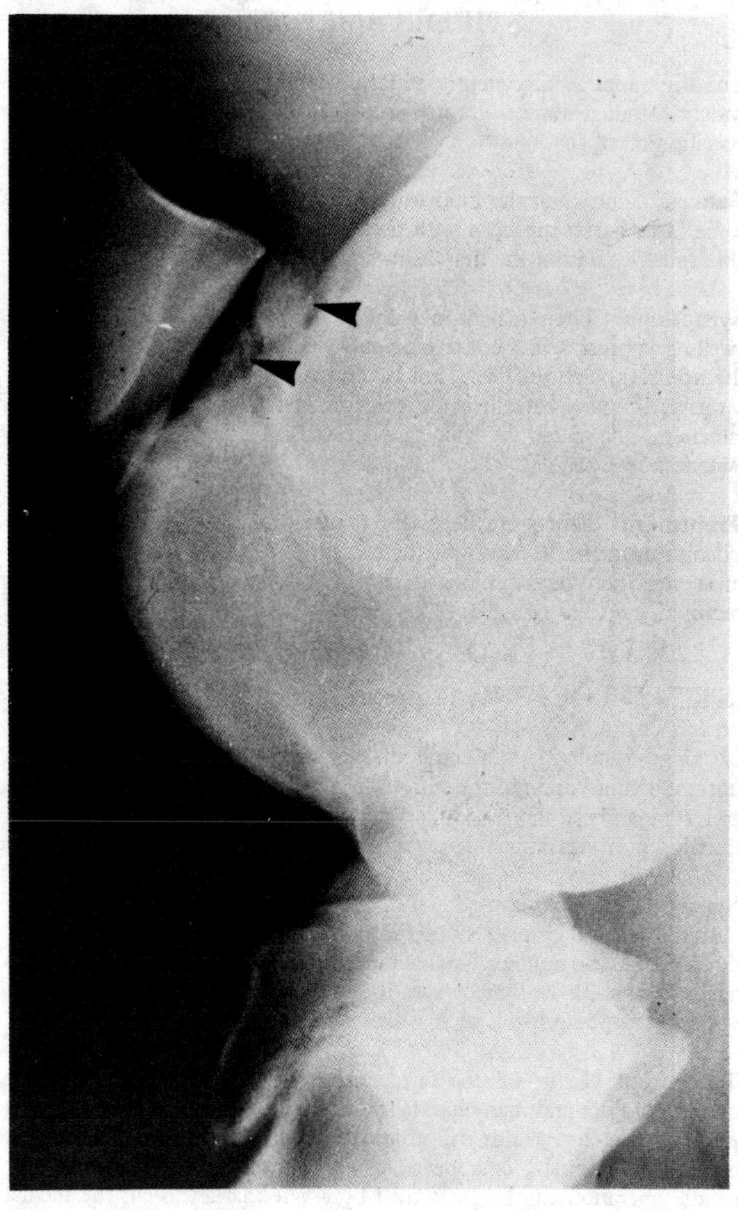

Fig. 93
X-ray of the stifle of a 2-year-old horse showing chips of bone (arrows) just above the patella (see *Stifle lameness,* p. 206).

STIFLE LAMENESS

The stifle joint is infrequently afflicted by injury, but has become more widely studied since improvement in x-ray machines allowed visualisation of the joint.

Causes Injuries to the hind leg may result in stifle lameness, but in some cases horses are born with problems in the stifle joint or develop abnormalities within the first 12 months of life.

Symptoms There may or may not be signs of swelling of the stifle. If swelling is present it is most commonly found between the ligaments at the front of the stifle. There will be a hind leg lameness which varies in severity. In many cases it is difficult to distinguish a hock from a stifle lameness. The spavin test will aggravate a stifle lameness as well as a hock lameness.

Treatment X-rays are necessary to determine the type of problem existing in the stifle. However there is little treatment that is useful for most conditions and prolonged rest periods of up to 12 months are required.

STIFLE LOCKING (Upward fixation of the patella)

Locking of the stifle is a condition usually seen in horses with a very upright conformation of the stifle. It is very common in Shetland ponies and standardbred horses. It is due to the ligaments of the kneecap catching over a prominence at the end of the femur.

Symptoms Locking of the stifle is most common first thing in the morning when the horse is moved out of its stable. It will be noted that the horse has the hind leg fixed out behind it in extension and is unable to bring it forward. In some horses the ligament slips back into a normal position and the horse is able to flex its leg and bring it forward.

Treatment In its mildest form, locking of the stifle may worry the horse very little and many horses showing symptoms of the condition as yearlings and 2 year olds will grow out of it. However, if the condition occurs continuously, or appears to worry the horse, then a relatively simple operation can be performed by a veterinarian to cut the medial patella ligament. This operation is very effective, although some horses are left with a small scar or swelling on the inside of the stifle.

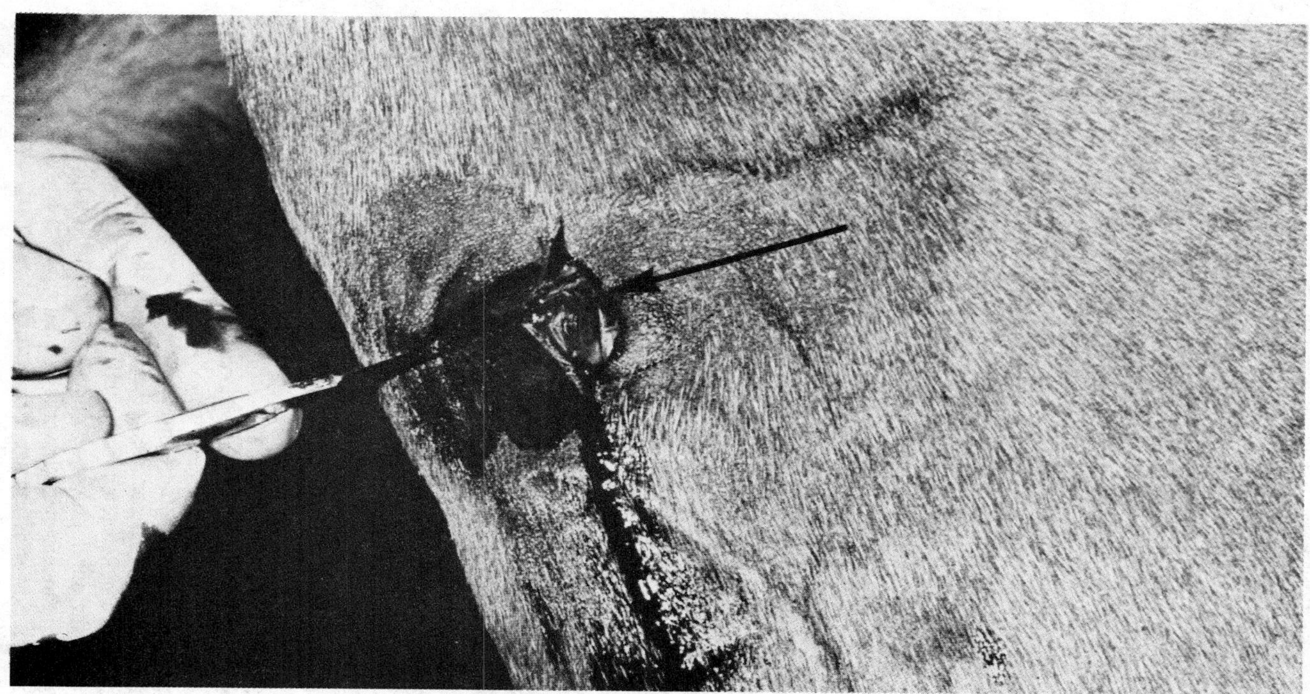

Fig. 94
Surgery to cut the medical patella ligament of the stifle to correct locking of the stifle.

STOMACH — RUPTURE OF

Rupture of the stomach is not a common condition in the horse. Nevertheless, it has occurred either from over-distension, when horses have been fed large quantities of bulky food, or have had unrestricted access to grain. It may also occur as a sequel to flatulent colic when there is great distension with gas, and has been known to occur following violent exertion such as jumping, or following a sudden fall when the stomach is distended with food or gas. Diseases of the mucous membranes of the stomach, calculi ("stones") and tumours may also be responsible.

Symptoms The general symptoms of distension of the stomach are colicky pains, which are not of much diagnostic value. Rapid and difficult breathing, sweating, trembling and staggering are common symptoms, and the horse may sit up like a dog for considerable periods and attempt to vomit. Actually some vomiting may occur, although this is difficult for the horse. The strong contractions of the abdominal muscles subject the stomach to severe pressure, which contributes to stomach rupture.

When the rupture has occurred, the attempts at vomiting cease and the horse is temporarily relieved. Cold patchy sweating and trembling continue, and there is severe congestion of the visible mucous membranes. The temperature, which is at first raised, becomes subnormal. A slimy food-stained liquid may come through the nostrils and mouth. Death follows in a few hours but may be delayed longer.

Treatment There is, of course, no treatment for rupture of the stomach.

STONES IN THE KIDNEYS, URETERS AND BLADDER

See *Urinary Calculi*

STRANGLES

Strangles, referred to in the United States of America as "distemper", is an acute contagious disease of equines, namely the horse, ass and mule. It is characterised by fever, a catarrhal inflammation of the nasal cavities and throat, and the development of abscesses in the lymph glands, especially between the branches of the lower jaw. Young horses are most commonly affected, but horses of any age can contract the disease, especially those which have not previously had it. One attack usually confers immunity for life, but sometimes the immunity breaks down and the animal can suffer a second attack. Naturally, an epidemic of strangles is more likely to occur when a number of horses are kept together, such as on stud horse farms and riding schools. The disease caused much trouble in mounted units of the armed forces in both world wars, but, although it can still be troublesome, it is now of minor importance in most countries.

Cause An organism known as *Streptococcus equi* is considered to be the main cause of strangles and, although it may be associated with other organisms, *S. equi* is always present in the nasal discharges and pus during the course of the disease. Exposure to cold, overwork, poor feeding and other factors which lower the animal's resistance are predisposing causes of the disease.

Horses most commonly become infected from the nasal or pus discharges from infected horses which contaminate the feed and watering troughs and pasture. Infection can also occur by inhalation of droplets coughed or breathed out by infected animals. The portal of entry of the germs is through the mucous membranes of the nose and pharynx. Recently recovered animals can spread infection for at least 4 weeks after an attack.

The organism is fairly resistant to environmental influences. Stables which have housed diseased animals and in which discharges will have been coughed on to the floor, walls and into the manger are sources of infection. Likewise, harness, nosebags, grooming utensils and the clothes of attendants can spread the infection.

The period of incubation — the time from exposure to infection until the development of symptoms of the disease—is 4 to 8 days.

Symptoms The main symptoms shown in typical or uncomplicated cases of strangles are fever with temperatures of 39 to 41°C, nasal catarrh, and swelling of the submaxillary lymph glands between the branches of the lower jaw, the pharyngeal (throat) lymph glands and sometimes the parotid lymph glands below the ear. There is often a varying degree of pharyngitis and laryngitis.

Attention is first drawn to the presence of the disease by a nasal discharge, difficulty in swallowing due to sore throat, cough, loss of appetite and general depression. The nasal discharge is at first watery but subsequently becomes thickened and pus-like. Within a few days, evidence of the germs having become arrested in the lymphatic glands about the head is shown by swelling of certain of these glands. Pus accumulates within the swollen glands which become hot and painful. In the course of another few days to a week, a soft fluctuating point is noticed at the peak of the swelling, and rupture of the abscess at this point commonly occurs. This is usually followed by a fall in temperature to normal, general improvement in the animal and, provided there are no complications, recovery in 2 to 4 weeks.

Atypical forms of strangles occur as a result of metastasis — a spread from the original site of the disease — and abscess formation in other organs including the lungs, liver, spleen, kidneys, brain, and the mesenteric lymph glands in the peritoneal attachment of the intestines. When these occur, the symptoms vary a great deal, depending on the location of the abscesses. For example, an abscess in the lung is likely to result in acute pneumonia. When the mesenteric lymph glands are involved, there are symptoms of colic or general abdominal pain, constipation, loss of appetite and fluctuating temperature. Such animals fall away in condition and death may occur from peritonitis due to rupture of an internal abscess some weeks or months later.

Treatment Since strangles is a highly contagious disease, affected animals should be immediately isolated, and care taken that the disease is not spread to other horses by feeding utensils or the hands and clothing of the attendants. Complete rest and good nursing are important in treatment of an affected animal. No attempt should be made to drench the horse, since, owing to the difficulty of swallowing, there is a risk that some of the drench may pass to the lungs and cause a fatal pneumonia.

Provided the weather is not too cold, a horse not accustomed to being stabled is best left in the open in a small convenient paddock and kept warm by rugging. Feed should be given from a box on the ground, because the nasal discharges come away more freely when the horse has its nose well down while feeding. Clean drinking water should be provided and repeatedly changed before it becomes fouled with nasal discharges. Sponging of the nose and eyes will frequently prevent "scalding" of the skin and is part of the general care of the patient.

The most effective antibiotic to be used to treat strangles is penicillin. A veterinarian will advise on the dose rate and a course of 5 to 10 days is usually given, depending on the severity of the symptoms. When abscesses develop in the lymph glands these may need drainage and a veterinarian should be called to perform minor surgery. There are many vital structures in the same region as the lymph glands and an unskilled person may damage these. Once the abscess has been drained of pus the wound should not be allowed to heal for at least 5 to 7 days as the infection will result in further pus accumulation. The abscess cavity should be syringed out daily with a weak solution of an antiseptic such as *Cetavlon, Dettol* or *Hibitane*.

Prevention Horses can be vaccinated for the prevention of strangles.

Whilst not always conferring an absolute immunity, this reduces the severity of the disease should it occur.

STRINGHALT

Stringhalt is an obscure condition in the horse in which there is an involuntary movement of one or both hind legs. The foot is suddenly and spasmodically lifted from the ground much higher than it is normally carried, with excessive flexion of the leg, sometimes up to the belly. The disease does not seem to be influenced by the horse's age, young and old horses of any breed being affected, but the condition does seem to become worse with age.

Cause There has been much theorising as to the cause of stringhalt, but the actual cause is very much in doubt. It has been suggested that the seat of the trouble is in the spinal cord, or that it may be due to degeneration of the tibial nerves. In Australia it has been found to be associated with horses grazing pastures where dandelions are dominant.

Symptoms The first manifestations of the condition are sometimes very slight. It may be noticeable when the horse is backed out of a stable when cold, or on turning the animal round to one side and then to the other. Again, it may be apparent only at the trot, or at a walk, and at other times only when the animal is turned around.

The usefulness of the horses may not be greatly diminished when mildly affected with stringhalt, but, as the peculiar action interferes with movement, the condition must be classified as an unsoundness. In most cases the amount of flexion is worse for the first few steps and improves as the horse continues to move. In severe cases stringhalt will interfere with the horse's ability to graze effectively.

Treatment If associated with the grazing of dandelions, the movement of the horse to another paddock may result in a gradual return to a normal gait over several months. If no improvement is seen with this treatment, surgery can be performed to remove a portion of the lateral extensor tendon and muscle from each hind leg. This usually results in great improvement or even return to a normal gait.

(See Fig. 95 on p. 212)

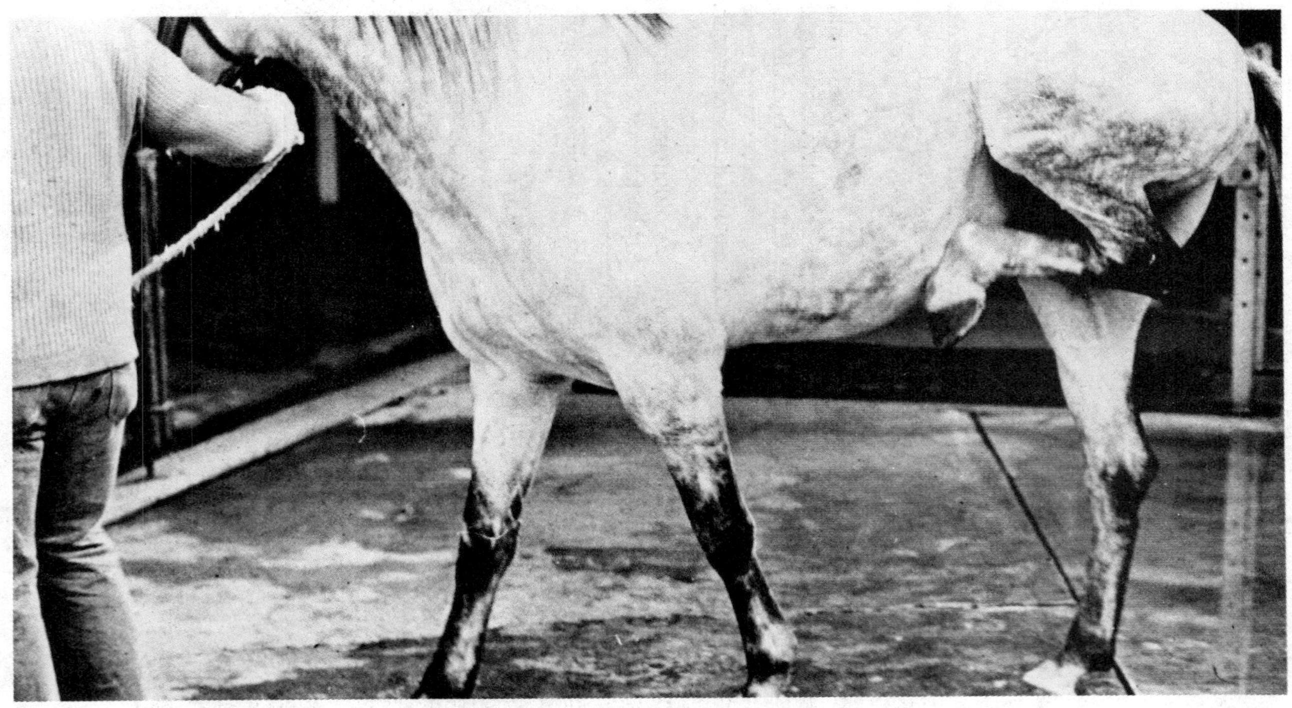

Fig. 95
Severe stringhalt in a standard-bred horse. This was completely resolved by removal of the lateral digital extensor tendon.

SUMMER SORES — CUTANEOUS HABRONEMIASIS

See *Parasites — Stomach Worms*

SUNSTROKE

See *Heatstroke*

TEETH — IRREGULARITIES OF MOLARS

Molar teeth are required both to cut and to grind the feed. The bearing surfaces of the upper and lower teeth are worn by the movements of the jaws so that they meet with a surface which slopes downwards and outwards. This results in the formation of a sharp edge along the outer border of the upper teeth and the inner border of the lower teeth. These edges are kept sharp by the grinding of the teeth and such sharpness must not be regarded as abnormal. Sometimes, however, due to malformation of the jaws, softness of the teeth or the direction of the teeth, there may be abnormal wear and sharp projections occur which can abrade or cut the tongue and cheeks. The bottom last molars sometimes grow up behind

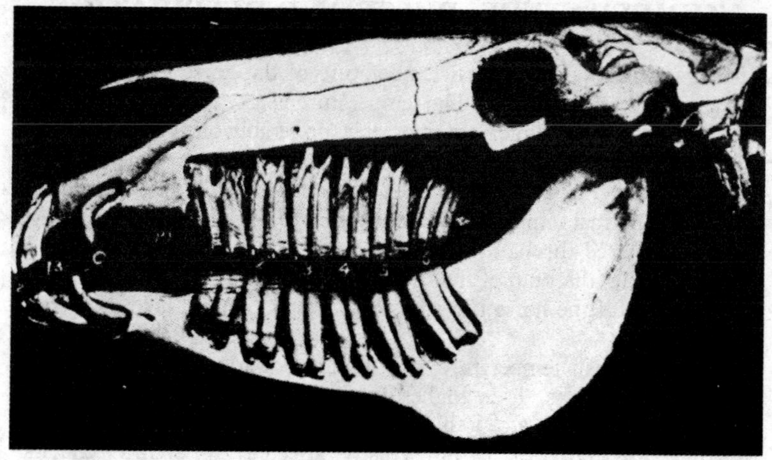

Fig. 96
Skull of horse, 5 years old, sculptured to show embedded parts of teeth.
(from Sisson-Grossman, "Anatomy of the Domestic Animals," 4th edition, Philadelphia, W.B. Saunders Co., 1953)

the top ones and penetrate the jaw. Injuries to other molar teeth may cause them to have broken sharp edges. Evidence of such irregularities of the molar teeth is usually shown by the horse "quidding" its feed, or slobbering while feeding. Sometimes there may be evidence of pain during mastication, the head being held to one side while chewing. A horse being ridden may pull to one side and toss the head if there are sharp projections or edges on the front premolars, as these may abrade the cheeks or tongue from the action of the bit.

Irregularities of the molar teeth can be discovered by backing the horse into a corner, grasping the tongue with the left hand and using the tip of the tongue as a gag against the upper jaw. The back teeth may now be looked at or felt with safety. A mouth-gag, of course, facilitates an examination of the mouth.

Molar teeth may be rasped if they have unduly sharp edges or projections, or minor irregularities on the table surfaces which are incompatible with the opposing teeth. It is preferable to have a veterinary surgeon do this, to ensure that it is carried out correctly. General irregularity of the molars in old age is not as common as is generally supposed, and, in the past, there has been much unnecessary filing of teeth.

Misplaced or malformed teeth should be extracted by a veterinarian.

See also *Dentition and Ageing*

TEMPERATURE, PULSE AND RESPIRATION

Temperature The normal temperature of the horse averages 37 °C, varying from 37.5 to 38 °C. The temperature is taken in the rectum with an ordinary human clinical thermometer, preferably one with a stub end, and it should be held in the rectum for at least double the time indicated on its register (1 to 2 minutes). The thermometer should be shaken down below the normal temperature, then wetted or oiled to make its passage easy, and passed through the anus into the rectum and held there. It is important that the bulb of the thermometer be kept in contact with the rectal lining. If the horse is restless, an assistant should hold up a front foot.

The normal temperature of the horse varies somewhat under different conditions. It is higher in foals and yearlings, which may register up to 38 °C, and is higher after severe exercise or in very hot weather. Generally, it is not greatly affected by average climatic variations.

A rise of temperature to 38.5 °C indicates a mild fever; if it reaches 39.5 °C, the fever is moderate; 41 °C is a high fever, and above this is regarded as very high.

Before putting the thermometer away, wash it in water or cold antiseptic solution and shake the mercury down.

Pulse The pulse rate of the healthy adult horse varies from 26 to 40 per minute, but is much higher in young animals, being up to 70 per minute in foals. The pulse may be counted and its character may be determined at any point where a large artery is close to the skin and passes over a hard surface such as a bone, cartilage or tendon. A convenient place is at the angle of the jaw where an artery crosses the bone. Its throb can be felt just before it turns around the lower border of the jawbone. The pulse may also be taken inside the fore-arm at the level of the elbow joint, where an artery crosses immediately over the bone.

The first and second fingers should be pressed lightly on the skin over the artery.

The animal should be at perfect rest when the pulse is taken, as exercise and excitement quicken it. Experience is necessary to obtain important information from the pulse rate. It is faster in fevers and slower and weaker in non-febrile debilitating diseases. The pulse rate and its character (whether it is stronger or weaker than it should be) is important in the diagnosis of disease, especially when considered together with other diagnostic aids, such as temperature and respiration.

Respiration The normal respiration of a 6 year old, healthy horse, observed by viewing the flank movements, is 8 to 12 inspirations per minute. It is usual to count the inspirations for half a minute and then to double the result. The respiration rate is greater in young horses and may be up to 14 or 15 inspirations per minute.

The type of respiration is very important in the diagnosis of disease. In normal breathing there is movement of the thorax and abdomen. Heavy, laboured breathing, confined chiefly to the abdominal wall with the thorax participating but little in the movements, signifies a painful condition of the chest, such as acute pleurisy and pneumonia. Exaggerated movements of the walls of the chest, on the other hand, are seen in disorders of the organs of the abdomen, such as in certain types of colic, peritonitis or other painful affections, when an attempt is made to limit the movements of the abdomen as much as possible.

Difficult or laboured breathing is known as dyspnoea and may occur when, for any reason, it is difficult for the animal to obtain the amount of oxygen it requires. This may be due to congestion or consolidation of the lungs as in pneumonia, to pleurisy, to tumours of the nose, to paralysis or swelling of the throat, foreign bodies and other causes. When chronic, it is seen in chronic obstructive pulmonary disease ("heaves").

In severe dyspnoea, the horse stands with its front feet apart, the neck straight out, and the head extended upon the neck. The nostrils are widely dilated, the face has an anxious expression, the eyeballs protrude, there is mouth breathing and increased movements of the thoracic and abdominal walls. Grunting may be heard.

TENDONS — CONTRACTED, WEAK FLEXOR

See *Foals — Limb Deformities*

TENDONS — SPRAINED ("Bowed tendons")

The fibrous structures situated below the knee and hock behind the cannon bones are often the seat of sprains, and are a very common cause of lameness in light horses. The most commonly injured tendon is the superficial flexor tendon, a broad flat tendon that can be felt at the back of the cannon region. Underneath this lies the deep flexor tendon and in between the cannon bone and the deep flexor tendon is the suspensory ligament.

Cause Prolonged exertion, particularly at the gallop, and violent efforts or sudden jerks, especially in young or poorly conditioned animals, are common causes of sprain of the back tendons. Muscular fatigue plays an important part in sprain as this allows greater movement of joints, and stress of tendons and ligaments. This commonly occurs when a horse is forced to prolonged effort and becomes tired. Sprained tendons may also result from improper shoeing; allowing the toes of the feet to grow too long, as occurs when horses are allowed to wear their shoes for too long a period; poor conformation (particularly long pasterns tied in behind the knee) or over-training of young animals.

The flexor tendons, the suspensory ligament and the check ligament are more frequently involved than the extensor tendons. The tendons of the fore leg are more commonly affected than those of the hind. The differential diagnosis between the various forms and situations of tendon sprains is very important as the site and type of sprain will affect the ultimate use of the horse.

Symptoms Heat, swelling, tenderness and lameness are the usual symptoms of sprained tendons. However, in the early stages of tendon sprain there may be no lameness seen. Other symptoms are: stumbling even when walking; digging the toe into the ground; knee and fetlock bent, with later thickening and "gumminess" of the leg. The degree of lameness varies according to the extent of the injury to the tendon fibres and the amount of haemorrhage and effusion. It is important to keep in

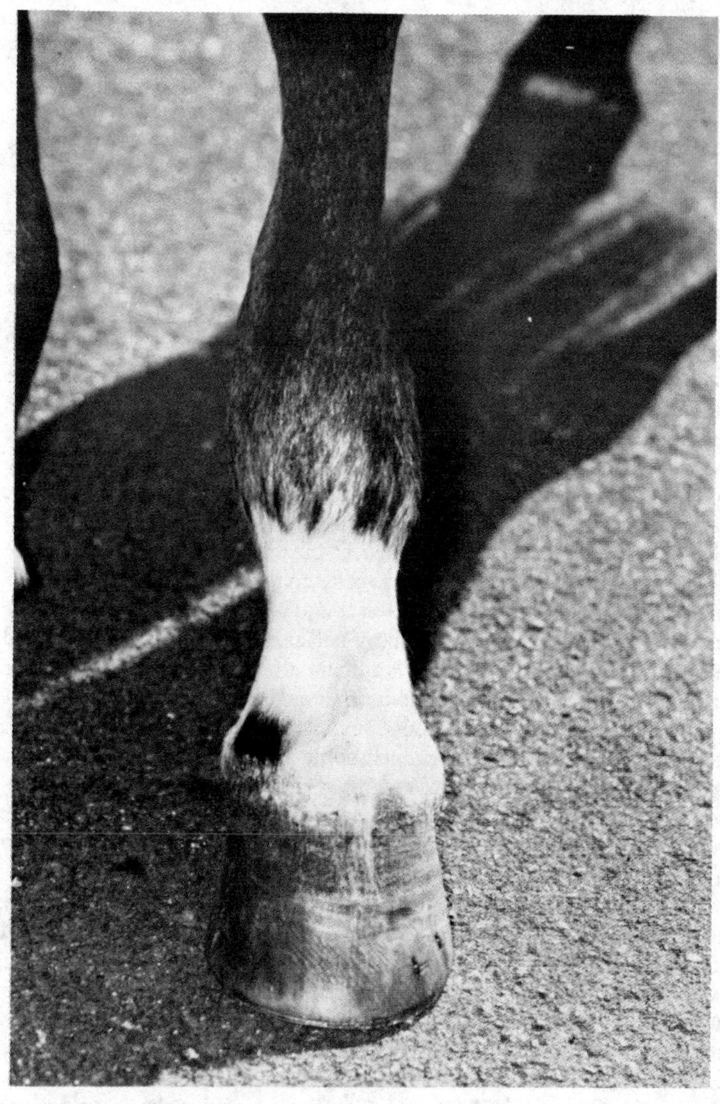

Fig. 97
Bowed tendon. Sprain of the suspensory ligament on the inside of the cannon bone of the left foreleg.

mind that all heat and swelling in the region of the back tendons is not necessarily due to sprain of the tendons. Such a condition can be caused by an infection in the foot or mechanical injury to the part, such as a blow from the opposite foot. It is possible to decide which tendon is involved by palpating each tendon with weight off the leg. Where the tendon is sprained the horse will show a painful response to gentle palpation.

Treatment It is advisable to obtain the services of a veterinarian, at least for diagnosis and advice on the initial treatment of the sprained tendons. There are various methods of treatment, but the essential factor is rest. The shoes should be removed. Cold water applications from a hose have some merit when used sufficiently early, but treatment should include continued pressure on the tendons. The application of a pressure bandage straight away will probably give the best results. The object of the pressure is to promote reabsorption of the fluid which has formed in the tendon sheath, and to prevent further fluid forming. Special pads are available for binding evenly along the sides of the tendons. Alternatively, cotton wool or cotton wadding is placed evenly round the leg, care being taken to have it so thick that subsequent pressure of the bandage will not injure the skin. Over this is wound a long crepe bandage as tightly and as evenly as possible, so that it will exert even pressure over the whole of the injured surface and extend well above and below it. The padding should also project at each end to ensure that there is no cutting of the skin by the edges of the bandage. This pressure bandage should remain on for 24 hours. If it becomes loose, it should be removed, the leg massaged and the bandage re-applied. Such pressure should be maintained for at least a week, the bandage being removed night and morning, the leg rubbed, and the bandage re-applied. Anti-inflammatory drugs, such as *phenylbutazone*, can be used during the acute stage of tendon sprain to aid in relief of the inflammatory response and the swelling.

After the acute inflammatory response has subsided, which usually takes 2 to 3 weeks, a programme of passive movement of tendon will aid in preventing restrictive adhesions. To achieve this the horse should be swum for periods beginning at 1 to 2 minutes and gradually increasing over a period of a month to 10 to 15 minutes a day. During swimming the tendons are mobilised but bear no weight. This mobilisation prevents the development of scar tissue, which results in reduction of the range of movement in the tendon, which will ultimately affect the future of the horse. Following this period the horse should then be turned out into a paddock for at least 9 to 10 months as tendon tissue heals very slowly. Various forms of surgery have been tried but only a new treatment involving insertion of carbon fibres into the tendon appears promising. No matter which form of treatment is tried it should be appreciated that once the tendon is sprained there is a strong possibility of recurrence.

TETANUS

Tetanus, sometimes known as "lockjaw", is an acute infectious disease of all domestic animals and man. Horses, sheep and goats are particularly susceptible, but cattle, pigs, dogs and cats less so. The disease has a world-wide distribution, particularly in closely settled areas, and occurs mainly in horses as individual sporadic cases. The disease, which usually originates from infection of a wound, is characterised by spasms affecting the muscles of the face, neck, body and limbs, and all muscles supplied by the cerebro-spinal nerves. It is essentially an affliction of the nervous system and is not a blood infection.

Cause The disease is caused by a toxin which is elaborated by the organism *Clostridium tetani*, when it gains entrance to deep punctured wounds, or any wound which seals over quickly and from which the air is excluded.

The tetanus germs form spores which are capable of living in the soil for long periods. When these spores gain entrance to a wound in which conditions are suitable for their propagation, they start to proliferate and at the same time produce a powerful toxin which affects the nervous system. Tetanus organisms occur quite commonly in the intestinal tract of animals without doing any harm, and are passed out in the droppings. This is the reason why infection is more likely to occur on heavily manured soils, or in horse yards, or wherever there is an accumulation of animal manure.

Predisposing Causes When a horse develops tetanus, there is generally a history of injury. Wounds most prone to be infected are those which come in contact with the ground, or those which penetrate deeply into the tissues. Nails, splinters, stakes and other sharp objects are common causes. Infection may also occur from contaminated dust, which has blown on to a superficial wound, which scabs over quickly. Tetanus may also occur following fractures of bones, castration, tail docking, injuries to the mouth (sharp teeth) or injuries to the genital passages (from aid given in difficult foaling) and infection of the navel cord in foals.

Incubation Period Although tetanus spores may lie dormant in the tissues for some months, and clinical symptoms of the disease may not be produced until the conditions are favourable for their propagation, it is common, if the germ has been introduced, for symptoms to develop after an incubation period which varies in different animals. In the horse it is between 1 and 3 weeks.

Symptoms The main symptoms are stiffness of the muscles and tremors. The muscles of the neck and along the spine become involved, and the legs are moved in a stiff manner. The head is extended and the third eyelid (or haw) protrudes over the inner portion of the eye with a characteristic movement. This movement is very quick as the third eyelid moves out over the eye, but very slow on return. This occurs especially when the animal is disturbed. Noise or disturbance throws the animal into increased spasms of the affected muscles. The tail is usually slightly elevated and stiff and the ears are erect. The jaws become set (locked), the animal is unable to eat and saliva may drool from the mouth. As the disease progresses, the horse adopts a characteristic attitude with fore and hind legs extended (saw-horse stance). Breathing becomes difficult, the lips are drawn tightly over the teeth, the nostrils are dilated and the animal, which has an anxious expression, may sweat profusely. Constipation sets in early in the attack. Temperature is not much changed at first, but may rise to 40 °C just before death. In severe attacks, recovery seldom occurs and death takes place in 3 to 5 days or a little longer. The mortality rate is about 80 per cent.

Those cases that set in slowly after a long incubation period, and in which the symptoms are not severe, may recover if carefully nursed in proper surroundings. A convalescent period of several months is required before the horse is worked again.

Tetanus may possibly be confounded with other disease conditions, such as strychnine poisoning, spinal meningitis and forage poisoning. The typical muscular spasms of tetanus, the movement of the third eyelid across the eye, coupled with the possible history of a wound, should assist in diagnosis.

Treatment If the horse is a valuable animal, or if for sentimental reasons it is desired to do everything possible to save the animal, a veterinary surgeon should be called in. He will treat the animal with large doses of tetanus antitoxin and will administer antibiotic drugs and muscle-relaxing agents. The treatment is costly and the results uncertain.

As already pointed out, mild cases of tetanus may recover with good nursing. The horse should be kept quiet in a darkened, roomy stall, away from the other animals, the floor being bedded with sawdust, sand or short straw. It is important to reduce any external stimuli (noise, light, etcetera), which will precipitate the muscle spasms. A fresh supply of cool drinking water should be placed in a convenient position on a level with the horse's head.

Prevention When a horse has sustained a severe or punctured wound, arrangements should be made for a veterinary surgeon to administer tetanus antitoxin, which is of far greater value as a preventive than as a curative agent. The preventive action lasts only for 10 to 14 days which is, however, usually sufficient to prevent the disease developing.

As a routine procedure, tetanus toxoid is used to immunise animals against the disease, and horse owners are advised to give serious consideration to having their horses protected against tetanus in this manner. Immunity is conferred in approximately 2 weeks after the initial injections, given at intervals of a month, when the horse will be immune to tetanus for at least a year. If annual "booster" injections are given, horses will remain immune from tetanus.

THOROUGHPIN

This unusual term is applied to a chronic synovitis (or inflammation of the synovial sheath) of the deep flexor tendon at the back of the hock, and distension of the membrane by fluid. It should be differentiated from bog spavin which is an effusion of fluid in the hock joint with distension of the joint capsule. In thoroughpin, the swelling is seen on either side of the hock in front of the hamstring about the level of the "point of the hock". It varies in size and may be more noticeable on the inside or on the outside. Pressure with the fingers on the swelling at one side of the leg causes a corresponding or even greater filling on the opposite side.

Cause A thoroughpin usually results from excessive strain on the flexor tendon as it passes around the hock. This results in inflammation and "filling" of the tendon sheath. The condition was formerly more commonly seen in draught horses, when it was associated with excessive exertion when backing heavy loads, especially on a slippery surface. It is also seen in light horses, in which the condition may result from jumping, pulling up suddenly when galloping, and from other forms of sudden strain on the tendons such as kicks and other injuries. On the other hand, thoroughpin is seen in horses in which there is no history of excessive strain and, as in the case of bog spavin, may be associated with defective conformation. The condition is sometimes seen in young horses, and may disappear spontaneously.

Symptoms Slight lameness may be evident when the condition first occurs, but this is not severe unless the flexor tendon has been severely sprained. After the lesion becomes chronic, it causes no inconvenience to the horse and does not interfere with its work. The blemish is, of course, unsightly and depreciates the value of the animal.

Treatment In those cases which arise gradually, without causing any inconvenience, and where the swelling is often quite small, no treatment is warranted. The swelling may slowly increase in size or it may diminish

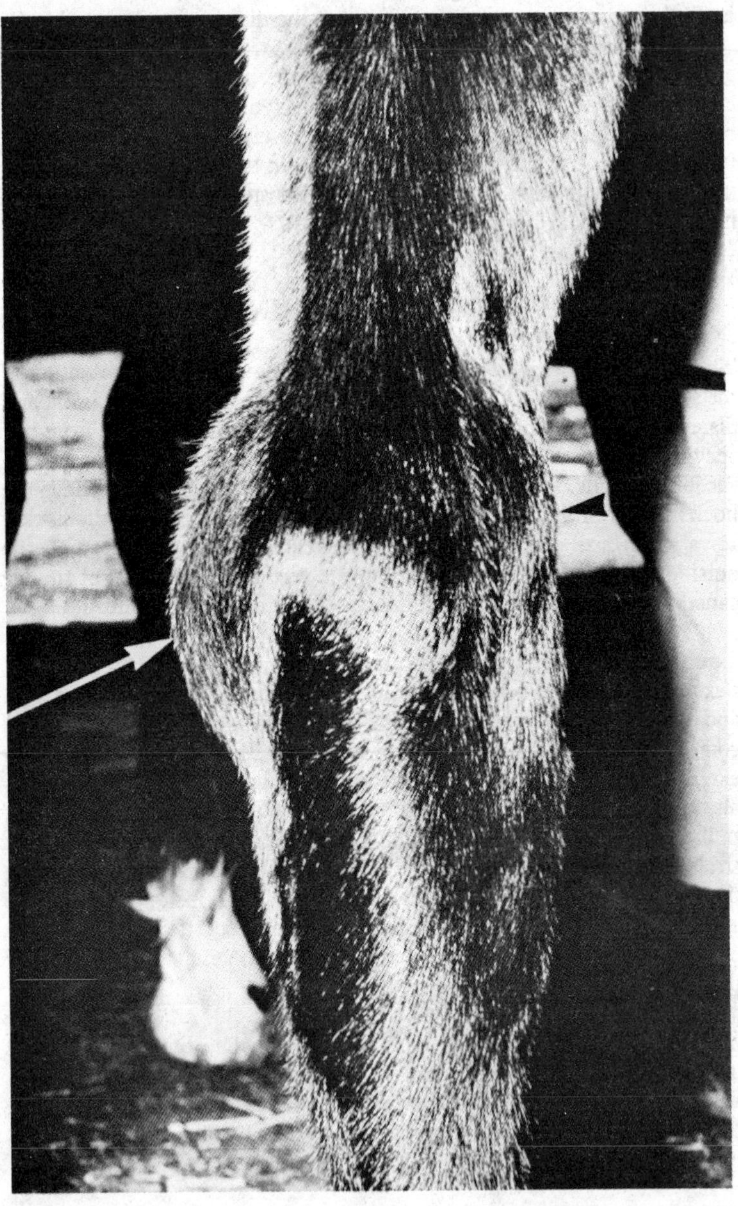

Fig. 98
Thoroughpin (arrow) in the hock of a horse.

and, especially in the case of young horses, disappear. For acute cases which have followed sprain of the flexor tendon, cold water applications with a hose are beneficial in reducing inflammation. Cooling astringent lotions may also be used. A pressure bandage with cotton wool, as recommended for the treatment of bog spavin, is useful in reducing the swelling if it can be well applied. Rest is, of course, essential. Any break in the skin must be treated as an open wound.

If the condition becomes chronic, it is doubtful if any treatment will be entirely successful, but as the usefulness of the horse is not impaired by the swelling, the only disadvantage is the blemish.

Aspiration of the fluid and corticosteroid injections by a veterinarian, if carried out early, may bring about lasting reduction of the swelling.

THRUSH

In horses the term "thrush" is applied to a disease affecting the cleft of the frog in which there is a degenerative condition of the horn, characterised by a black and offensive discharge from the cleft.

Cause The condition results from a bacterial infection and catarrhal inflammation of the glands deep in the cleft of the frog.

The frog is normally resistant to bacterial invasion, but may deteriorate and become susceptible as the result of long-continued exposure to excessively wet or filthy stable floors and yards.

Thrush can also occur under dry conditions in horses with contracted feet and where there is little or no frog pressure.

Symptoms Attention is usually drawn first to the condition of thrush by the characteristic foul smell of the discharge from the affected frog. The frog may be wasted and fissured, and the horn soft and easily detachable in the depth of the cleft. Mild thrush rarely causes lameness. In more advanced cases of the disease, the sensitive structures become involved, the frog is hot and tender to pressure, and there may be tenderness of the heels and coronet. Under such circumstances, lameness occurs.

Treatment Attention to stable hygiene and cleanliness of the foot is, of course, essential. When the condition has arisen as the result of lack of frog pressure, this should be rectified. Remove the shoes and rasp down the heels and walls as low as possible, without making the foot tender, the object being to obtain frog pressure as soon as possible. Good frog pressure is essential for a healthy foot.

As far as the actual treatment of lesions is concerned, the first step is to clean out the cleft of the frog with a stiff brush and warm soap and water and then to trim away any loose pieces of the frog. Subsequent treatment will depend on the seriousness of the condition. Poulticing may be of value at this stage, followed by the application of some suitable astringent antiseptic dressing, such as *white lotion.*

It may be necessary to syringe out suppurating areas with very weak solutions of antiseptics, such as *Dettol, Savlon, Cetavlon* etcetera. Aerosol sprays such as *Chloropel* are also useful in drying out infected areas, and occasionally antibiotic injections may be necessary if prescribed by a veterinarian.

With restoration, as far as possible, of frog pressure, and with general cleanliness and careful dressing, a cure is nearly always obtained.

TUMOURS

See *Cancer*

TWISTED BOWEL

Under this heading is included also strangulation and intussusception—telescoping—of the bowel. All these conditions are very serious, and lead to intestinal obstruction, which generally terminates in death of the animal.

A twisting of the bowel upon itself is referred to as a volvulus. It is most likely to occur during strenuous exercise, such as violent rolling, jumping, or other sudden bodily movements, or be associated with a severe attack of colic.

Intestinal strangulation is seen in cases of inguinal or umbilical hernia, or may result from a twist of the bowel. Long-necked tumours in the mesentery sometimes become twisted around a part of the small intestine and cause strangulation.

Intussusception of the bowel is a slipping or telescoping of a portion of the intestine into another portion immediately adjoining, like a partially turned-in glove finger. This may occur at any part of the bowels, but is more frequent in the small intestines. The telescoped portion may be small—5 or 7 cm only—or extensive, measuring up to a metre. The causes include irregular or excessive peristaltic movements, as may result from profuse diarrhoea, inflammation of the bowels and worm infection. Foals are most commonly affected by this condition.

Symptoms The symptoms of all the above conditions are similar, and a non-professional person is unlikely to be able to make a definite diagnosis. There is a sudden onset of acute colicky pain. The horse rolls, paws the ground, breaks out in a sweat, and shows increased respiration and heart rate. The mucous membranes of the eyes and nose are usually congested. A little dung may be passed at first, followed by constipation. Severe straining occurs in some cases of intussusception and this may be regarded with suspicion when it occurs. As death approaches, the horse sweats profusely, presents an anxious countenance, the legs and ears become cold, and there is often freedom from pain just before death. Most cases end fatally within 12 to 24 hours.

Treatment There should be no delay in obtaining the services of a veterinarian. Surgery may save the life of the patient.

UDDER — INFLAMMATION OF

See *Mastitis*

ULCER

Black's Veterinary Dictionary defines an ulcer as "a breach on the surface of the skin, or on the surface of any mucous or other membrane of a cavity of the body, which does not tend to heal". It is a process of destruction involving the death of small portions of healthy tissue around the edge, which causes the ulcer to spread. This is called ulceration.

There are various types of ulcers, and specific ulcers occur in association with a number of diseases.

Spontaneous or primary ulcers, such as those that follow injury anywhere on the surface of the skin, in the mouth and on the tongue, are due to a continuous irritant on the wound, which prevents healing.

Such irritation may be caused by bacteria, the use of strong antiseptics, constant rubbing of the wound by harness or, in the case of the mouth, by the irritating influence of infected, loose or irregular teeth on the cheek or tongue. Debility and disturbances of circulation are predisposing causes.

Treatment Specific ulcers associated with various diseases usually heal under general treatment or when the disease has run its course.

In the case of spontaneous ulcers, the first thing is to remove the exciting cause. The ulcer should be cleaned up with some weak antiseptic solution and any pieces of dead tissue on the surface removed. It may now be treated with a stimulating healing lotion, such as *white lotion,* or dusted with sulphonamide or antibiotic powders. The horse should be rested, preferably in a well-grassed paddock, kept under observation and treated as required.

A seriously-inflamed or chronic ulcer requires professional attention.

URINARY CALCULI — ("STONE" OR "GRAVEL") (Urolithiasis)

The horse is not uncommonly affected by urinary calculi, either in the kidneys, ureters (tubes leading from kidneys to the bladder), bladder, or urethra. These calculi or "stones", as they are commonly called, are formed from various salts normally excreted in the urine. The more common calculi found in the horse consist of calcium carbonate, calcium phosphate and magnesium carbonate.

Although calculi may occur anywhere along the urinary tract, they are most commonly found in the bladder of the horse. Here they occur as egg-shaped or flat, hard, yellowish grey concretions, the surfaces of which are either smooth or mulberry-like, and they vary in size from a small stone up to a concretion the size of a man's fist. In addition to these stone-like concretions, there may also be present a "gravel" or sand-like sediment commonly referred to as "urinary gravel" or "urinary sand".

Several small calculi or one large calculus may sometimes occur in the pelvis of the kidney, and be undiagnosed until death of the animal, when they are seen at post-mortem examination.

Those calculi which are found in the passages leading from the kidney to the bladder are simply small renal calculi that have escaped from the pelvis of the kidney. If they completely block the ureter, the retained urine causes destructive pressure in the kidney.

Urethral calculi are less frequent in horses than in sheep and cattle because of the larger size of the urethra in the horse, and the absence of the S-shaped curve which occurs in the penis of the former animals. The calculi which are arrested in the urethra are not formed there, but consist of cystic calculi which have been small enough to pass through the neck of the bladder, but which are too large to pass through the whole length of the urethra (in the male) and so escape. This trouble is most unlikely to occur in the mare.

Still other calculi occur in the horse, namely concretions in the sheath, and these are known as preputial calculi. Within the sheath, the concretions are usually of soft, cheese-like sebaceous matter and not true calculi, but the latter do occur. Both may interfere with the flow of urine, but are easily removed by the fingers.

Cause The underlying causes of urinary calculi (or urolithiasis) are not fully understood and are still the subject of scientific investigation.

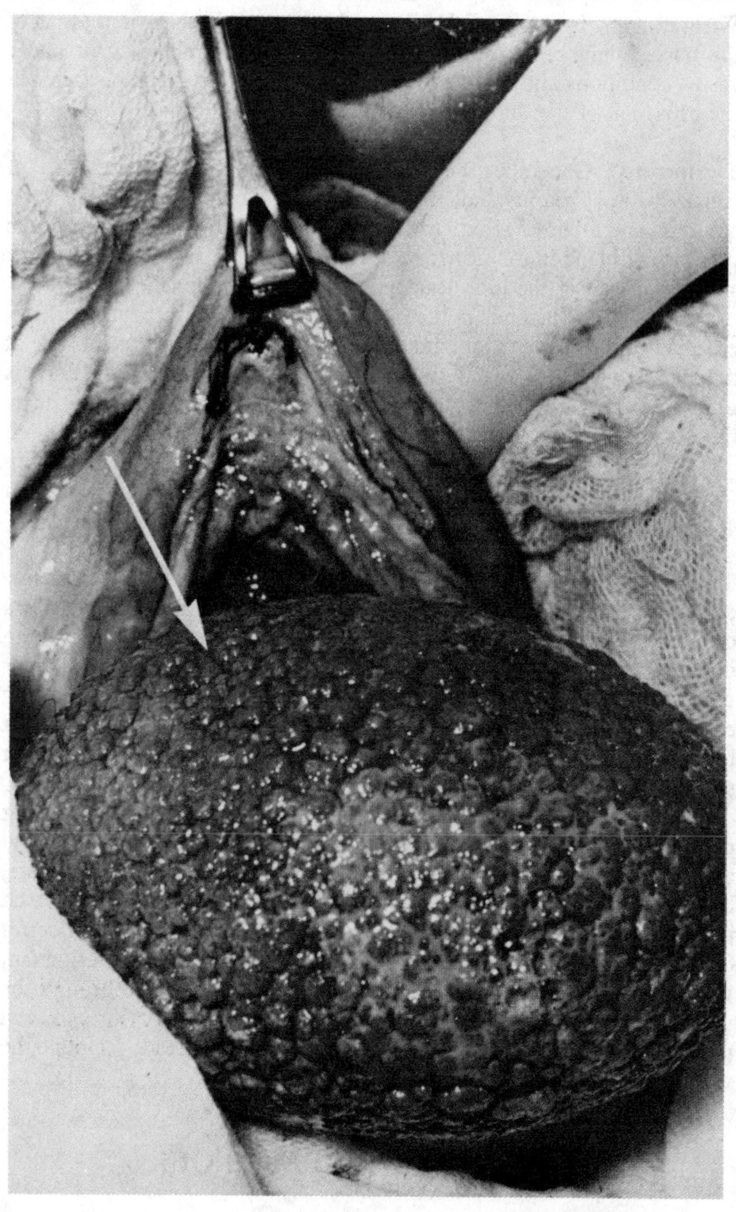

Fig. 99
Large calculus shown being surgically removed from the bladder.

Without going into a lot of detail as to how calculi in the urinary tract of the horse might be formed, it can be said that the calculi occur under varied conditions and it seems unlikely that there is a common factor in the causation of the different types of calculi.

Symptoms Generally, the symptoms of urinary calculi are those of colicky pain, appearing suddenly, very often following exhausting work; straining and reported efforts to urinate; interruption in the flow of urine; presence of blood in the urine; presence of sand-like deposit in the urine; stiffness of gait of the hind legs and movement of the tail.

In the case of "stone" in the bladder, the rough mulberry-like calculi, especially, lead to irritation and wounding of the mucous membrane of the bladder with bleeding. This occurs most commonly when the horse is ridden or driven. When the horse is pulled up and proceeds to urinate, there follows the passage of bloodstained urine.

The presence of a stone or stones in the bladder can be readily ascertained by a veterinarian who can place a gloved arm into the rectum and palpate the stone in the bladder.

Treatment It will be appreciated that the treatment for obstructive calculi in various positions in the urinary tract is difficult, and is usually a case for surgery by an experienced veterinarian. It is not practicable to dissolve the calculi by medical means, but veterinarians have at their disposal certain drugs which may prevent increase in the size of existing calculi and the development of new ones. Drugs are also available to relax the urethral muscle and allow the obstructing stone to pass on, but success depends on very early treatment.

The removal of a large stone in the bladder, whilst presenting great difficulties and the necessity for a major operation under a general anaesthetic in the case of a stallion or gelding, can, in the case of a mare, be comparatively easily carried out through the short female urethra which is only 5 to 7 cm in length. The female urethra opens on to the floor of the vagina about 10 cm from the outside. It is possible for a veterinarian, with his hand in the vagina, to remove the stone by hand through the urethra, which is capable of remarkable dilation if sufficient care and patience are exercised in the process. Special forceps greatly facilitate the work.

UTERUS — DISEASES OF

See *Metritis*

WARTS (Equine Cutaneous Papillomatosis)

Warts, or cutaneous papillomas as they are technically called, are solid outgrowths of epidermis, which appear as small, elevated, horny masses, usually on the muzzle, nose, and lips. They seldom occur elsewhere on the body. They may remain flat and small, but some increase greatly in size or become pendulous. They are more common in young horses and may be few in number or quite numerous.

When not complicated by other conditions, warts are non-inflammatory and painless and usually cause little inconvenience. Around the mouth they may interfere with feeding and, when occurring around the nostrils, they may obstruct breathing.

Warts usually disappear spontaneously after a few months but may persist for 6 months and sometimes longer, when they can be responsible for loss of condition.

Cause The disease is caused by a virus, and is infectious. The disease has been transmitted experimentally to young horses by injection, or by application of a suspension of wart tissue to scarified skin. Under natural conditions, transmission of the disease is believed to take place by direct contact with infected horses through a break in the skin, or when animals with an abrasion of the skin rub against rails, posts or other objects which have become contaminated with the virus. Halters, headstalls and grooming equipment can spread the disease.

Although the virus is relatively resistant, it is not known how long it will remain alive on inanimate objects.

Treatment As already indicated, the disease is self-limiting and eventually disappears. After recovery, the horse is immune to further infection. Vaccines are used, both for the treatment and prevention of the disease, but, unless the vaccine is prepared from the virus of equine cutaneous papillomatosis, it is likely to be ineffective. Vaccines prepared from wart tissue of the affected animal give better results.

Other treatments include the injection of proprietary preparations containing antimony and bismuth, local application of glacial acetic acid or a caustic potash stick. When the latter 2 are used, care should be taken that only the warts are treated, and that the skin around them is protected with petroleum jelly. Several applications will be necessary, at intervals of a few days.

The tendency for spontaneous recovery to occur makes assessment of the results of treatment difficult.

Warts may also be removed surgically, but the operation should not be carried out in the early stage of development, as this will often stimulate the growth of remaining warts and cause others to appear.

Pendulous warts, which are not common in horses, may sometimes be successfully removed by ligation with a strong thread close to the base.

Bearing in mind that the disease is infectious, efforts should be made to keep affected horses apart from healthy animals.

WATERING

A horse requires a daily average of between 20 to 40 litres of water. In very hot weather, or when the horse has diarrhoea, up to 80 to 100 litres of water may be consumed per day. The quantity varies not only with the weather and the amount of work performed, but also with the character of the feed. Stabled horses should be watered at least 3 times a day before feeding, and paddocked horses should have an ample supply of good clean water available to them at all times.

Water obtained from pools or shallow wells contaminated with surface drainage or decomposing organic matter frequently leads to digestive upsets, while water containing a large amount of sediment causes mechanical irritation of the mucous membrane of the stomach and intestines and may cause the condition known as sand colic.

A horse may be permitted to drink when hot if the quantity allowed is not too great. After prolonged exertion or fast work, the body fluids are depleted. The animal will not eat sufficiently until its thirst has at least been partially satisfied. Water should be given first, and while the animal is still warm is the best time to give it. However, after hard or fast work, drinking should not be permitted until the breathing has returned to normal. It is preferable to provide small quantities at intervals than to allow unlimited water, particularly if the water is very cold. Small quantities of water can be given if desired an hour after the completion of feeding.

After a long trek, it is a good plan to water a kilometre or so before the journey's end and take the horse in slowly afterwards. This prevents chills and colic due to the ingestion of a large quantity of water when in an exhausted state.

Girths should always be loosened before watering, and horses allowed ample time to drink. They should not be led away the first time they raise their heads from the water.

WEAVING

Weaving is a vice or nervous habit acquired by many wild animals in captivity and sometimes by horses, especially those that are stabled for long periods. The animal rocks itself to and fro continually, swinging the head and neck and front part of the body, sometimes lifting each fore foot in turn as the body is swayed to the opposite side. Some horses practise the vice occasionally while others do it constantly. A constant weaver wears itself out to the extent that its working capacity is affected.

Idleness and boredom appear to predispose to weaving and, as with other vices, the habit is likely to be copied by other horses in a stable. It is advisable, therefore, to keep a weaver away from other horses, so that they will not be disturbed and learn the trick from observation. It has been suggested that an uneven stable floor will start a horse weaving.

Once acquired, the habit of weaving is difficult to break. Various devices are adopted to control the weaving, but the confirmed weaver usually overcomes these and continues to weave even if in a restricted manner. A simple method of controlling weaving is to tie the horse to side rings. The horse should be given plenty of exercise or regular work and be turned out into a grass paddock, rather than being stabled. If the horse has to be stabled, care should be taken that the stable floor is even, and plenty of good bedding should be provided to encourage the horse to lie down.

WHISTLING

See *Roaring and Whistling*

WHEAT — ENGORGEMENT WITH

See *Colic*

WHITE LOTION

White lotion is an astringent-antiseptic preparation which is particularly useful for controlling proud-flesh and drying up moist sores. It is prepared by taking 30 g of lead acetate plus 20 g of zinc sulphate and making this up to 500 ml with water. In this mixture the ingredients settle out quickly and, therefore, the solution should be well shaken immediately prior to use.

WIND — BROKEN

See *Broken-wind*

WINDGALLS

A windgall is defined as a soft fluid-filled swelling in the region of the fetlock joint of the horse. The common types of windgalls recognised are articular windgall, in which the bursa of the fetlock joint is involved, and tendinous windgall, when the swelling occurs in the tendon sheath surrounding the flexor tendon at the back of the leg. Independent bursae also develop between bone and tendon. Windgalls appear in the form of soft puffy swellings, varying in size from a pea to a walnut or larger. They occur at the back of the fetlock joint and are most commonly seen in the fore leg.

Cause Windgalls occur as the result of sudden or sustained strain thrown upon the fetlock joint or the tendons at the back of the leg with resultant inflammation of the bursa of the joint or the tendon sheath. They occur in young animals that are put to work too soon, and are quite common in old horses. They are not uncommonly seen in trotters and jumpers. Faulty conformation, such as short pasterns and upright shoulders, are contributing causes. An articular windgall can indicate the start of damage to the joint and the early stages of arthritis.

Symptoms Usually windgalls are painless and only cause lameness under certain conditions. Lameness occurs if there is damage to the fetlock joint as in the case of arthritis or chip fractures. In these conditions the horse would usually show pain when the joint is flexed.

Treatment As most windgalls are of little consequence except for being unsightly, and rarely cause lameness, treatment is not very important. When the condition occurs in young animals, it frequently clears up without treatment as the animal grows older. However, if there are any signs of lameness or pain associated with the condition a veterinarian should attend the horse.

X-rays are usually necessary to determine if there is damage to the bone or joint and, if so, injections of certain medications may be made directly into the joint. If there is a chip fracture in the fetlock joint this can be moved surgically.

WIND-SUCKING

See *Crib-biting and Wind-sucking*

WITHERS — FISTULOUS

See *Fistulous Withers and Poll Evil*

WOBBLER SYNDROME

This condition, which is thought to be hereditary, is found in young growing horses and results in unsteadiness and a wobbly gait in the fore and hind limbs.

Cause Due to malformation of the vertebrae in the neck there is excessive mobility of these vertebrae so that undue pressure is placed on parts of the spinal cord. This excessive spinal cord pressure leads to interference with various neural pathways and so results in the typical wobbly gait. In other cases there may be no abnormalities of the neck vertebrae and the primary lesion may be within the spinal cord itself.

Symptoms The wobbler gait is quite characteristic and is most severe in the hind limbs. Affected horses will frequently cross-over their hind limbs and sometimes drag their toes as they bring their legs forward. In other cases the fore limbs will also be affected.

Treatment A definite diagnosis is important and this can sometimes be made by x-raying the neck. This can rule out traumatic lesions, such as fracture of the neck vertebrae, which can give similar symptoms. In most cases little can be done in the way of treatment and severely affected horses will have to be destroyed.

In the United States research is currently under way in examining the use of surgery to stabilise the vertebrae of the neck as a means of treating this disorder. This treatment is still experimental and may not turn out to be useful.

(See Fig. 100 on p. 234)

WOMB — INFLAMMATION OF

See *Metritis*

WORMS

See *Parasites — Internal*

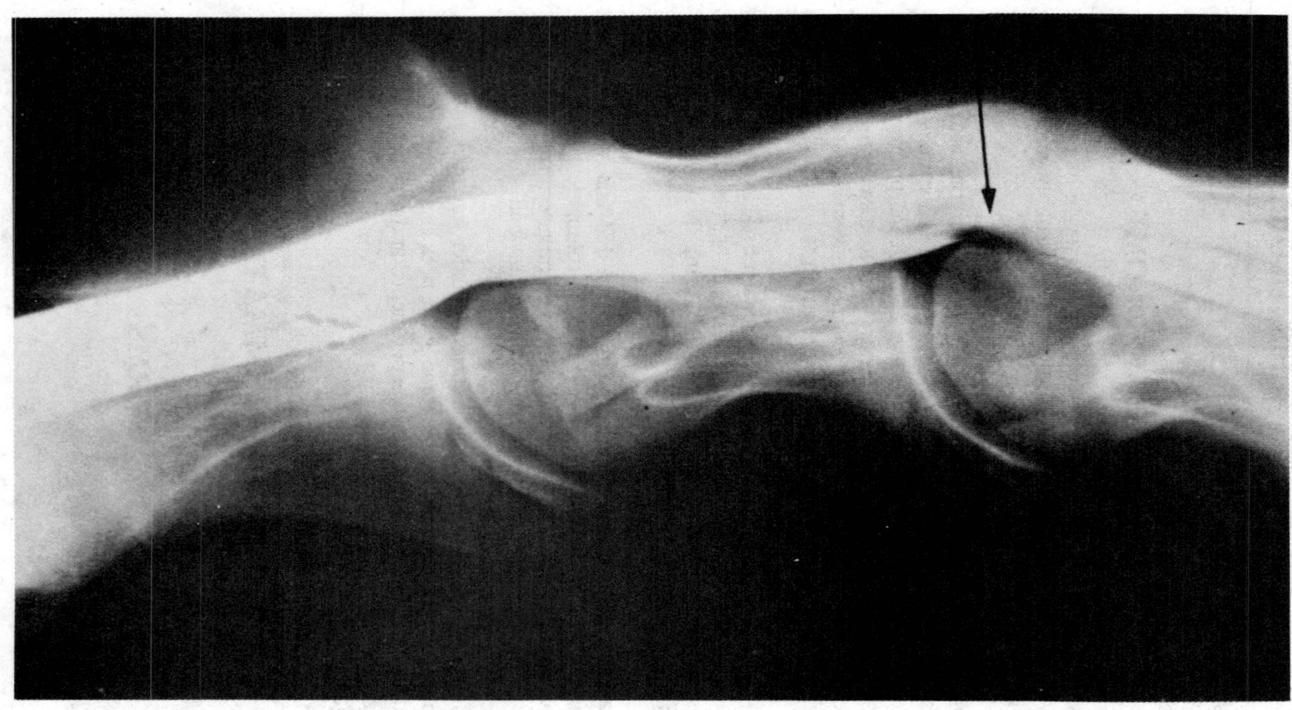

Fig. 100
X-ray of the neck of a "wobbler" yearling showing narrowing (arrow) of the spinal cord.

WOUNDS

Of all domestic animals, the horse is probably the most subject to accidental wounds. Horse owners, particularly in the country, are often called upon to use their own ingenuity in treating animals which have been injured from a variety of causes. In this connection, the owner frequently places great reliance on the value of some particular ointment or dressing with which he is familiar. Not only are these dressings of very little benefit in the healing of wounds but they frequently retard the healing processes.

In the usual rural environment in Australia, 2 factors favour the healing of wounds in stock: (1) the relatively large area over which the animal may roam with low risk of exposure to heavily-contaminated areas, and (2) the clear dry climate which keeps the surface of the wound dry, which is very important. The free movement of the animal also mechanically brings about natural drainage of the wound, and drainage is perhaps the most important factor in wound treatment.

Classification of Wounds For convenience, wounds may be classified under 5 main headings:

1. Simple incised wounds—clean cut edges.
2. Abrasions—surface layers of skin destroyed by friction.
3. Lacerated wounds—torn edges; portions of skin, muscle and other tissue torn away.
4. Puncture wounds—deep penetration by pointed slender objects, frequent in horse's feet, such as nail pricks, and always dangerous because of the possibility of tetanus and other germ infection.
5. Contused wounds or bruises—diffuse damage about actual wound, blood and lymph invading neighbouring parts.

Healing Processes There are four processes of healing: (1) healing by first intention; (2) healing by granulation; (3) healing under a scab; (4) wound contraction.

Healing by first intention is the immediate healing of 2 clean cut surfaces without complication. In large animals, other than in the case of surgical wounds, this seldom occurs. Most wounds in large animals can be looked upon as infected or septic, that is contamination of the wound by germs has taken place. This may not be serious, and is commonly controlled by natural processes.

Healing by granulation is the most common way by which wound repair in the horse takes place. Granulation tissue is newly-developed tissue composed of minute blood-vessels and cells producing fibrous tissue. This may be seen initially as tiny greyish-white flecks which appear over the surface of the wound. These spots gradually extend to

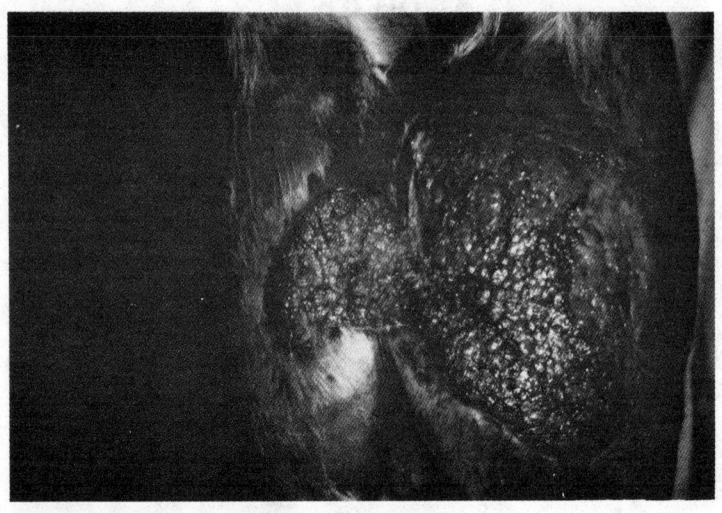

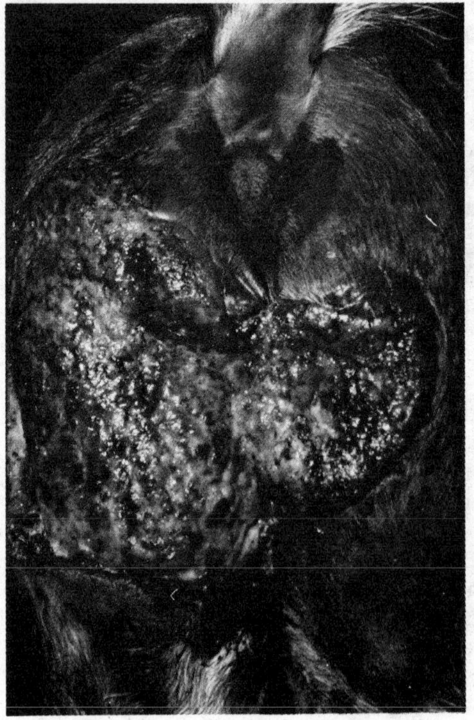

Fig. 101
Wound to the buttocks of a 3-week-old foal 10 days after initial injury.

Fig. 102
The same wound 3 weeks after the injury.

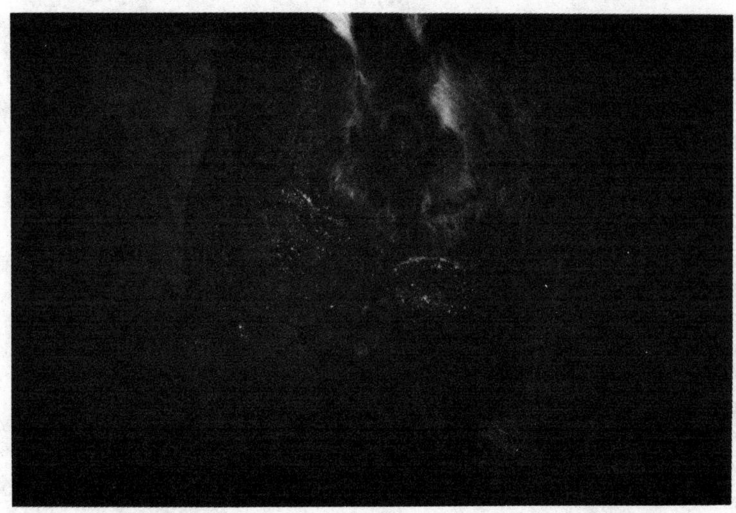

Fig. 103
The same wound 5 weeks after injury.

Fig. 104
The same wound 2½ months after injury.

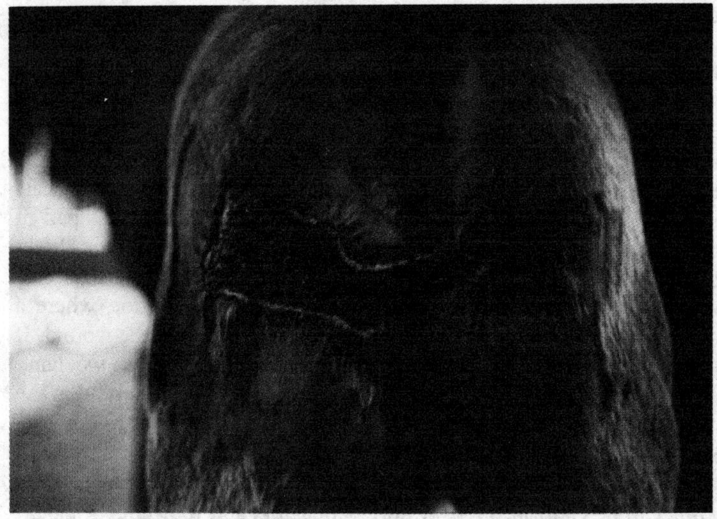

cover the surface of the exposed area. This new tissue is richly supplied with blood vessels and bleeds freely if damaged but has no pain sensation. The granulation tissue then grows together, filling up the gap in the wounded area. The wound is now impervious to bacterial invasion and infection is prevented. Healing proceeds by an outgrowth of skin cells which gradually cover the area. If, however, the surface of the wound is interfered with by rubbing, irritant dressings or other over-zealous treatment, excessive granulation tissue is formed, growing freely above the surface. This is the so called "proud-flesh" which can also occur under other unfavourable conditions, particularly in areas of the body where there is poor wound contraction. Wound contraction is the movement of the 2 skin surfaces towards each other. This is one of the most important factors in wound healing in horses, as the great skin mobility in many areas of the body can cover extensive initial defects. However, in certain areas of the body, particularly the head, the croup and the lower limb, wound contraction is very poor due to the lack of skin mobility.

Treatment of Wounds Serious wounds call for the services of a veterinarian. There may be severe bleeding which, although temporarily arrested by pressure packs, must be permanently stopped by tying-off the blood vessels. Deep punctured wounds, in addition to local treatment, will call for the injection of tetanus antitoxin and possibly an antibiotic.

In various types of wounds, haemorrhage is likely to occur from the cutting of arteries or veins, the former being the more serious. Bleeding from an artery can be recognised by the manner in which the blood spurts in jets. The blood is also of a brighter red colour than that from the veins. When veins only are cut, the blood pours out in a continuous stream. Bleeding must be arrested before any attempt is made to dress the wound.

The loss of up to 10 litres of blood by a robust horse is not dangerous, but if bleeding is long continued, severe weakening, and eventually death, will result. Whilst awaiting the arrival of the veterinarian, it may be possible to stop the flow of blood, at least temporarily, by the application of pressure over the part with a pad of sterile gauze, or clean cloth preferably sterilised by boiling. Direct pressure on the wound for 5 to 10 minutes will allow clotting to occur. Should this not be effective and the wound be in a position where a bandage can be applied, a sterile pad may be bandaged over the wound. If this is not possible, pack the wound with sterile gauze or cotton wool and insert 1 or 2 large safety-pins through the skin of the wound to hold in the gauze, and then wind some fine string around the safety-pins in a figure-of-eight fashion to exert pressure. This should be removed carefully in 12 to 24 hours if professional assistance has not been available. Most bleeding can be controlled by pressure bandaging, and tourniquets should not be applied as they frequently increase the amount of bleeding by blocking off only the venous part of blood supply.

Any irritating substance, such as kerosene, turpentine, stockholm tar, or any other favourite wound remedy, should not be applied to the wound. Most of the substances used on wounds are irritant and it should be remembered that this applies to disinfectant and antiseptic solutions.

If there is a foreign body, such as a stake, in the wound, it may be necessary to withdraw it to save further injury, otherwise it is preferable to leave it until the veterinarian arrives. If the stake must be removed, care should be taken not to break it off and leave a fragment deeply embedded in the tissues.

When bleeding has been arrested it will be necessary to remove any dirt, clots of blood and other foreign material very carefully. This may be done by syringing the affected area with normal saline solution (1 teaspoonful of salt to 600 ml of boiled water) which has been allowed to cool to blood heat. A human enema syringe is very useful in applying a continuous stream of solution of salt or weak antiseptic solution to the wound. The hands should be kept away from the wound as much as possible and, if it is necessary to sponge the wound or to remove foreign matter, clean cotton wool, or preferably gauze swabs soaked in salt or weak antiseptic solution, should be used. Common ways of infecting a wound are by dirty hands and contaminated material such as cotton wool. Most wounds, especially puncture wounds and extensive lacerations, should not be stitched. Stitching of a wound is the best way of keeping harmful germs in, or of introducing them if not already there. Any suturing of wounds should be left to a veterinarian who has been trained in the art of correct wound treatment and can decide whether a wound should be stitched or not.

Penetrating abdominal and thoracic wounds, and open joints, also require professional attention.

A fundamental principle underlying all wound treatment is to endeavour to provide suitable downward drainage for discharges from the wound. If such drainage is provided, most wounds tend to heal satisfactorily. Wounds which penetrate in an upward direction need little interference beyond ensuring that they remain open while healing from their deepest part and that they are reasonably clean on the surface.

Deep wounds penetrating downwards, and which form pockets, heal badly, as discharges collect within them and cannot get away. In the case of down-penetrating wounds it is necessary for a veterinarian to provide drainage at the lower-most point. This can be done by the use of a stab incision and insertion of special sterile drainage tubes.

When a wound persists in discharging and will not heal, it is a sign that infection, or a foreign body, such as a piece of wood, splinter of bone or a piece of dead tissue is present. Such a wound should be opened right to the bottom, preferably by a veterinarian, and the offending material removed, or infection treated.

Systemic administration of antibiotics by intramuscular injection may be prescribed by a veterinarian to enable control of the more serious wound infections. In the majority of wounds, antibiotics are not necessary and, in fact, may be harmful as they can cause adverse reactions.

Puncture wounds are particularly liable to be contaminated deeply by tetanus spores and gas gangrene organisms, which find themselves in a favourable situation, namely with the absence of air, to multiply and elaborate their powerful toxins (see *Tetanus*).

Wounds open to the air, or only covered by a light protection, heal better than those heavily bandaged. It is sometimes necessary to use bandages to immobilise the injured area or to prevent further contamination or fly strike.

Where necessary, wounds may be protected to some extent from flies by smearing a fly-repellant dressing, such as 10 per cent *citronella* or *dibutyl phthalate,* around but not on the wound.

The application of stockholm tar is undesirable even around the wound; it is not a safe repellant; dust and dirt adhere to it, and it may retard healing of the wound. Should excess granulation tissue (proud-flesh) occur, it may be checked by the application of 5 per cent bluestone solution or *white lotion.*

It is again stressed that strong, irritating antiseptics should not be used in the treatment of wounds, as they only damage the tissues and lower the resistance of the wound to germ infection, and actually delay the healing process. When the horse has sustained a severe wound, or suturing has been carried out, complete rest for 5 to 7 days will be necessary.

The majority of wounds will heal gradually by wound contraction under good nursing and a minimum of interference to the wound. However, serious complications, such as cellulitis, may occur as a result of virulent infection, and will require prompt treatment by a veterinarian. Shock is sometimes a complication of severe and extensive wounds, and will require professional treatment, as also will great loss of blood.

Contused Wounds or Bruises These are injuries to the deeper parts of the skin and the underlying tissues and commonly occur with only minor abrasions of the skin, although considerable swelling may occur from effusion of blood. They usually result from kicks from other horses, hitting an obstruction, or a fall. The importance of these bruises depends on the amount of damage to underlying tissue and on body location. A small contusion on a limb can be serious, owing to damage to the periosteum covering the bones, whereas a large bruise on the more fleshy parts of the body usually heals readily by resolution and absorption of the damaged tissue and blood which escapes from damaged vessels.

Treatment Simple bruises, if treated early, respond very well to cold water applications with a hose. Alternatively, a pad of cotton wool or a cloth soaked in cold or ice water may be held over the bruise or applied with a bandage. The cold applications cause the blood vessels to contract and prevent further effusion of blood. This cold water treatment should be carried out for the first day, after which hot fomentations should be applied to the bruise and gentle massage given. Light exercise is beneficial. If the skin has been broken, the wound should be cleaned with salt solution or a very weak antiseptic and otherwise treated as an open wound. Serious contusions will require veterinary attention.

Appendix

COLOURS AND MARKINGS OF HORSES FOR IDENTIFICATION PURPOSES

The following are the names of body colours and markings as approved by the British Royal College of Veterinary Surgeons in 1954, together with a few minor additions applicable in Australia.

Body Colours The principal colours are black, brown, bay, chestnut and grey. Where there is any doubt as to the colour, the muzzle and eyelids should be carefully examined for guidance.

Black: Where black pigment is general throughout the coat, limbs, mane and tail, with no pattern factor present other than white markings. Brown-black is also recognised.

Black-brown: Where the predominating colour is black, with muzzle, and sometimes flanks, brown or tan.

Brown: Where there is a mixture of black and brown pigment in the coat, with black limbs, mane and tail. Brown-bay is recognised.

Bay-brown: Where the predominating colour is brown, with muzzle bay, black limbs, mane and tail.

Bay: Bay varies considerably in shade from dull red approaching brown, to a yellowish colour approaching chestnut, but it can be distinguished from the chestnut by the fact that the bay has a black mane and tail and almost invariably has black on the limbs.

Chestnut: This colour consists of yellow-coloured hair in different degrees of intensity, which may be noted if thought desirable. A "true" chestnut has a chestnut mane and tail which may be lighter or darker than the body colour. Lighter coloured chestnuts may have flaxen manes and tails. There are various shades from light washy to deep liver. Limbs are never black.

Blue Dun: The body colour is a dilute black evenly distributed. The mane and tail are black. There may or may not be a dorsal band (list) and/or a withers stripe. The skin is black.

Yellow Dun: Where there is a diffuse yellow pigment in the hair. There may or may not be a dorsal band (list), withers stripe, and bars on the legs. The striping is usually associated with black pigment on the head and limbs. The skin is black.

Cream: The body coat is of a cream colour, with unpigmented skin. The iris is deficient in pigment and is often devoid of it, giving the eye a pinkish or bluish appearance.

Grey: Where the body coat is a varying mosaic of black and white hairs, with the skin black. With increasing age the coat grows lighter in colour. As there are many variations according to age and season, all of them should be described by the general term "grey". The flea-bitten grey may contain 3 colours or the 2 basic colours, and should be so described.

Roans: Roans are distinguished by the ground or body colours, all of which are permanent.

Blue Roan: Where the body colour is black or black-brown, with an admixture of white hair, which gives a blue tinge to the coat. On the limbs from the knees and hocks down the black hairs usually predominate; white markings may be encountered.

Bay or Red Roan: Where the body colour is bay or bay-brown with an admixture of white hairs which gives a reddish tinge to the coat. On the limbs from the knees and hocks down the black hairs usually predominate; white markings may be encountered.

Strawberry or Chestnut Roan: Where the body colour is chestnut with an admixture of white hairs.

Piebald: Where the body coat consists of large irregular patches of black and of white. The line of demarcation between the 2 colours is generally well defined.

Skewbald: Where the body coat consists of large irregular patches of white and of any definite colour except black. The line of demarcation between the colours is generally well defined.

Odd Coloured: Where the body coat consists of large irregular patches of more than 2 colours, which may merge into each other at the edges of the patches.

Note: The term "whole coloured" is used where there are no hairs of any other colour on the body, head or limbs.

Markings The variations in markings of horses are infinite and cannot be accurately described by a limited number of terms without certain arbitrary groupings. In some cases a combination of the terms given below must be employed. It is stressed again that all certificates of identification should, in conformity with later remarks, be accompanied by a diagram on which the markings are indicated accurately.

Head *Star:* Any white mark on the forehead. Size, shape, intensity, position and coloured markings (if any) on the white to be specified. Should the marking in the region of the centre of the forehead consist of a few white hairs only it should be so described and not referred to as a star.

Stripe: Many terms have been used to describe the narrow white marking down the face, not wider than the flat anterior surface of the nasal bones, for example, rase, race, rache, reach, streak, stripe, strip, etcetera.

The Sub-Committee recommend for the sake of uniformity that one term only be used and they select as being most useful for the purpose the term "stripe". In the majority of cases the star and stripe are continuous and should be described as "star and stripe conjoined"; where the stripe is separate and distinct from the star it should be described as "interrupted stripe"; where no star is present the point or origin of the stripe should be indicated. The termination of the stripe and any variation in breadth, direction and any markings on the white should be stated, for example, "broad stripe", "narrow stripe", "inclined to left/right".

Blaze: A white marking covering almost the whole of the forehead between the eyes and extending beyond the width of the nasal bones and usually to the muzzle. Any variation in direction, termination and any markings on the white should be stated.

White Face: Where the white covers the forehead and front of the face, extending laterally towards the mouth. The extension may be unilateral or bilateral, in which cases it should be described accordingly.

Snip: An isolated white marking, independent of those already named, and situated between or in the region of the nostrils. Its size, position and intensity should be specified.

Lip Markings: Should be accurately described, whether embracing the whole or a portion of either lip. (See *Flesh Marks.)*

White Muzzle: Where the white embraces both lips and extends to the region of the nostrils.

Wall-eye: This term should be used exclusively where there is such a lack of pigment — whether partial or complete — in the iris, that it appears pinkish-white or bluish-white.

Showing the White of the Eye: Where some part of the sclera of the eye appears unpigmented (white).

Whorls: See Note 3.

Body *Grey-Ticked:* Where white hairs are sparsely distributed through the coat in any part of the body.

Flecked: Where small collections of white hairs occur distributed irregularly in any part of the body. The degrees of flecking may be described by the terms "heavily flecked", "lightly flecked".

Black Marks: This term should be used to describe small areas of black hairs among white or any other colour.

Spots: Where small, more or less circular, collections of hairs differing from the general body colour occur, distributed in various parts of the body. The position and colour of the spots must be stated.

Patch: This term should be used to describe any larger well-defined irregular area (not covered by previous definitions) of hairs differing from the general body colour. The colour, shape, position and extent should be described.

Zebra Marks: Where there is striping on the limbs, neck, withers or quarters.

Mane and Tail: The presence of differently coloured hairs in mane and tail should be specified.

Whorls: See Note 3.

Limbs *Hoofs:* Any variation in the colour of the hoofs should be noted.

White Markings on Limbs: It is recommended that any white markings on the limbs should be accurately defined and the extent precisely stated, for example, "white to half pastern", "white to below the fetlock", etcetera. The use of such terms as "sock" and "stocking" should be discontinued.

General *Mixed:* To be used to describe a white marking which contains varying amounts of hairs of the general body colour.

Bordered: To be used where any marking is circumscribed by a mixed border, for example, "bordered star", "bordered stripe".

Flesh Marks: Patches where the pigment of the skin is absent should be described as "flesh marks".

Notes 1. *Acquired Marks:* There are many adventitious marks (that is, not congenital marks) which are permanent, for example saddle marks, bridle marks, collar marks, girth marks, and other harness marks, permanent bandage marks, firing and branding marks, scars, tattoo marks. Wherever these occur they should be described. If a horse should happen to be docked this fact should be mentioned.

2. *Congenital Abnormalities:* Any congenital marks or other abnormalities which cannot be included in the description under other headings should be clearly described in the certificate and indicated on the diagram where possible.

3. *Whorls, etcetera:* The location of whorls or irregular setting of coat hairs should be precisely indicated on the diagram accompanying the certificate. Whorls should be shown by the use of a small circle with a central dot, indicating the centre of the whorl.

Routine The Sub-Committee recommended that the following order of certification should be adopted:

Colour, Breed, Sex, Age, Height; marks on head (including eyes) in the order described above; marks on the limbs, fore first, then hind, commencing from below; marks on body, including mane and tail; acquired marks, congenital abnormalities, whorls or any other features of note.

In Australia brands (if present) are always noted.

Extra Terms The following additional terms have been introduced with specific Breed Societies. They have been extracted from a paper presented at a conference of the New Zealand Thoroughbred and Standardbred Breeders Association, at Christchurch, New Zealand in June 1973 by Dr D. Zartmann of Albuquerque, New Mexico, United States.

Breeds

(1) *Appaloosa:* Pattern, white patch over rump with spots in it or a leopard-like arrangement of spots. Sometimes carry a roan type of spotting.

(2) *Palomino:* A golden to light creamy body with white mane and tail.

(3) *The Paint or Pinto Horse:* Has a pattern with extensive white patches over a darker body colour. Varieties of pinto are piebald and skewbald.

Synonyms are paint, calico, and particoloured.

Two types of inheritance are *overo* and *tobiano* with characteristic spotting differences.

Overo is a pinto pattern with white patches which spread irregularly upward from the belly. The base colour is frequently roaned; mane and tail are usually dark. The legs are seldom white. The face is commonly bald (all white).

Tobiano is a pinto pattern with white patches which spread down from the back with borders which are usually clean-cut. Mane and tail may be white spotted or white and white legs are usual. The head is coloured but may have a blaze.

Colour Terms Only

Buckskin: A light yellowish coat with black legs, mane, and tail. Usually no black stripe.

Claybank: A type of dun but carries brown points instead of black.

Cremello (cream): Very pale diluted sorrel or yellow colour; may be nearly white and called pseudo-albino. Blue eyes.

Mouse: A mousy, diluted black. Basic tone is grey or yellow.

Seal Brown: Brownish black with traces of light areas on muzzle and flanks.

Sorrel: Light red or golden shades of body colour. Coat may be uniform in colour, or the legs, mane, and tail be lighter.

White: A true white is born white. Albino, in the technical sense, has never been documented in horses. Pure albino is an animal that due to its genetic composition cannot transmit to any offspring a factor for pigment production. Apparently all so called "albino" horses have some pigment (dark eyes) or transmit a pigment factor to their offspring.

Bibliography

REFERENCE BOOKS CONSULTED

F. ANDRIST, *Mares, Foals and Foaling,* J. A. Allen & Co., 6th impression 1962.

D. C. BLOOD and J. A. HENDERSON, *Veterinary Medicine,* Bailliere, Tindall & Cox, 3rd edition 1968.

J. F. BONE, E. J. CATCOTT, A. A. GABEL, L. E. JOHNSON and W. F. RILEY, Jr. (editors), *Equine Medicine and Surgery,* American Veterinary Publications, Inc., 1st edition 1963.

R. J. GARNER, *Veterinary Toxicology,* Bailliere, Tindall & Cox, 2nd edition 1961.

T. E. GIBSON, *Veterinary Anthelmintic Medication,* Commonwealth Agricultural Bureau, England, 1962.

M. HORACE HAYES, *Veterinary Notes for Horse Owners,* revised by J. F. D. Tutt, Stanley Paul & Co. Ltd, 1965.

MERCK AND CO., INC., *The Merck Veterinary Manual,* Merck & Co., 3rd edition 1967.

W. C. MILLER and G. P. WEST, *Black's Veterinary Dictionary,* Adam and Charles Black, 6th edition 1962.

NEW ZEALAND DAIRY EXPORTER, *The Veterinary Handbook,* 1949.

NEW ZEALAND VETERINARY ASSOCIATION INC., Technical Committee, *Diseases of Domestic Animals in New Zealand,* Editorial Services Ltd., Wellington, 3rd edition 1971.

H. CAULTON REEKS, *Diseases of the Horse's Foot,* Bailliere, Tindall & Cox, 1906.

F. H. S. ROBERTS, *Insects Affecting Livestock,* Angus & Robertson, 1952.

J.A. SPRINGHALL, *Elements of Horseshoeing,* University of Queensland Press, 1964.

THE VETERINARY DEPARTMENT OF THE WAR OFFICE, LONDON, *Animal Management,* Her Majesty's Stationery Office, 1933.

UNITED STATES DEPARTMENT OF AGRICULTURE, *Diseases of the Horse,* 1942.

UNITED STATES DEPARTMENT OF AGRICULTURE, Yearbook of Agriculture, *Keeping Livestock Healthy,* Part 3, 1942.

JOURNALS CONSULTED

Agricultural Gazette of New South Wales.
Australian Veterinary Journal.

INDEX

A PERSONAL WORD FROM MELVIN POWERS
PUBLISHER, WILSHIRE BOOK COMPANY

Dear Friend:

My goal is to publish interesting, informative, and inspirational books. You can help me accomplish this by answering the following questions, either by phone or by mail. Or, if convenient for you, I would welcome the opportunity to visit with you in my office and hear your comments in person.

Did you enjoy reading this book? Why?

Would you enjoy reading another similar book?

What idea in the book impressed you the most?

If applicable to your situation, have you incorporated this idea in your daily life?

Is there a chapter that could serve as a theme for an entire book? Please explain.

If you have an idea for a book, I would welcome discussing it with you. If you already have one in progress, write or call me concerning possible publication. I can be reached at (213) 875-1711 or (213) 983-1105.

Sincerely yours,
MELVIN POWERS

12015 Sherman Road
North Hollywood, California 91605

MELVIN POWERS SELF-IMPROVEMENT LIBRARY

ASTROLOGY

____ ASTROLOGY: HOW TO CHART YOUR HOROSCOPE *Max Heindel* 3.00
____ ASTROLOGY: YOUR PERSONAL SUN-SIGN GUIDE *Beatrice Ryder* 3.00
____ ASTROLOGY FOR EVERYDAY LIVING *Janet Harris* 2.00
____ ASTROLOGY MADE EASY *Astarte* 3.00
____ ASTROLOGY MADE PRACTICAL *Alexandra Kayhle* 3.00
____ ASTROLOGY, ROMANCE, YOU AND THE STARS *Anthony Norvell* 4.00
____ MY WORLD OF ASTROLOGY *Sydney Omarr* 5.00
____ THOUGHT DIAL *Sidney Omarr* 4.00
____ WHAT THE STARS REVEAL ABOUT THE MEN IN YOUR LIFE *Thelma White* 3.00

BRIDGE

____ BRIDGE BIDDING MADE EASY *Edwin B. Kantar* 7.00
____ BRIDGE CONVENTIONS *Edwin B. Kantar* 7.00
____ BRIDGE HUMOR *Edwin B. Kantar* 5.00
____ COMPETITIVE BIDDING IN MODERN BRIDGE *Edgar Kaplan* 4.00
____ DEFENSIVE BRIDGE PLAY COMPLETE *Edwin B. Kantar* 10.00
____ GAMESMAN BRIDGE—Play Better with Kantar *Edwin B. Kantar* 5.00
____ HOW TO IMPROVE YOUR BRIDGE *Alfred Sheinwold* 5.00
____ IMPROVING YOUR BIDDING SKILLS *Edwin B. Kantar* 4.00
____ INTRODUCTION TO DECLARER'S PLAY *Edwin B. Kantar* 5.00
____ INTRODUCTION TO DEFENDER'S PLAY *Edwin B. Kantar* 3.00
____ KANTAR FOR THE DEFENSE *Edwin B. Kantar* 5.00
____ SHORT CUT TO WINNING BRIDGE *Alfred Sheinwold* 3.00
____ TEST YOUR BRIDGE PLAY *Edwin B. Kantar* 5.00
____ VOLUME 2—TEST YOUR BRIDGE PLAY *Edwin B. Kantar* 5.00
____ WINNING DECLARER PLAY *Dorothy Hayden Truscott* 4.00

BUSINESS, STUDY & REFERENCE

____ CONVERSATION MADE EASY *Elliot Russell* 3.00
____ EXAM SECRET *Dennis B. Jackson* 3.00
____ FIX-IT BOOK *Arthur Symons* 2.00
____ HOW TO DEVELOP A BETTER SPEAKING VOICE *M. Hellier* 3.00
____ HOW TO MAKE A FORTUNE IN REAL ESTATE *Albert Winnikoff* 4.00
____ INCREASE YOUR LEARNING POWER *Geoffrey A. Dudley* 3.00
____ MAGIC OF NUMBERS *Robert Tocquet* 2.00
____ PRACTICAL GUIDE TO BETTER CONCENTRATION *Melvin Powers* 3.00
____ PRACTICAL GUIDE TO PUBLIC SPEAKING *Maurice Forley* 5.00
____ 7 DAYS TO FASTER READING *William S. Schaill* 3.00
____ SONGWRITERS' RHYMING DICTIONARY *Jane Shaw Whitfield* 5.00
____ SPELLING MADE EASY *Lester D. Basch & Dr. Milton Finkelstein* 3.00
____ STUDENT'S GUIDE TO BETTER GRADES *J. A. Rickard* 3.00
____ TEST YOURSELF—Find Your Hidden Talent *Jack Shafer* 3.00
____ YOUR WILL & WHAT TO DO ABOUT IT *Attorney Samuel G. Kling* 4.00

CALLIGRAPHY

____ ADVANCED CALLIGRAPHY *Katherine Jeffares* 7.00
____ CALLIGRAPHER'S REFERENCE BOOK *Anne Leptich & Jacque Evans* 7.00
____ CALLIGRAPHY—The Art of Beautiful Writing *Katherine Jeffares* 7.00
____ CALLIGRAPHY FOR FUN & PROFIT *Anne Leptich & Jacque Evans* 7.00
____ CALLIGRAPHY MADE EASY *Tina Serafini* 7.00

CHESS & CHECKERS

____ BEGINNER'S GUIDE TO WINNING CHESS *Fred Reinfeld* 4.00
____ CHECKERS MADE EASY *Tom Wiswell* 2.00
____ CHESS IN TEN EASY LESSONS *Larry Evans* 3.00
____ CHESS MADE EASY *Milton L. Hanauer* 3.00
____ CHESS PROBLEMS FOR BEGINNERS *edited by Fred Reinfeld* 2.00
____ CHESS SECRETS REVEALED *Fred Reinfeld* 2.00
____ CHESS STRATEGY—An Expert's Guide *Fred Reinfeld* 2.00
____ CHESS TACTICS FOR BEGINNERS *edited by Fred Reinfeld* 3.00
____ CHESS THEORY & PRACTICE *Morry & Mitchell* 2.00
____ HOW TO WIN AT CHECKERS *Fred Reinfeld* 3.00
____ 1001 BRILLIANT WAYS TO CHECKMATE *Fred Reinfeld* 4.00

____ 1001 WINNING CHESS SACRIFICES & COMBINATIONS *Fred Reinfeld* 4.00
____ SOVIET CHESS *Edited by R. G. Wade* 3.00

COOKERY & HERBS

____ CULPEPER'S HERBAL REMEDIES *Dr. Nicholas Culpeper* 3.00
____ FAST GOURMET COOKBOOK *Poppy Cannon* 2.50
____ GINSENG The Myth & The Truth *Joseph P. Hou* 3.00
____ HEALING POWER OF HERBS *May Bethel* 4.00
____ HEALING POWER OF NATURAL FOODS *May Bethel* 4.00
____ HERB HANDBOOK *Dawn MacLeod* 3.00
____ HERBS FOR COOKING AND HEALING *Dr. Donald Law* 2.00
____ HERBS FOR HEALTH—How to Grow & Use Them *Louise Evans Doole* 3.00
____ HOME GARDEN COOKBOOK—Delicious Natural Food Recipes *Ken Kraft* 3.00
____ MEDICAL HERBALIST *edited by Dr. J. R. Yemm* 3.00
____ NATURAL FOOD COOKBOOK *Dr. Harry C. Bond* 3.00
____ NATURE'S MEDICINES *Richard Lucas* 3.00
____ VEGETABLE GARDENING FOR BEGINNERS *Hugh Wiberg* 2.00
____ VEGETABLES FOR TODAY'S GARDENS *R. Milton Carleton* 2.00
____ VEGETARIAN COOKERY *Janet Walker* 4.00
____ VEGETARIAN COOKING MADE EASY & DELECTABLE *Veronica Vezza* 3.00
____ VEGETARIAN DELIGHTS—A Happy Cookbook for Health *K. R. Mehta* 2.00
____ VEGETARIAN GOURMET COOKBOOK *Joyce McKinnel* 3.00

GAMBLING & POKER

____ ADVANCED POKER STRATEGY & WINNING PLAY *A. D. Livingston* 5.00
____ HOW NOT TO LOSE AT POKER *Jeffrey Lloyd Castle* 3.00
____ HOW TO WIN AT DICE GAMES *Skip Frey* 3.00
____ HOW TO WIN AT POKER *Terence Reese & Anthony T. Watkins* 3.00
____ SECRETS OF WINNING POKER *George S. Coffin* 3.00
____ WINNING AT CRAPS *Dr. Lloyd T. Commins* 3.00
____ WINNING AT GIN *Chester Wander & Cy Rice* 3.00
____ WINNING AT POKER—An Expert's Guide *John Archer* 3.00
____ WINNING AT 21—An Expert's Guide *John Archer* 5.00
____ WINNING POKER SYSTEMS *Norman Zadeh* 3.00

HEALTH

____ BEE POLLEN *Lynda Lyngheim & Jack Scagnetti* 3.00
____ DR. LINDNER'S SPECIAL WEIGHT CONTROL METHOD *P. G. Lindner, M.D.* 2.00
____ HELP YOURSELF TO BETTER SIGHT *Margaret Darst Corbett* 3.00
____ HOW TO IMPROVE YOUR VISION *Dr. Robert A. Kraskin* 3.00
____ HOW YOU CAN STOP SMOKING PERMANENTLY *Ernest Caldwell* 3.00
____ MIND OVER PLATTER *Peter G. Lindner, M.D.* 3.00
____ NATURE'S WAY TO NUTRITION & VIBRANT HEALTH *Robert J. Scrutton* 3.00
____ NEW CARBOHYDRATE DIET COUNTER *Patti Lopez-Pereira* 1.50
____ QUICK & EASY EXERCISES FOR FACIAL BEAUTY *Judy Smith-deal* 2.00
____ QUICK & EASY EXERCISES FOR FIGURE BEAUTY *Judy Smith-deal* 2.00
____ REFLEXOLOGY *Dr. Maybelle Segal* 3.00
____ REFLEXOLOGY FOR GOOD HEALTH *Anna Kaye & Don C. Matchan* 3.00
____ YOU CAN LEARN TO RELAX *Dr. Samuel Gutwirth* 3.00
____ YOUR ALLERGY—What To Do About It *Allan Knight, M.D.* 3.00

HOBBIES

____ BEACHCOMBING FOR BEGINNERS *Norman Hickin* 2.00
____ BLACKSTONE'S MODERN CARD TRICKS *Harry Blackstone* 3.00
____ BLACKSTONE'S SECRETS OF MAGIC *Harry Blackstone* 3.00
____ COIN COLLECTING FOR BEGINNERS *Burton Hobson & Fred Reinfeld* 3.00
____ ENTERTAINING WITH ESP *Tony 'Doc' Shiels* 2.00
____ 400 FASCINATING MAGIC TRICKS YOU CAN DO *Howard Thurston* 4.00
____ HOW I TURN JUNK INTO FUN AND PROFIT *Sari* 3.00
____ HOW TO WRITE A HIT SONG & SELL IT *Tommy Boyce* 7.00
____ JUGGLING MADE EASY *Rudolf Dittrich* 2.00
____ MAGIC FOR ALL AGES *Walter Gibson* 4.00
____ MAGIC MADE EASY *Byron Wels* 2.00
____ STAMP COLLECTING FOR BEGINNERS *Burton Hobson* 3.00

HORSE PLAYERS' WINNING GUIDES

____ BETTING HORSES TO WIN *Les Conklin* 3.00
____ ELIMINATE THE LOSERS *Bob McKnight* 3.00

____	HOW TO PICK WINNING HORSES *Bob McKnight*	3.00
____	HOW TO WIN AT THE RACES *Sam (The Genius) Lewin*	5.00
____	HOW YOU CAN BEAT THE RACES *Jack Kavanagh*	5.00
____	MAKING MONEY AT THE RACES *David Barr*	3.00
____	PAYDAY AT THE RACES *Les Conklin*	3.00
____	SMART HANDICAPPING MADE EASY *William Bauman*	3.00
____	SUCCESS AT THE HARNESS RACES *Barry Meadow*	3.00
____	WINNING AT THE HARNESS RACES—An Expert's Guide *Nick Cammarano*	3.00

HUMOR

____	HOW TO BE A COMEDIAN FOR FUN & PROFIT *King & Laufer*	2.00
____	HOW TO FLATTEN YOUR TUSH *Coach Marge Reardon*	2.00
____	HOW TO MAKE LOVE TO YOURSELF *Ron Stevens & Joy Grdnic*	3.00
____	JOKE TELLER'S HANDBOOK *Bob Orben*	3.00
____	JOKES FOR ALL OCCASIONS *Al Schock*	3.00
____	2000 NEW LAUGHS FOR SPEAKERS *Bob Orben*	4.00
____	2,500 JOKES TO START 'EM LAUGHING *Bob Orben*	4.00

HYPNOTISM

____	ADVANCED TECHNIQUES OF HYPNOSIS *Melvin Powers*	2.00
____	BRAINWASHING AND THE CULTS *Paul A. Verdier, Ph.D.*	3.00
____	CHILDBIRTH WITH HYPNOSIS *William S. Kroger, M.D.*	5.00
____	HOW TO SOLVE Your Sex Problems with Self-Hypnosis *Frank S. Caprio, M.D.*	5.00
____	HOW TO STOP SMOKING THRU SELF-HYPNOSIS *Leslie M. LeCron*	3.00
____	HOW TO USE AUTO-SUGGESTION EFFECTIVELY *John Duckworth*	3.00
____	HOW YOU CAN BOWL BETTER USING SELF-HYPNOSIS *Jack Heise*	3.00
____	HOW YOU CAN PLAY BETTER GOLF USING SELF-HYPNOSIS *Jack Heise*	3.00
____	HYPNOSIS AND SELF-HYPNOSIS *Bernard Hollander, M.D.*	3.00
____	HYPNOTISM *(Originally published in 1893) Carl Sextus*	5.00
____	HYPNOTISM & PSYCHIC PHENOMENA *Simeon Edmunds*	4.00
____	HYPNOTISM MADE EASY *Dr. Ralph Winn*	3.00
____	HYPNOTISM MADE PRACTICAL *Louis Orton*	3.00
____	HYPNOTISM REVEALED *Melvin Powers*	2.00
____	HYPNOTISM TODAY *Leslie LeCron and Jean Bordeaux, Ph.D.*	5.00
____	MODERN HYPNOSIS *Lesley Kuhn & Salvatore Russo, Ph.D.*	5.00
____	NEW CONCEPTS OF HYPNOSIS *Bernard C. Gindes, M.D.*	5.00
____	NEW SELF-HYPNOSIS *Paul Adams*	4.00
____	POST-HYPNOTIC INSTRUCTIONS—Suggestions for Therapy *Arnold Furst*	3.00
____	PRACTICAL GUIDE TO SELF-HYPNOSIS *Melvin Powers*	3.00
____	PRACTICAL HYPNOTISM *Philip Magonet, M.D.*	3.00
____	SECRETS OF HYPNOTISM *S. J. Van Pelt, M.D.*	5.00
____	SELF-HYPNOSIS A Conditioned-Response Technique *Laurence Sparks*	5.00
____	SELF-HYPNOSIS Its Theory, Technique & Application *Melvin Powers*	3.00
____	THERAPY THROUGH HYPNOSIS *edited by Raphael H. Rhodes*	4.00

JUDAICA

____	MODERN ISRAEL *Lily Edelman*	2.00
____	SERVICE OF THE HEART *Evelyn Garfiel, Ph.D.*	4.00
____	STORY OF ISRAEL IN COINS *Jean & Maurice Gould*	2.00
____	STORY OF ISRAEL IN STAMPS *Maxim & Gabriel Shamir*	1.00
____	TONGUE OF THE PROPHETS *Robert St. John*	5.00

JUST FOR WOMEN

____	COSMOPOLITAN'S GUIDE TO MARVELOUS MEN Fwd. by *Helen Gurley Brown*	3.00
____	COSMOPOLITAN'S HANG-UP HANDBOOK Foreword by *Helen Gurley Brown*	4.00
____	COSMOPOLITAN'S LOVE BOOK—A Guide to Ecstasy in Bed	4.00
____	COSMOPOLITAN'S NEW ETIQUETTE GUIDE Fwd. by *Helen Gurley Brown*	4.00
____	I AM A COMPLEAT WOMAN *Doris Hagopian & Karen O'Connor Sweeney*	3.00
____	JUST FOR WOMEN—A Guide to the Female Body *Richard E. Sand, M.D.*	5.00
____	NEW APPROACHES TO SEX IN MARRIAGE *John E. Eichenlaub, M.D.*	3.00
____	SEXUALLY ADEQUATE FEMALE *Frank S. Caprio, M.D.*	3.00
____	SEXUALLY FULFILLED WOMAN *Dr. Rachel Copelan*	5.00
____	YOUR FIRST YEAR OF MARRIAGE *Dr. Tom McGinnis*	3.00

MARRIAGE, SEX & PARENTHOOD

____	ABILITY TO LOVE *Dr. Allan Fromme*	5.00
____	ENCYCLOPEDIA OF MODERN SEX & LOVE TECHNIQUES *Macandrew*	5.00
____	GUIDE TO SUCCESSFUL MARRIAGE *Drs. Albert Ellis & Robert Harper*	5.00

____ HOW TO RAISE AN EMOTIONALLY HEALTHY, HAPPY CHILD *A. Ellis* 4.00
____ SEX WITHOUT GUILT *Albert Ellis, Ph.D.* 5.00
____ SEXUALLY ADEQUATE MALE *Frank S. Caprio, M.D.* 3.00
____ SEXUALLY FULFILLED MAN *Dr. Rachel Copelan* 5.00

MELVIN POWERS' MAIL ORDER LIBRARY

____ HOW TO GET RICH IN MAIL ORDER *Melvin Powers* 10.00
____ HOW TO WRITE A GOOD ADVERTISEMENT *Victor O. Schwab* 15.00
____ MAIL ORDER MADE EASY *J. Frank Brumbaugh* 10.00
____ U.S. MAIL ORDER SHOPPER'S GUIDE *Susan Spitzer* 10.00

METAPHYSICS & OCCULT

____ BOOK OF TALISMANS, AMULETS & ZODIACAL GEMS *William Pavitt* 5.00
____ CONCENTRATION—A Guide to Mental Mastery *Mouni Sadhu* 4.00
____ CRITIQUES OF GOD *Edited by Peter Angeles* 7.00
____ EXTRA-TERRESTRIAL INTELLIGENCE—The First Encounter 6.00
____ FORTUNE TELLING WITH CARDS *P. Foli* 3.00
____ HANDWRITING ANALYSIS MADE EASY *John Marley* 4.00
____ HANDWRITING TELLS *Nadya Olyanova* 5.00
____ HOW TO INTERPRET DREAMS, OMENS & FORTUNE TELLING SIGNS *Gettings* 3.00
____ HOW TO UNDERSTAND YOUR DREAMS *Geoffrey A. Dudley* 3.00
____ ILLUSTRATED YOGA *William Zorn* 3.00
____ IN DAYS OF GREAT PEACE *Mouni Sadhu* 3.00
____ LSD—THE AGE OF MIND *Bernard Roseman* 2.00
____ MAGICIAN—His Training and Work *W. E. Butler* 3.00
____ MEDITATION *Mouni Sadhu* 5.00
____ MODERN NUMEROLOGY *Morris C. Goodman* 3.00
____ NUMEROLOGY—ITS FACTS AND SECRETS *Ariel Yvon Taylor* 3.00
____ NUMEROLOGY MADE EASY *W. Mykian* 3.00
____ PALMISTRY MADE EASY *Fred Gettings* 3.00
____ PALMISTRY MADE PRACTICAL *Elizabeth Daniels Squire* 4.00
____ PALMISTRY SECRETS REVEALED *Henry Frith* 3.00
____ PROPHECY IN OUR TIME *Martin Ebon* 2.50
____ PSYCHOLOGY OF HANDWRITING *Nadya Olyanova* 5.00
____ SUPERSTITION—Are You Superstitious? *Eric Maple* 2.00
____ TAROT *Mouni Sadhu* 6.00
____ TAROT OF THE BOHEMIANS *Papus* 5.00
____ WAYS TO SELF-REALIZATION *Mouni Sadhu* 3.00
____ WHAT YOUR HANDWRITING REVEALS *Albert E. Hughes* 3.00
____ WITCHCRAFT, MAGIC & OCCULTISM—A Fascinating History *W. B. Crow* 5.00
____ WITCHCRAFT—THE SIXTH SENSE *Justine Glass* 5.00
____ WORLD OF PSYCHIC RESEARCH *Hereward Carrington* 2.00

SELF-HELP & INSPIRATIONAL

____ DAILY POWER FOR JOYFUL LIVING *Dr. Donald Curtis* 5.00
____ DYNAMIC THINKING *Melvin Powers* 2.00
____ EXUBERANCE—Your Guide to Happiness & Fulfillment *Dr. Paul Kurtz* 3.00
____ GREATEST POWER IN THE UNIVERSE *U. S. Andersen* 5.00
____ GROW RICH WHILE YOU SLEEP *Ben Sweetland* 3.00
____ GROWTH THROUGH REASON *Albert Ellis, Ph.D.* 4.00
____ GUIDE TO DEVELOPING YOUR POTENTIAL *Herbert A. Otto, Ph.D.* 3.00
____ GUIDE TO LIVING IN BALANCE *Frank S. Caprio, M.D.* 2.00
____ GUIDE TO PERSONAL HAPPINESS *Albert Ellis, Ph.D. & Irving Becker, Ed. D.* 5.00
____ HELPING YOURSELF WITH APPLIED PSYCHOLOGY *R. Henderson* 2.00
____ HELPING YOURSELF WITH PSYCHIATRY *Frank S. Caprio, M.D.* 2.00
____ HOW TO ATTRACT GOOD LUCK *A. H. Z. Carr* 4.00
____ HOW TO CONTROL YOUR DESTINY *Norvell* 3.00
____ HOW TO DEVELOP A WINNING PERSONALITY *Martin Panzer* 5.00
____ HOW TO DEVELOP AN EXCEPTIONAL MEMORY *Young & Gibson* 4.00
____ HOW TO LIVE WITH A NEUROTIC *Albert Ellis, Ph. D.* 5.00
____ HOW TO OVERCOME YOUR FEARS *M. P. Leahy, M.D.* 3.00
____ HOW YOU CAN HAVE CONFIDENCE AND POWER *Les Giblin* 3.00
____ HUMAN PROBLEMS & HOW TO SOLVE THEM *Dr. Donald Curtis* 4.00
____ I CAN *Ben Sweetland* 5.00
____ I WILL *Ben Sweetland* 3.00
____ LEFT-HANDED PEOPLE *Michael Barsley* 4.00

____ MAGIC IN YOUR MIND *U. S. Andersen* 5.00
____ MAGIC OF THINKING BIG *Dr. David J. Schwartz* 3.00
____ MAGIC POWER OF YOUR MIND *Walter M. Germain* 5.00
____ MENTAL POWER THROUGH SLEEP SUGGESTION *Melvin Powers* 3.00
____ NEW GUIDE TO RATIONAL LIVING *Albert Ellis, Ph.D. & R. Harper, Ph.D.* 3.00
____ OUR TROUBLED SELVES *Dr. Allan Fromme* 3.00
____ PSYCHO-CYBERNETICS *Maxwell Maltz, M.D.* 3.00
____ SCIENCE OF MIND IN DAILY LIVING *Dr. Donald Curtis* 5.00
____ SECRET OF SECRETS *U. S. Andersen* 5.00
____ SECRET POWER OF THE PYRAMIDS *U. S. Andersen* 5.00
____ STUTTERING AND WHAT YOU CAN DO ABOUT IT *W. Johnson, Ph.D.* 2.50
____ SUCCESS-CYBERNETICS *U. S. Andersen* 5.00
____ 10 DAYS TO A GREAT NEW LIFE *William E. Edwards* 3.00
____ THINK AND GROW RICH *Napoleon Hill* 3.00
____ THINK YOUR WAY TO SUCCESS *Dr. Lew Losoncy* 5.00
____ THREE MAGIC WORDS *U. S. Andersen* 5.00
____ TREASURY OF COMFORT *edited by Rabbi Sidney Greenberg* 5.00
____ TREASURY OF THE ART OF LIVING *Sidney S. Greenberg* 5.00
____ YOU ARE NOT THE TARGET *Laura Huxley* 5.00
____ YOUR SUBCONSCIOUS POWER *Charles M. Simmons* 5.00
____ YOUR THOUGHTS CAN CHANGE YOUR LIFE *Dr. Donald Curtis* 5.00

SPORTS

____ BICYCLING FOR FUN AND GOOD HEALTH *Kenneth E. Luther* 2.00
____ BILLIARDS—Pocket • Carom • Three Cushion *Clive Cottingham, Jr.* 3.00
____ CAMPING-OUT 101 Ideas & Activities *Bruno Knobel* 2.00
____ COMPLETE GUIDE TO FISHING *Vlad Evanoff* 2.00
____ HOW TO IMPROVE YOUR RACQUETBALL *Lubarsky Kaufman & Scagnetti* 3.00
____ HOW TO WIN AT POCKET BILLIARDS *Edward D. Knuchell* 4.00
____ JOY OF WALKING *Jack Scagnetti* 3.00
____ LEARNING & TEACHING SOCCER SKILLS *Eric Worthington* 3.00
____ MOTORCYCLING FOR BEGINNERS *I. G. Edmonds* 3.00
____ RACQUETBALL FOR WOMEN *Toni Hudson, Jack Scagnetti & Vince Rondone* 3.00
____ RACQUETBALL MADE EASY *Steve Lubarsky, Rod Delson & Jack Scagnetti* 4.00
____ SECRET OF BOWLING STRIKES *Dawson Taylor* 3.00
____ SECRET OF PERFECT PUTTING *Horton Smith & Dawson Taylor* 3.00
____ SOCCER—The Game & How to Play It *Gary Rosenthal* 3.00
____ STARTING SOCCER *Edward F. Dolan, Jr.* 3.00
____ TABLE TENNIS MADE EASY *Johnny Leach* 2.00

TENNIS LOVERS' LIBRARY

____ BEGINNER'S BUIDE TO WINNING TENNIS *Helen Hull Jacobs* 2.00
____ HOW TO BEAT BETTER TENNIS PLAYERS *Loring Fiske* 4.00
____ HOW TO IMPROVE YOUR TENNIS—Style, Strategy & Analysis *C. Wilson* 2.00
____ INSIDE TENNIS—Techniques of Winning *Jim Leighton* 3.00
____ PLAY TENNIS WITH ROSEWALL *Ken Rosewall* 2.00
____ PSYCH YOURSELF TO BETTER TENNIS *Dr. Walter A. Luszki* 2.00
____ SUCCESSFUL TENNIS *Neale Fraser* 2.00
____ TENNIS FOR BEGINNERS, *Dr. H. A. Murray* 2.00
____ TENNIS MADE EASY *Joel Brecheen* 3.00
____ WEEKEND TENNIS—How to Have Fun & Win at the Same Time *Bill Talbert* 3.00
____ WINNING WITH PERCENTAGE TENNIS—Smart Strategy *Jack Lowe* 2.00

WILSHIRE PET LIBRARY

____ DOG OBEDIENCE TRAINING *Gust Kessopulos* 5.00
____ DOG TRAINING MADE EASY & FUN *John W. Kellogg* 4.00
____ HOW TO BRING UP YOUR PET DOG *Kurt Unkelbach* 2.00
____ HOW TO RAISE & TRAIN YOUR PUPPY *Jeff Griffen* 3.00
____ PIGEONS: HOW TO RAISE & TRAIN THEM *William H. Allen, Jr.* 2.00

The books listed above can be obtained from your book dealer or directly from Melvin Powers. When ordering, please remit 50¢ per book postage & handling. Send for our free illustrated catalog of self-improvement books.

Melvin Powers

12015 Sherman Road, No. Hollywood, California 91605

Notes

Notes